T0318741

Advanced Food Analysis Tools

Advanced Food Analysis Tools
Biosensors and Nanotechnology

Edited by

Rovina Kobun

Senior Lecturer, Faculty of Food Science and Nutrition,
Universiti Malaysia Sabah

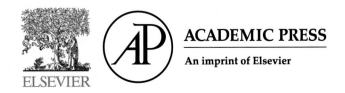

ACADEMIC PRESS
An imprint of Elsevier

Academic Press is an imprint of Elsevier
125 London Wall, London EC2Y 5AS, United Kingdom
525 B Street, Suite 1650, San Diego, CA 92101, United States
50 Hampshire Street, 5th Floor, Cambridge, MA 02139, United States
The Boulevard, Langford Lane, Kidlington, Oxford OX5 1GB, United Kingdom

Library of Congress Cataloging-in-Publication Data
A catalog record for this book is available from the Library of Congress

British Library Cataloguing-in-Publication Data
A catalogue record for this book is available from the British Library

ISBN: 978-0-12-820591-4

For information on all Academic Press publications
visit our website at https://www.elsevier.com/books-and-journals

Publisher: Charlotte Cockle
Acquisitions Editor: Patricia Osborn
Editorial Project Manager: Hilary Carr
Production Project Manager: Kiruthika Govindaraju
Cover Designer: Alan Studholme

Typeset by SPi Global, India

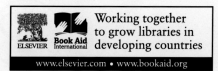

Contents

Biosensor and nanotechnology

Introduction

Nanotechnology is an interdisciplinary field of study that plays a significant role in the advancement of biosensors. Nanotechnology-enabled products are increasingly ubiquitous and one of the most exciting future innovations that have led to a significant advancement in current nutrition and food sciences. It has already implemented some of its applications in analytical techniques and other technologies (Weiss, Takhistov, & McClements, 2006). In this new era, nanotechnology has a significant impact on many areas, particularly in the food industry, such as the advancement of novel food packaging materials into nanodelivery systems, along with analytical control of the entire food chain. Nanotechnology is an alternative technique because the increasingly urgent demand for new, fast, efficient, and accurate information on the quality and safety of food products has led to more selective and sensitive analytical methods (Hosnedlova, Sochor, Baron, Bjørklund, & Kizek, 2019; Peng, Zhang, Aarts, & Dullens, 2018).

Biosensors and nanotechnologies are evolving rapidly in current fields, including food, agricultural, biomedical, medicinal, and pharmaceutical sciences, as well as catalysis and environmental remediation. Biosensors are analytical devices that convert the biological response to electrical signals, which are considered promising devices because of their unique properties such as high sensitivity, ease of miniaturization, and fast response. The sensitivity and efficiency of biosensors are enhanced by the use of nanomaterials (NSMs) that have made it possible to implement a range of new signal transduction technologies in biosensors.

In recent years, the application of NSMs in sensor technology and the evolution of analytical tools has significantly increased the portability of the analytical instrument. Sensing techniques based on NSMs such as the employment of nanoparticles (NPs) and other nanostructures to improve efficiency and specificity measurement, as well as facilitate sample preparation (Bulbul, Hayat, & Andreescu, 2015). Portable tools capable of analyzing different elements due to their submicron dimensions, nanosensors, nanoprobes, and other nanosystems have made it possible to test in vivo easily and quickly (Jianrong, Yuqing, Nongyue, Xiaohua, & Sijiao, 2004). This widespread use of nanotechnology and biosensors continues to drive the need to consider potential relationships on human and environmental health to assure efficient advancement. This chapter reviews the general principles and application of biosensors and nanotechnology that influence different aspects of human life.

Advanced Food Analysis Tools. https://doi.org/10.1016/B978-0-12-820591-4.00001-3

Nanotechnology

Nanotechnology can be defined as manufacture or technology that interacts with nanoscale materials and clusters of nanoscale matter in the various aspects of life that occur from a minimal scale range from specific atoms or molecules to submicron dimensions and the incorporation of the resulting nanostructures into larger systems (Bhushan, 2017; Gago, Llorente, Junquera, & Domingo, 2009). Nanotechnology involves interdisciplinary research, NSMs, and the use of physical, chemical, and biological processes in conjunction with material engineering, biotechnology, and industrial processing technology. Nanotechnology has now emerged as a multidisciplinary area in our society, where gaining a basic knowledge of the electrical, optical, magnetic, biological, medicinal, and mechanical properties of nanostructures expects to provide the next generation of functional materials with broad applications (Schaming & Remita, 2015). Due to their unique mechanical, optoelectronic, and physicochemical characteristics, NSMs can boost today's technology or open the way for new technologies in different areas such as electrochemical biosensing (Howes, Chandrawati, & Stevens, 2014; Vasilescu, Hayat, Gáspár, & Marty, 2018).

Nanotechnology is a new and emerging innovation that introduces novel ways for developing new products, formulating new chemicals and materials, and updating current equipment generation with better performance equipment, leading in lower material and energy consumption and diminished environmental damage, and also promising environmental remediation (Thiruvengadam, Rajakumar, & Chung, 2018). Over the year, several new technologies focused on nanotechnology have been developed to detect a wide range of targets, such as infectious agents, protein biomarkers, nucleic acids, drugs, and cancer cells. Nanotechnology represents an innovative road to technical advancement that relates to nanometer-scale material management. This has the power to transform our perspectives and perceptions and allow us to overcome global problems. The development and use of carbon NSMs have encouraged the development of many new fields like nanomedicine, biosensors, and bioelectronics technology. The application of nanotechnology may also provide approaches to technical and environmental problems in the fields of catalysis, medicine, solar energy conversion, and water treatment(Lv et al., 2018).

Moreover, nanotechnology has become one of the most important inventions and significant developments in reinventing the standard food science and food industry (He & Hwang, 2016). Nanotechnology devices have become extremely useful in biomedicine, and a hybrid science called nanobiotechnology has emerged (Saji, Choe, & Yeung, 2010). Therefore, nanotechnology offers a solution to environmental issues, steps to tackle the relevant issues of materials and energy exchange with the environment as well as potential risks associated with nanotechnology (Lee, Mahendra, & Alvarez, 2010). Nanotechnology has provided excellent tools that allow the processes to be defined in complex biological processes to a degree previously impossible. Nanotechnology has multidimensional impacts on society, which will undoubtedly be discussed for future decades (Baker, Brent, & Thomas, 2009).

Nanomaterials

NSMs are unequivocally classified as a material with an externally and internally dimensioned structure or surface of 100 nm and less. According to this concept, most of the substances around us will classify as NSMs, as nanoscale modulation of their internal structure (Buzea, Pacheco, & Robbie, 2007). They can derive either from combustion, manufacturing, or formed naturally. Many NSMs are NSMs engineered (EN) specifically for several consumer products and processes, some of which have been available for many years or decades (Alagarasi, 2013). The range of commercial products currently available is extensive, including fabrics, cosmetics, sunscreens, appliances, paints, and varnishes that are stain-resistant and wrinkle-free. Additionally, the large surface-to-volume ratio of NSMs is particularly useful in their use in the medical field, which enables cells and active ingredients to bind together.

NSMs composed of metal or nonmetal atoms are classified as metal, organic, or semi-conductive particles smaller than a micrometer. The morphological properties in at least one external dimension or with an internal nanoscale structure. In this way, NSMs, including NPs, nanowires, and nanotubes, have gained interest. NSMs used in nanobiosensors not only helped to deal with issues centered on the sensitivity and detection limit of the instruments but also increased the interfacial reaction due to enhanced immobilization of molecules for biorecognition (Bhattarai & Hameed, 2020).

Hybrid NSMs have lately been looked at as potential therapeutic platforms. This class of NSMs maintains beneficial characteristics of both inorganic and organic components and provides a way to change the nanohybrid properties by combining functional components (García & Uberman, 2019). The hybridization of nanomaterial-based strategies with a microscale system has permitted a new form of biomolecular research along with a high degree of sensitivity that can exploit nanoscale binding processes to distinguish the analytes (Kelley et al., 2014). NSMs with excellent electrical, optical, mechanical, and thermal characteristics have been acknowledged as one of the most innovative technologies in the production of next-generation biosensors for opening new gates (Lan, Yao, Ping, & Ying, 2017). Besides, NSMs also apply in plant security, nutrition, control of farm systems due to their small size, high surface to volume ratio, and unique optical features (Duhan et al., 2017).

Classification and production of nanomaterials

NSMs can be divided into various groups according to structures such as sizes or dimensions; and four types of NSMs are available, including zero-dimensional, one dimensional, two dimensional, and three dimensional (Malhotra & Ali, 2017). Moreover, emerging NSMs and NPs can also be categorized into four categories of materials, including carbon-based materials, metal-based materials, dendrimers, and composites (Jeevanandam, Barhoum, Chan, Dufresne, & Danquah, 2018).

The reactivity, strength, and fundamental physical and chemical characteristics of NPs rely on their specific size, shape, and structure, making them suitable for a variety of commercial and domestic applications (Khan, Saeed, & Khan, 2019). NPs can be differentiated by their chemical properties, their ability to carry various ingredients, and their ability to react to either organic or inorganic environmental conditions.

There are also several types of NPs, including nanofibers, nanoemulsions, and nanoclay. The diameter for nanofibers is around 5 nm long and about 15 µm long and is used as a thickener in food and filtering substances. Diversely, nanoemulsions have a diameter ranging from 50 to 500 nm per droplet, giving them rheological properties and differing stability. They are used for stabilizing certain materials, improving viscosity, and encapsulating components for release afterward. On the other hand, nanoclay is generally made of phosphosilicate and used mainly in food packaging, which functions as a barrier against oxygen and carbon dioxide. This nanoclay helps to make the plastic lighter, thinner, and more durable (Zhang & Wei, 2016). The classification of NSMs is summarized in Table 1.1.

Biosensor

Biosensors are categorized according to the elements of the bioreceptor involved in the investigation and the elements of the physicochemical transduction. The biosensor function can be clarified by the bioreceptor recognizing the target analyte. The desired biological material will be immobilized by traditional methods and will interact with the transducer intimately. The analyte binds to the biological material to form a bound analyte, and the transducer converts the corresponding biological responses into electrical equivalents. A significant output signal will be provided, which contains requisite frequency elements of an input signal as the amplifier responds to the small input signal. The signal processor must additionally store, view, and analyze the amplified signal. In some cases, the analyte is transformed into a product that may be correlated with heat, gas (oxygen), electrons, or hydrogen ions released (Velusamy, Arshak, Korostynska, Oliwa, & Adley, 2010). Fig. 1.1 shows the schematic diagram of the biosensor.

Usually, bioreceptors can be classed into five main groups, including enzymes, antibodies, nucleic acid, cells, and bacteriophages. Fig. 1.2 shows a biosensor configuration. The bioreceptors can be identified as the target analytes and corresponding biologically responses then translated them into an equivalent electrical signal by the transducer/electrode. The amplifier in the biosensor reacts to the transducer's small input signal and produces a large output signal that contains an input signal's crucial frequency characteristics. A processor will process the amplified signal where the signal can be stored, displayed, and analyzed.

Generally, biosensors are classified into three main categories, which are based on receptors, transducers, and nanobiosensors. Biosensors are the preferred tools in the current scenario because of their high sensitivity, safe handling, accuracy,

Table 1.1 Classification of nanomaterials.

Types	Description
Zero dimensional	Materials are available in nanoscales such as gold, palladium, platinum, silver, or quantum dots. Nanoparticles are available in spherical sizes with a diameter of 1–50 nm and some in cube and polygon shapes are zero-dimensional nanomaterials
One dimensional	These nanomaterials with one dimension are in the range of 1–100 nm and the other two dimensions can be in the microscale. Examples include nanowires, nanotubes, and nanotubes. Some metals, such as Au, Ag, Si, or quantum dots, can be provided as one-dimensional nanostructures
Two dimensional	Nanomaterials in nanoscale and one dimension are in microscale. Nanothin-films, thin-film multilayer, nanosheets, or nanowalls are two-dimensional nanomaterials. Also, several square micrometers can be used to keep the thickness within the nanoscale range
Three dimensional	Nanomaterials with no dimension in nanoscale and all dimensions are in macroscale. Bulk materials are three-dimensional, consisting of individual blocks that may be of a nanometer or more size
Carbon-based nanomaterial	Consist of carbon that found in morphologies, including hollow tubes, ellipsoids, or spheres. Other examples of carbon-based NMs include fullerenes, carbon nanotubes, carbon nanotubes, carbon black, graphene, and carbon onions. Laser ablation, arc discharge, and chemical vapor deposition are the crucial production techniques for these carbon-based materials (Kumar & Kumbhat, 2016)
Inorganic-based nanomaterials	Consists of metal and metal oxide nanoparticles and nanomaterials and can be synthesized into metals such as gold or silver nanoparticles, metal oxides such as tin oxide and zinc nanoparticles, and semiconductors including silicone and ceramics. Gold nanoparticles have a unique interaction between nanoparticle-free electrons and light. When a gold nanoparticle is exposed to an external optical field, the electrical portion of the light acts on and displaces the electrons in the conduction band. Uncompensated charges will be created on the surface of nanoparticles (Buzea et al., 2007; Khlebtsov & Dykman, 2010)
Organic-based nanomaterials	Mostly made from organic matter, excluding carbon-based or inorganic-based nanomaterials. The use of non-covalent interactions for self-assembly and molecular design enables NMs to be transformed into ideal structures, including nanoparticle dendrimers, mice, liposomes, and polymers
Composite-based nanomaterials	Composite nanomaterials are multi-nanoparticles and nanomaterials with a single-phase nanoscale dimension that can be combined either with other nanoparticles or with bulk- materials or with more complex structures. The composites may be any mixture of carbon, metal, or organic-nanomaterials with any type of metal, ceramic, or polymer bulk materials. Nanomaterials are produced in various morphologies, based on the properties needed for the specific application

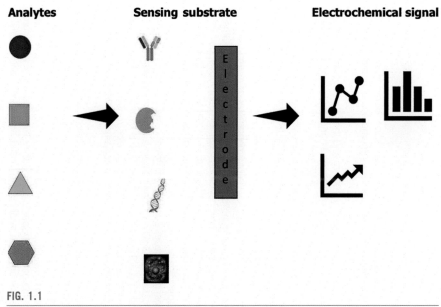

FIG. 1.1

The schematic diagram of biosensors.

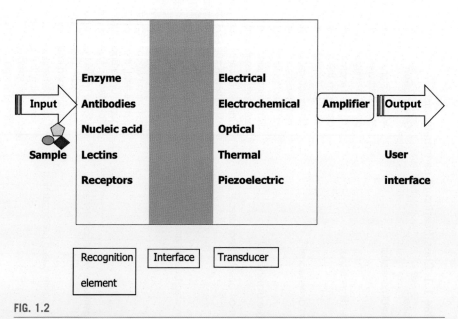

FIG. 1.2

The configuration of biosensors.

precision, and quick response time (Narsaiah, Jha, Bhardwaj, Sharma, & Ramesh, 2012). Knowledge of chemical and physical changes during the handling, preparing, processing, and storage of food is the basis for the layout and invention of different biosensors. The constructs utilize optical, electrochemical, thermometric, piezoelectric, magnetic, or micromechanical methods to convey the relevant information in the form of a signal (Shandilya et al., 2019).

Classification of biosensors

Biosensors have been broadly used in various scientific areas due to their excellent performance. Biosensors usually can be classified into two major groups based on bioreceptors and transducers as shown in Fig. 1.3. Firstly is a bioreceptor, which refers to the molecular species and acts by utilizing a biochemical mechanism and binds to the target analytes. Bioreceptors are assorted into five major groups, namely, an enzyme, an antibody, biomimetic, nucleic acid, cells, and bacteriophage, which typically used to identify foodborne pathogens (Velusamy et al., 2010).

Secondly, transducer-based biosensors can be divided into four main classes such as electrochemical, optical, piezoelectric, and thermometric that extensively practiced in the food industry (Velusamy et al., 2010). Previously, the electrochemical biosensors method showed rapid and ease of miniaturization, cost-effective, compliant with present microfabrication technologies, and have entered numerous markets specifically in antioxidant research (Su, Jia, Hou, & Lei, 2011; Ye, Ji, Sun, Shen, & Sun, 2019). Besides, optical sensors are also the most popular biosensors after electrochemical sensors because of their high detection speed, sensitivity, durability, and the ability to detect multiple analytes (Yoo & Lee, 2016). Surface plasmon resonance

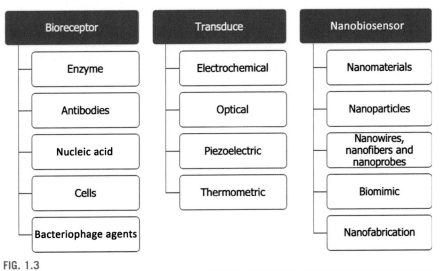

FIG. 1.3

Classification of the biosensors.

(SPR) is an example of the optical techniques that commonly used in biosensor production that can determine the presence of a chemical and does not require molecules labeled during the analysis (Alhadrami, 2018; Ziegler & Göpel, 1998).

Besides, nanobiosensors are virtually sensors consisting of NSMs or nanoscaled analytical structures composed of nanoconjugated biological materials such as transduction systems for detecting minuscule amounts of any biological, physical, or chemical analytes. Nanobiosensors performed a significant development intervention in the field of biosensors, which was achievable only because of the wonders of the nanotechnological ramifications of the matter. In many studies, a wide range of biosensing systems using NPs or nanostructures have been investigated (Malik et al., 2013).

From previous work, nanobiosensor reported as nanoscaled analytical frameworks that comprise nanoconjugated biological materials and better suited to identify the miniscule interacting process due to the SPR mechanism that makes a much higher and far more accurate degree of estimation of biological interactions via a nanobiosensor compared to a biosensor (Malik et al., 2013; Shandilya et al., 2019). Besides, nanobiosensor technology is pioneering the healthcare sector, and the food industry even plays a significant role in environmental fields (Pandit, Dasgupta, Dewan, & Prince, 2016). Additionally, advanced nanoscaled sensors can help to achieve higher sensitivity, precision, and multiplexing to clarify the stage and cancer type completely. It will take advantage of all systems such as photoacoustic tomography, Raman spectroscopic imaging, and multimodal imaging.

Application of biosensor and nanotechnology

Biosensors and nanotechnology have been widely used in various research fields such as enzyme-based, tissue-based, immunosensors, DNA biosensors, and thermal and piezoelectric biosensors (Mehrotra, 2016). Until now, in every walk of life, this growing field of biosensors has almost got a stronghold. The current innovations and advancements in this biosensing method are applied in the primary fields of agriculture, medicine, biomedicine, health, and environmental studies and offer better stability and sensitivity compared to conventional techniques (Ali, Najeeb, Ali, Aslam, & Raza, 2017; Ensafi, 2019; Karunakaran, Bhargava, & Benjamin, 2015). Some of the popular fields, including the food industry, used biosensors to monitor their quality and health, to help distinguish between natural and artificial, and biosensors used in the fermentation and saccharification industries to monitor specific concentrations of glucose; in metabolic engineering to permit in vivo control of cell metabolism.

Food industry

Research has contributed to the full benefit of this food industry worldwide, to meet the consumer demands of fresh and nutritious foods (Ali et al., 2017). To ensure the protection of processed foods, the food companies have implemented different methods to overcome the problems that lead to food spoilage and identification and destruction of certain chemicals or biological agents that are responsible for causing specific significant health-related issues. The food industry is the leading group concerned with the existence of pathogenic microorganisms, where failure to detect a pathogen may lead to a terrible impact. Conventional techniques conducting chemical experiments and spectroscopy have human fatigue deficiencies, which are expensive and time-consuming (Amit, Uddin, Rahman, Islam, & Khan, 2017). The nanotechnological strategy can be implemented in the food industry to improve food quality (Dumitriu, de Lerma, Luchian, Cotea, & Peinado, 2018), health, shelf-life, cost, food packaging (Duncan, 2011; Vilarinho, Sanches Silva, Vaz, & Farinha, 2018), nutritional benefits (Sozer & Kokini, 2009), taste characteristics (Duncan, 2011), and the delivery of natural antimicrobials in food (Pinilla, Norena, & Brandelli, 2017).

Biosensors play a significant role in the food industry once it comes to tracking nutrients and screening off biological and chemical pollutants. Throughout the food processing industry, biosensors can be used in the fermentation process; and they can also be employed to identify heavy metals in food and to detect pesticides in juices and wine. Fermentation is an integral part of the food, feed, and biofuels production since the fermentation industries concentrate on process protection and product quality (Mehrotra, 2016). Besides, biosensor has been used in fermentation industries to track the existence of products, biomass, enzymes, antibodies, or by-products from the fermentation process and can indirectly calculate the process state.

Nanotechnology enhances the shelf-life of certain forms of food resources and also ensures a reduction in the amount of food wastage due to microbial infestation (Pradhan et al., 2015). An optical biosensor is a versatile and sensitive tool capable of identifying defective rates of chemicals and biologics and of measuring molecular interactions in situ and in real-time (Nath & Chilkoti, 2002; Rovina, Shaeera, Vonnie, & Yi, 2019). This approach is used in the food industry to detect bacteria directly in foods to detect changes in refractive indices as the cell attaches to the transducer's immobilized receptor (Pirinçci et al., 2018). Furthermore, Lu and Gunasekaran (2019) developed and manufactured an electrochemical immunosensor for simultaneous identification of two mycotoxins due to the widespread co-contamination of mycotoxins in raw food materials. Besides, Ghasemi-Varnamkhasti et al. (2012) researched on detecting the aging of beer utilizing enzymatic biosensors based on cobalt phthalocyanine, where a strong potential to track the aging of beer throughout storage could be demonstrated. Additionally, enzymatic biosensors are often used in the dairy industry, where a biosensor based on a screen-printed carbon electrode was incorporated into a flow cell to quantify the three organophosphate pesticides in milk (Mishra, Dominguez, Bhand, Muñoz, & Marty, 2012).

Biosensors are used to identify pathogens in foodstuffs. For example, *Escherichia coli* (*E. coli*) was detected in vegetables using a potentiometric alternating biosensing method by evaluating changes in the pH caused by ammonia (Arora, Ahmed, Khubber, & Siddiqui, 2018). Additionally, intelligent nutrient control and rapid inspection of biological and chemical contamination are of vital importance for the quality and health of the food. Material science, nanotechnology, electrochemical, and microfluidic systems are moving towards the imminent use of sensing technology on the market (Mehrotra, 2016). For example, glucose control during storage may be altered due to food quality and composition. A luminol electrochemiluminescence-based flow-injection optical fiber biosensor for glucose was identified. The sol–gel process is used to immobilize glucose oxidase (GOx) on a glassy carbon electrode surface (2012). The electrochemistry of immobilized GOx was studied by German, Ramanaviciene, Voronovic, and Ramanavicius (2010) on a graphite chain, altered by gold NPs (AuNPs), which enhanced its sensitivity. Furthermore, sunset yellow (SY) belongs to the azo group, which can contribute to toxicity and photogenic to human health through a high intake of SY in the food industry. To quantify the degree of SY in commercial food products, a simple and highly sensitive electrochemical sensor was developed based on the modified glassy carbon electrode (GCE) with graphene (GO), multiwall carbon nanotubes (MWCNTs), gold NPs (AuNPs), and nanocomposite chitosan membrane (CHIT) (Rovina, Siddiquee, & Shaarani, 2017).

Biomedical fields

Within the medical community, diagnostics are central to successful disease prevention or treatment, and the ability to recognize molecular markers linked to diseases is increasingly being researched and significantly extended. Biologic substances such as blood, saliva, or urine are rich in physiological data. Biosensors that can track multiple analytes at the same time would, therefore, be useful for accurate analysis of one's physiological state (Mazur, Bally, Städler, & Chandrawati, 2017). Enzyme-linked immunosorbent assay (ELISA) represents the global gold standard in science and clinical diagnostics because of its high specificity, standard configuration, and legibility. Biosensors are the analytical devices that allow molecular interactions to be sensed and converted into an electrical signal which can be detected. Across medical sciences, biosensors are prevalently used to detect infectious diseases. Recent advances in nanotechnology and its applications in the field of biomedicine have led to the development of new technologies in clinical diagnostics (Medawar-Aguilar et al., 2019).

Medically, biosensors are devised to detect tumors, bacteria, toxins, and biomarkers reliably and precisely, to recognize the onset of different disorders at an initial stage. Biosensors have gained prominence because of their low production costs, rapid response times, convenience, the ability to measure biological elements at a tiny scale, high specificity, and sensitivity (Solaimuthu, Vijayan, Murali, & Korrapati, 2020). Nanotechnology advances have recently stimulated the creation of multiple types of ZnO nanostructures such as nanolayers, NPs, nanowires, and others. Because of their improved sensing properties, enhanced binding capability with biomolecules as well as biological activities has allowed them to be suitable candidates for the manufacture of biomedical devices. Early cancer detection in patients is a continuing challenge and can provide an important starting point for developing new tumor treatment strategies. Low-cost, fast, and label-free detection and portability are some of the obstacles to defeat. For early detection of mucin 16, an electrochemical approach based on the structures of ZnO nanorod-AuNPs was used in which hydrothermal synthesis was used to produce ZnO nanorods on the surface of gold and silver surfaces for use as a working electrode, accompanied by sputtering AuNPs (Shetti, Bukkitgar, Kakarla, Reddy, & Aminabhavi, 2019).

Furthermore, it is necessary to classify end-stage heart failure patients who are vulnerable to adverse effects during the early stages of implantation of the left ventricular assist system. A novel hafnium-based biosensor oxide (HfO2), was used to detect human interleukin (IL)-10 early in the cycle. Enzymes are also especially important for biosensing applications due to its active catalysts that can very precisely and selectively transform substrates into products (Mazur et al., 2017). Previous research has developed liposome-enzyme receptors for the detection of biomarkers of disease, thrombin, or C-reactive proteins (CRP). In this process, liposomes are used to trap amyloglucosidase or invertase non-covalently for signal transduction and amplification (Lin et al., 2016).

On the other hand, 3D printing has also achieved the fabrication of medical devices with integrated electronics and circuits. 3D printers are used as production tools for a broad range of devices, from diagnostics to sensors to external prostheses. The simplicity of use, accessibility of 3D-design software, and cheapness have made 3D printing an open method for development and production in many bioanalytical research labs. 3D printers can print materials of varying density, optical character, power, and chemical properties and provide a wide range of strategic alternatives for the consumer (Sharafeldin, Jones, & Rusling, 2018).

Environment fields

The causes of pollution in the environment may be attributed to acts by humans or nature. Contamination has become a vital concern for health and environmental safety. The need for disposable tools or environmental management methods has stimulated the emergence of new technology and more appropriate techniques, the ability to control the number of environmental significance analyses as rapidly and as cheaply as possible, and also the potential of on-site analysis of the environment (Rodriguez-Mozaz, de Alda, & Barceló, 2006). Previously, the scientist has focused on the identification of environmental threats or pollution. Biosensors have gained enormous interest in recent times in monitoring pollutants that need high specificity and sensitivity (Sarkar, Sarkar, Amrutha, & Dutta, 2019). Unlike traditional analytical methods, the biosensor is beneficial in terms of its cost-effectiveness, usability, eco-friendliness, convenience, and the potential to provide online monitoring in real-time (Daverey, Dutta, & Sarkar, 2019). As well as identifying large amounts of contaminants, the entire cell-based biosensor has opened the gates to identify and analyze real-life conditions. The eukaryotic cell-based biosensor is also available to analyze for analysis of water toxicity for real-time.

Biosensors based on enzymes such as urease, trypsin, or biosensor based on phosphatase have been used for the detection of heavy metals. Also, the whole cell-based biosensors were designed for heavy metal analysis. Whole cell-based biosensors are more potent than enzyme-based biosensors since the use of enzymes causes the loss of activity after immobilization and gives the wrong result (Suryan, 2017). Besides, the immunosensors technique that is used to detect the environmental control system (ECs) in the environment are immunochemical techniques, such as ELISA. The immunosensors are highly selective and can be used to determine the toxicity of a specific contaminant (Verma & Bhardwaj, 2015).

Another form of the biosensor, called a phage sensor, was invented to track food and environmental pathogens and pollutants (Van Dorst et al., 2010). The primary contaminant that can be identified and extracted progressively with biosensors includes heavy metals, pesticides, biochemical oxygen demand (BOD), nitrogen compounds, and various pathogens such as viruses and bacteria (Ali et al., 2017). Similarly, industrial biosensors were also effectively implemented and used to detect dioxins, nitrates, and *E. coli*, and chemicals identical to dioxins. Biosensors focused on microbes can also be used to track airborne pollutants and pathogenic agents. Phage sensors can be used to identify pathogenic microbes carried by air (Van Dorst et al., 2010).

Agriculture

Agriculture is a source of income and opportunities to a large proportion of the population, where it plays a crucial role in the self-sustaining economic development of a country by providing humanity with nutritious food and raw material for industrialization. After the industrial revolution, the production of different agricultural technology incorporating chemical pesticides and herbicides led to further increases in crop yields by effectively managing weeds and the infestation of pests. Biosensors are now gaining prominence in all fields, from farm to fork amongst the new novel patterns and streams in agriculture (Kundu, Krishnan, Kotnala, & Sumana, 2019). Nanotechnology developments in the field of materials science and biomass conversion technologies used in agriculture are the basis for supplying food, feed, fiber, fire, and fuels. Recently, nanosized lignocellulosic materials have been collected from crops and trees that have opened up a new opportunity for advanced nanosized materials and goods with added value. For example, nanosized cellulosic crystals were used in the polymer matrix as lightweight reinforcement (Lucia & Rojas, 2009). Use of a variety of NSMs in agriculture that helps to minimize agrochemical use by using innovative delivery systems, reduce nutrient losses, and increase yield by optimizing water and nutrient control.

Due to leaching, degradation, and long-term assimilation by soil microorganisms, nanofertilizers should be used to reduce the nitrogen loss. A biosensor could be linked to this nanofertilizer, which helps the selective release of nitrogen connected to the conditions of time, the environment, and the soil. Slow-controlled release of fertilizers can also boost soil by minimizing fertilizer-related harmful effects over implementation (Rai, Acharya, & Dey, 2012). Zeolites are normal, aluminum silicates that are ideally suited to plant growth not only to enhance performance, fertilizer quality, water absorption, and retention, but also to boost yield, maintain long-term soil quality nutrients, and minimize soil nutrient degradation. Moreover, when zeolites are connected to a nanobiosensor that can technologize agriculture to sense the shortage in either plant or soil and monitor, water or nutrient release is maintained in the zeolite (Singh, 2017).

It can be potentially helpful in improving professionalism for farmers because of weather, temperature, and strain, nanodevices sense toxins, biomolecules, pests, nutrients, and plant stress. Nanodevices such as electronic noses (*E*-nose) are NPs-based gas sensors; the resistance changes as the gas passes over it and induces a change in the electrical signal, eventually detecting gas. Seeds produce volatile aldehydes during storage, which trigger aging and are also hazardous to other seeds (Prasad, Bhattacharyya, & Nguyen, 2017).

Tissue engineering

Tissue engineering is an extremely demanding and flexible field that plays an essential role in integrating the concepts of alternative materials to replace the damaged tissue or facilitate endogenous regeneration (Ali et al., 2017). In tissue engineering, biosensors play an essential role in the applicability of different applications such as producing organ-specific and clinical trial on-chip, microfluidic designs, genetic modification, restoring damaged tissue and preserving the configuration of cell cultures where tissue fate is directly correlated with the content of small biomolecules in the medium. Throughout the new scientific century, the tissue engineering method was prevalent throughout addressing the shortcomings of organ transplantation, graft rejection, difficulties in functional tissue reconstruction, and specificities at the regeneration site.

Current tissue engineering approaches face difficulties involving lack of adequate biomaterials, weak cell growth, and a shortage of procedures to capture correct physiological architectures, as well as unstable and insufficient growth factor output to promote cell contact and proper reaction. NPs are at the center of nanotechnology, and their inherent size-dependent abilities have demonstrated promise in resolving many of today's tissue engineering barriers. The surface combination and conducting characteristics of gold NPs (GNPs), the antimicrobial properties of silver and other metallic NPs and metal oxides, the fluorescence features of quantum dots, and the unique electro-mechanical properties of carbon nanotubes (CNTs) have rendered them quite valuable in many tissue engineering technologies (Hasan et al., 2018).

Conclusion and future perspectives

Biosensors have lately risen as the major players in many types of industrial or educational sectors. Development of nanotechnology in biosensors offers opportunities to improve a future generation of biosensor technologies that will enhance the mechanical, electrochemical, optical, and magnetic characteristics of biosensors with arrays of high-performance biosensors. Nanotechnology has created an outstanding chance to create advanced biosensors of the nanoscale that can be incorporated into lab-on-chip systems. Recent advances in biosensor technology over the last few years have opened the way for future researchers to strengthen these biosensing aspects further and enhance them to the degree that even the most dangerous diseases can be identified. The integration of nanotechnology and disease-specific molecular signatures provides comprehensive analysis and treatment opportunities. If all technological challenges are solved, it will be a massive achievement in humankind's history even though it is being used, but the rate of achievement still needs to be improved. In the future, biosensors will focus on cost minimization and the difficulties associated with moving technology from academics to industries. Besides, future research will also work on clarifying the principle of interaction on the surface of electrodes or nanofilms between NSMs and biomolecules and use novel materials to create a new generation of biosensors. Research work on biological agents may contribute to the production of new biosensors with potential advantages for human health. In summary, biosensors can be implemented in more fields with the advancement of technology. The identification of contagious diseases can be easily accomplished by improving biosensors.

References

Alagarasi, A. (2013). *Chapter-Introduction to nanomaterials*: (pp. 1–24). Indian Institute of Technology Madras.

Alhadrami, H. A. (2018). Biosensors: Classifications, medical applications, and future prospective. *Biotechnology and Applied Biochemistry*, *65*(3), 497–508.

Ali, J., Najeeb, J., Ali, M. A., Aslam, M. F., & Raza, A. (2017). Biosensors: Their fundamentals, designs, types and most recent impactful applications: A review. *Journal of Biosensors and Bioelectronics*, *8*(1), 1–9.

Amit, S. K., Uddin, M. M., Rahman, R., Islam, S. R., & Khan, M. S. (2017). A review on mechanisms and commercial aspects of food preservation and processing. *Agriculture & Food Security*, *6*(1), 51.

Arora, S., Ahmed, D. N., Khubber, S., & Siddiqui, S. (2018). Detecting food borne pathogens using electrochemical biosensors: An overview. *International Journal of Chemical Studies*, *6*(1), 1031–1039.

Baker, J. R., Brent, B. W., Jr., & Thomas, T. P. (2009). Nanotechnology in clinical and translational research. In *Clinical and translational science* (pp. 123–135). Academic Press.

Bhattarai, P., & Hameed, S. (2020). Basics of biosensors and nanobiosensors. In *Nanobiosensors: From design to applications* (pp. 1–22).

Bhushan, B. (2017). Introduction to nanotechnology. In *Springer handbook of nanotechnology* (pp. 1–19). Berlin, Heidelberg: Springer.

Bulbul, G., Hayat, A., & Andreescu, S. (2015). Portable nanoparticle-based sensors for food safety assessment. *Sensors*, *15*(12), 30736–30758.

Buzea, C., Pacheco, I. I., & Robbie, K. (2007). Nanomaterials and nanoparticles: Sources and toxicity. *Biointerphases*, *2*(4), MR17–MR71.

Daverey, A., Dutta, K., & Sarkar, A. (2019). An overview of analytical methodologies for environmental monitoring. In *Tools, techniques and protocols for monitoring environmental contaminants* (pp. 3–17). Elsevier.

Duhan, J. S., Kumar, R., Kumar, N., Kaur, P., Nehra, K., & Duhan, S. (2017). Nanotechnology: The new perspective in precision agriculture. *Biotechnology Reports, 15*, 11–23.

Dumitriu, G. -D., de Lerma, N. L., Luchian, C. E., Cotea, V. V., & Peinado, R. A. (2018). Study of the potential use of mesoporous nano-materials as fining agent to prevent protein haze in white wines and its impact in major volatile aroma compounds and polyols. *Food Chemistry, 240*, 751–758.

Duncan, T. V. (2011). The communication challenges presented by nanofoods. *Nature Nanotechnology, 6*(11), 683.

Ensafi, A. A. (2019). An introduction to sensors and biosensors. In *Electrochemical biosensors* (pp. 1–10). Elsevier.

Gago, J. M., Llorente, C., Junquera, E., & Domingo, P. (2009). *Nanociencia y Nanotecnología: Entre la ciencia ficción del presente y la tecnología del futuro.* Publicación de la Fundación Española para la Ciencia y la Tecnología http://www.fecyt.es.

García, M. C., & Uberman, P. M. (2019). Nanohybrid filler-based drug-delivery system. In *Nanocarriers for drug delivery* (pp. 43–79). Elsevier.

German, N., Ramanaviciene, A., Voronovic, J., & Ramanavicius, A. (2010). Glucose biosensor based on graphite electrodes modified with glucose oxidase and colloidal gold nanoparticles. *Microchimica Acta, 168*(3–4), 221–229.

Ghasemi-Varnamkhasti, M., Rodríguez-Méndez, M. L., Mohtasebi, S. S., Apetrei, C., Lozano, J., Ahmadi, H., … de Saja, J. A. (2012). Monitoring the aging of beers using a bioelectronic tongue. *Food Control, 25*(1), 216–224.

Hasan, A., Morshed, M., Memic, A., Hassan, S., Webster, T. J., & Marei, H. E. S. (2018). Nanoparticles in tissue engineering: Applications, challenges and prospects. *International Journal of Nanomedicine, 13*, 5637.

He, X., & Hwang, H. M. (2016). Nanotechnology in food science: Functionality, applicability, and safety assessment. *Journal of Food and Drug Analysis, 24*(4), 671–681.

Hosnedlova, B., Sochor, J., Baron, M., Bjørklund, G., & Kizek, R. (2019). Application of nanotechnology based-biosensors in analysis of wine compounds and control of wine quality and safety: A critical review. *Critical Reviews in Food Science and Nutrition,* 1–19. https://doi.org/10.1080/10408398.2019.1682965.

Howes, P. D., Chandrawati, R., & Stevens, M. M. (2014). Colloidal nanoparticles as advanced biological sensors. *Science, 346*(6205), 1247390.

Jeevanandam, J., Barhoum, A., Chan, Y. S., Dufresne, A., & Danquah, M. K. (2018). Review on nanoparticles and nanostructured materials: History, sources, toxicity and regulations. *Beilstein Journal of Nanotechnology, 9*(1), 1050–1074.

Jianrong, C., Yuqing, M., Nongyue, H., Xiaohua, W., & Sijiao, L. (2004). Nanotechnology and biosensors. *Biotechnology Advances, 22*(7), 505–518.

Karunakaran, C., Bhargava, K., & Benjamin, R. (2015). *Biosensors and bioelectronics.* Elsevier.

Kelley, S. O., Mirkin, C. A., Walt, D. R., Ismagilov, R. F., Toner, M., & Sargent, E. H. (2014). Advancing the speed, sensitivity and accuracy of biomolecular detection using multi-length-scale engineering. *Nature Nanotechnology, 9*(12), 969.

Khan, I., Saeed, K., & Khan, I. (2019). Nanoparticles: Properties, applications and toxicities. *Arabian Journal of Chemistry, 12*(7), 908–931.

Khlebtsov, N. G., & Dykman, L. A. (2010). Optical properties and biomedical applications of plasmonic nanoparticles. *Journal of Quantitative Spectroscopy and Radiative Transfer*, *111*(1), 1–35.

Kumar, N., & Kumbhat, S. (2016). *Essentials in nanoscience and nanotechnology*. Wiley Online Library.

Kundu, M., Krishnan, P., Kotnala, R. K., & Sumana, G. (2019). Recent developments in biosensors to combat agricultural challenges and their future prospects. *Trends in Food Science and Technology*, *88*, 157–178. https://doi.org/10.1016/j.tifs.2019.03.024.

Lan, L., Yao, Y., Ping, J., & Ying, Y. (2017). Recent advances in nanomaterial-based biosensors for antibiotics detection. *Biosensors and Bioelectronics*, *91*, 504–514.

Lee, J., Mahendra, S., & Alvarez, P. J. (2010). Nanomaterials in the construction industry: A review of their applications and environmental health and safety considerations. *ACS Nano*, *4*(7), 3580–3590.

Lin, B., Liu, D., Yan, J., Qiao, Z., Zhong, Y., Yan, J., Zhu, Z., Ji, T., & Yang, C. J. (2016). Enzyme-encapsulated liposome-linked immunosorbent assay enabling sensitive personal glucose meter readout for portable detection of disease biomarkers. *ACS Applied Materials & Interfaces*, *8*(11), 6890–6897.

Lu, L., & Gunasekaran, S. (2019). Dual-channel ITO-microfluidic electrochemical immunosensor for simultaneous detection of two mycotoxins. *Talanta*, *194*, 709–716.

Lucia, L. A., & Rojas, O. (Eds.), (2009). *The nanoscience and technology of renewable biomaterials*. John Wiley & Sons.

Lv, M., Liu, Y., Geng, J., Kou, X., Xin, Z., & Yang, D. (2018). Engineering nanomaterials-based biosensors for food safety detection. *Biosensors and Bioelectronics*, *106*, 122–128.

Malhotra, B. D., & Ali, M. A. (2017). *Nanomaterials for biosensors: Fundamentals and applications*. William Andrew.

Malik, P., Katyal, V., Malik, V., Asatkar, A., Inwati, G., & Mukherjee, T. K. (2013). Nanobiosensors: Concepts and variations. *ISRN Nanomaterials*, *2013*, 1–9. https://doi.org/10.1155/2013/327435.

Mazur, F., Bally, M., Städler, B., & Chandrawati, R. (2017). Liposomes and lipid bilayers in biosensors. *Advances in Colloid and Interface Science*, *249*, 88–99.

Medawar-Aguilar, V., Jofre, C. F., Fernández-Baldo, M. A., Alonso, A., Angel, S., Raba, J., ... Messina, G. A. (2019). Serological diagnosis of toxoplasmosis disease using a fluorescent immunosensor with chitosan-ZnO-nanoparticles. *Analytical Biochemistry*, *564*, 116–122.

Mehrotra, P. (2016). Biosensors and their applications—A review. *Journal of Oral Biology and Craniofacial Research*, *6*(2), 153–159.

Mishra, R. K., Dominguez, R. B., Bhand, S., Muñoz, R., & Marty, J. L. (2012). A novel automated flow-based biosensor for the determination of organophosphate pesticides in milk. *Biosensors and Bioelectronics*, *32*(1), 56–61.

Narsaiah, K., Jha, S. N., Bhardwaj, R., Sharma, R., & Ramesh, K. (2012). Optical biosensors for food quality and safety assurance—A review. *Journal of Food Science and Technology*, *49*(4), e383–e406.

Nath, N., & Chilkoti, A. (2002). A colorimetric gold nanoparticle sensor to interrogate biomolecular interactions in real time on a surface. *Analytical Chemistry*, *74*(3), 504–509.

Pandit, S., Dasgupta, D., Dewan, N., & Prince, A. (2016). Nanotechnology based biosensors and its application. *The Pharmaceutical Innovation*, *5*(6, Pt. A), 18.

Peng, B., Zhang, X., Aarts, D. G., & Dullens, R. P. (2018). Superparamagnetic nickel colloidal nanocrystal clusters with antibacterial activity and bacteria binding ability. *Nature Nanotechnology*, *13*(6), 478. https://doi.org/10.1038/s41565-018-0108-0.

Pinilla, C. M. B., Norena, C. P. Z., & Brandelli, A. (2017). Development and characterization of phosphatidylcholine nanovesicles, containing garlic extract, with antilisterial activity in milk. *Food Chemistry, 220*, 470–476.

Pirinçci, Ş. Ş., Ertekin, Ö., Laguna, D. E., Özen, F. Ş., Öztürk, Z. Z., & Öztürk, S. (2018). Label-free QCM immunosensor for the detection of ochratoxin A. *Sensors, 18*(4), 1161.

Pradhan, N., Singh, S., Ojha, N., Shrivastava, A., Barla, A., Rai, V., & Bose, S. (2015). Facets of nanotechnology as seen in food processing, packaging, and preservation industry. *BioMed Research International*, 1–17.

Prasad, R., Bhattacharyya, A., & Nguyen, Q. D. (2017). Nanotechnology in sustainable agriculture: Recent developments, challenges, and perspectives. *Frontiers in Microbiology, 8*, 1014.

Rai, V., Acharya, S., & Dey, N. (2012). Implications of nanobiosensors in agriculture. *Journal of Biomaterials and Nanobiotechnology, 3*, 1–10. https://doi.org/10.4236/jbnb.2012.322039.

Rodriguez-Mozaz, S., de Alda, M. J. L., & Barceló, D. (2006). Biosensors as useful tools for environmental analysis and monitoring. *Analytical and Bioanalytical Chemistry, 386*(4), 1025–1041.

Rovina, K., Shaeera, S. N., Vonnie, J. M., & Yi, S. X. (2019). Recent biosensors technologies for detection of mycotoxin in food products. In *Mycotoxins and food safety*. IntechOpen.

Rovina, K., Siddiquee, S., & Shaarani, S. M. (2017). Highly sensitive electrochemical determination of sunset yellow in commercial food products based on CHIT/GO/MWCNTs/AuNPs/GCE. *Food Control, 82*, 66–73.

Saji, V. S., Choe, H. C., & Yeung, K. W. (2010). Nanotechnology in biomedical applications: A review. *International Journal of Nano and Biomaterials, 3*(2), 119–139.

Sarkar, A., Sarkar, K. D., Amrutha, V., & Dutta, K. (2019). An overview of enzyme-based biosensors for environmental monitoring. In *Tools, techniques and protocols for monitoring environmental contaminants* (pp. 307–329). Elsevier.

Schaming, D., & Remita, H. (2015). Nanotechnology: From the ancient time to nowadays. *Foundations of Chemistry, 17*(3), 187–205.

Shandilya, R., Bhargava, A., Bunkar, N., Tiwari, R., Goryacheva, I. Y., & Mishra, P. K. (2019). Nanobiosensors: Point-of-care approaches for cancer diagnostics. *Biosensors and Bioelectronics, 130*, 147–165.

Sharafeldin, M., Jones, A., & Rusling, J. F. (2018). 3D-printed biosensor arrays for medical diagnostics. *Micromachines, 9*(8), 394.

Shetti, N. P., Bukkitgar, S. D., Kakarla, R. R., Reddy, C., & Aminabhavi, T. M. (2019). ZnO-based nanostructured electrodes for electrochemical sensors and biosensors in biomedical applications. *Biosensors and Bioelectronics*. https://doi.org/10.1016/j.bios.2019.111417.

Singh, R. P. (2017). Application of nanomaterials toward development of nanobiosensors and their utility in agriculture. In *Nanotechnology* (pp. 293–303). Singapore: Springer.

Solaimuthu, A., Vijayan, A. N., Murali, P., & Korrapati, P. S. (2020). Nano-biosensors and their relevance in tissue engineering. *Current Opinion in Biomedical Engineering, 13*, 84–93.

Sozer, N., & Kokini, J. L. (2009). Nanotechnology and its applications in the food sector. *Trends in Biotechnology, 27*(2), 82–89.

Su, L., Jia, W., Hou, C., & Lei, Y. (2011). Microbial biosensors: A review. *Biosensors and Bioelectronics, 26*(5), 1788–1799.

Suryan, S. K. (2017). Biosensors: A tool for environmental monitoring and analysis. In R. Kumar, A. Sharma, & S. Ahluwalia (Eds.), *Advances in environmental biotechnology*. Singapore: Springer.

Thiruvengadam, M., Rajakumar, G., & Chung, I. M. (2018). Nanotechnology: Current uses and future applications in the food industry. *3 Biotech*, *8*(1), 74.

Van Dorst, B., Mehta, J., Bekaert, K., Rouah-Martin, E., De Coen, W., Dubruel, P., ... Robbens, J. (2010). Recent advances in recognition elements of food and environmental biosensors: A review. *Biosensors and Bioelectronics*, *26*(4), 1178–1194.

Vasilescu, A., Hayat, A., Gáspár, S., & Marty, J. L. (2018). Advantages of carbon nanomaterials in electrochemical aptasensors for food analysis. *Electroanalysis*, *30*(1), 2–19.

Velusamy, V., Arshak, K., Korostynska, O., Oliwa, K., & Adley, C. (2010). An overview of foodborne pathogen detection: In the perspective of biosensors. *Biotechnology Advances*, *28*(2), 232–254.

Verma, N., & Bhardwaj, A. (2015). Biosensor technology for pesticides—A review. *Applied Biochemistry and Biotechnology*, *175*, 3093–3119. https://doi.org/10.1007/s12010-015-1489-2.

Vilarinho, F., Sanches Silva, A., Vaz, M. F., & Farinha, J. P. (2018). Nanocellulose in green food packaging. *Critical Reviews in Food Science and Nutrition*, *58*(9), 1526–1537.

Weiss, J., Takhistov, P., & McClements, D. J. (2006). Functional materials in food nanotechnology. *Journal of Food Science*, *71*(9), R107–R116. https://doi.org/10.1111/j.1750-3841.2006.00195.x.

Ye, Y., Ji, J., Sun, Z., Shen, P., & Sun, X. (2019). Recent advances in electrochemical biosensors for antioxidant analysis in foodstuff. *TrAC Trends in Analytical Chemistry*. https://doi.org/10.1016/j.trac.2019.115718.

Yoo, S. M., & Lee, S. Y. (2016). Optical biosensors for the detection of pathogenic microorganisms. *Trends in Biotechnology*, *34*(1), 7–25.

Zhang, Y., & Wei, Q. (2016). The role of nanomaterials in electroanalytical biosensors: A mini review. *Journal of Electroanalytical Chemistry*, *781*, 401–409.

Ziegler, C., & Göpel, W. (1998). Biosensor development. *Current Opinion in Chemical Biology*, *2*(5), 585–591.

Biosensor and nanotechnology: Past, present, and future in food research

Introduction

The market for biomolecules to be identified directly, low cost, rapidly, sensitively, and easily is massive. Modernization of technology nowadays allows biosensor and nanotechnology to be used for biomolecules recognition and generating results in real-time and on-site. Biosensors incorporate the elements of biological recognition and the elements of signal conversion into the detection system. These were designed for a wide variety of detection applications, providing the benefits of improved speed and ease of use compared to conventional methods of detection (Karunakaran, Rajkumar, & Bhargava, 2015). A biosensor acts as a detection tool that measures biological or chemical reactions by producing signals proportional to an analyte's concentration in the reaction (Bhalla, Jolly, Formisano, & Estrela, 2016). Hughes (1922) realized a linear manner between the potential differences with the logarithm of the hydrogen-ion concentration by using an electrode to measure pH. Clark Jr and Lyons (1962) invented the first recognized biosensor in 1962, which is used to monitor the blood gas tension during cardiovascular surgery. Since the development of biosensor by Clark Jr and Lyons (1962), several types of biosensors were established, containing a biological sensing element in the transducer of the biosensors.

Nanotechnology has been the latest frontier of this century; and is applied in studying the incredibly small structures to get extra high accuracy and ultra-fine dimensions on the order of the size of 0.1 to 100 nm (Theis et al., 2006; Sozer & Kokini, 2009). The first reference of intentionally developed and implemented technical processes and methods, which were later known as nanotechnology, is generally associated with Mr. Richard Feynman, a famous lecture, delivered a talk in 1959 on "There's plenty of room at the bottom" and suggested that atoms and molecules are possible to be manipulated precisely. The lecture is known as the root of the nanotechnological paradigm (Fanfair, Desai, & Kelty, 2007; Tolochko, 2009). Nanotechnology has been evolved around humanity and is used widely in many applications, including environmental, constructions, cosmetics, personal healthcare, and food aspects.

Biosensor and nanotechnology have been used widely in food research. From an essential pH measurement using an electrode to the invention of the biosensor to monitor blood gas tension, biosensor keeps on revolutionizing with the aid of modern

Advanced Food Analysis Tools. https://doi.org/10.1016/B978-0-12-820591-4.00002-5

technology. Biosensors also widely used in food industries as food allergen detection (Yman, Eriksson, Johansson, & Hellens, 2006), *E. coli* detection in vegetables (Ercole, Del Gallo, Mosiello, Baccella, & Lepidi, 2003), biogenic amines detection to evaluate the freshness of food products (Carelli, Centonze, Palermo, Quinto, & Rotunno, 2007), and also can detect food toxin present in food (Kalita et al., 2012; Srivastava et al., 2014). Biosensors are commonly paired with nanotechnology. Research conducted by Pilolli, Monaci, and Visconti (2013) developed a biosensor based on integrating nanotechnology and applied to food allergen management. Otles and Yalcin (2010) claimed a nanobiosensor as a tool for the detection of food quality and safety. On the other hand, biosensors also responsible as platforms for monitoring food traceability, quality, safety, and nutritional value (Bhalla et al., 2016).

The revolution of nanotechnology from the conventional methods lead to several applications of nanomaterials in food industries, including nanotechnology in developing food packaging with high barrier and nanomaterials such as silver nanoparticles as potent antimicrobial agents (Fig. 2.1). Besides, nanotechnology also applied as the detection method for sensing contamination of food-relevant analytes such as gasses, small organic molecules, and pathogens, which can ensure the safety of the

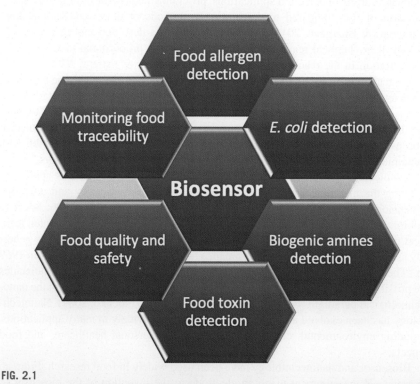

FIG. 2.1

Applications of biosensors in food industries.

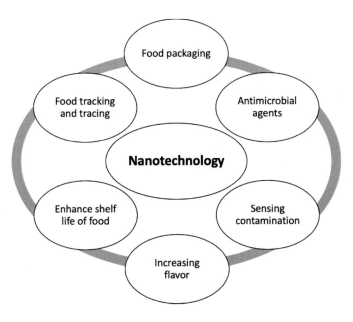

FIG. 2.2

Applications of nanotechnology in food industries.

food. Furthermore, nanotechnology involving nanoencapsulation of nutraceuticals also provides quick delivery of nutrients, increasing the flavor, enhance the shelf life of food products, and help in tracking, tracing, and brand protection (Duncan, 2011; Sozer & Kokini, 2009; Chellaram et al., 2014; Alfadul & Elneshwy, 2010). However, Fig. 2.2 shows the application of nanotechnology in food industries.

The past of biosensor and nanotechnology in food sector

Before the existence of biosensor and nanotechnology, monitoring of food quality had to be tested in the laboratory. Food quality testing mainly dealt with chemical, physical, and microbiological testing. Chemicals are commonly analyzed by using high-performance liquid chromatography (HPLC), gas chromatography (GC), or mass spectroscopy (MS). Undoubtedly, the implementation of that analytical method in chemical testing of food is considered as a right approach as those instruments provide high selectivity and sensitivity with reliable and accurate results. However, handling the analytical instruments requires a skilled workforce and is time-consuming too. Microbiological testing required conventional methods to grow the culture and is time-consuming for the detection of microorganisms present in the food as microbiologist needs to incubate the culture for the microorganisms to grow. The traditional way of detecting microbial contamination in food takes a long time and causing forward processing decisions, and confirming the manufacturing processes can be delayed and might cause loss to the companies as the processed food in the processing line might get contaminated as well (Adley, 2014). Neethirajan, Ragavan, Weng, and Chand (2018) reported that an average of $15 million loss per food recalls incident is recorded for the past few years causing harm to the credibility and reputations of the food brands. Meanwhile, contaminated food might cause foodborne illness, and it is recorded that there were 48 million sick cases that are responsible for 3000 fatalities annually.

Food industries should have technologies that have the ability of point-of-care testing for on-site, rapid diagnosis, and treatment for food productions. Food quality control is necessary and crucial as these departments are responsible for monitoring the nutrient contents, food safety, and security and food production control. The application of nanotechnology in biosensors makes biosensing technology into a rapid, simple, accurate, and portable device that can fulfill the demand of food industries to have point-of-care testing. Advancement of nanotechnology allows this technology to revolutionize food systems that can affect the safety, efficiency, bioavailability, better nutritional content, and molecular synthesis of new products and ingredients (Rashidi & Khosravi-Darani, 2011).

Applications of biosensor and nanotechnology in food sector

The revolution of biosensor and nanotechnology creates opportunities not only for food researchers but also for food industries. Incorporating modern technology in food production and processing line can improve the quality and safety of the food products from the aspects of food packaging, distribution, and storage, enhancement of sensory properties of food. Development of biosensor devices and applying nanotechnology had attracted the attention of many researchers for the past few years with specific numbers of devices are designed and reported in the scientific literature.

Biosensor composes of two main parts: (i) a bio-element or sensing element which undergoes biochemical reactions with the analyte particles (ii) a transducer that collects information from the biological part, amplifies and produces signal either in the form of electrical, thermal, or optical signal depending on the concentration of analyte present in the sample (Monošík, Stredanský, & Šturdík, 2012). Generally, bio-element or sensing element is immobilized onto the surface of a transducer that acts as a contact point between transducer and analyte. Bio-element or sensing element interacts accurately and efficiently towards analyte particles and causes a physicochemical change on the transducer surface and finally displaying the signal (Ayesha, 2015). Fig. 2.3 in the following section shows elements of biosensor:

A biosensor is classified according to the mode of signal transduction, biological specificity mechanisms, or a combination of the two characteristics. The signal transduction might either potentiometric sensors, amperometric sensors, piezoelectric, surface plasmon resonance (SPR), or magnetoelectric. Meanwhile, the bio-element or sensing elements might compose of antibody, enzyme, phage, or DNA. There are

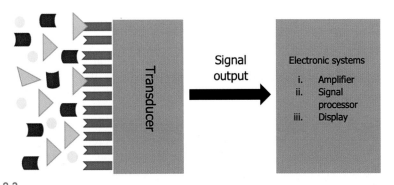

FIG. 2.3

Elements of biosensor.

several types of immobilization methods of biological components onto the transducer, namely, cross-linking, covalent binding, adsorption, microencapsulation, and inclusion (Korotkaya, 2014). Classification of biosensors according to the mode of signal transduction and the nature of the biological entity as the identification element (Mungroo & Neethirajan, 2014) is presented later in Fig. 2.4:

Optical and electrochemical biosensors are types of biosensors that are commonly used. An optical biosensor is performed by displaying visual changes by exploiting the interaction between analytes and biorecognition elements.

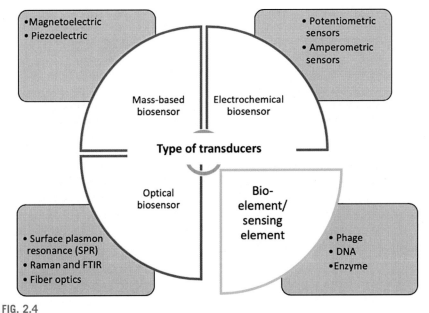

FIG. 2.4

Schematic diagram representing the classification of biosensors.

Visible result generating from the biochemical reaction of analytes and transducer depends on the concentration of analytes in the sample (Damborský, Švitel, & Katrlík, 2016). An electrochemical biosensor generates a measurable potential or charge accumulation or change of conductivity of a medium between electrodes. Both optical and electrochemical biosensors work under the same principle and generate output that is proportional to the logarithm of the electrochemically active analytes (Koyun, Ahlatcolu, Koca, & Kara, 2012). Broad applications involving biosensors had been applied in the food sector, including *E. coli* and *Salmonella* detection in food. Besides, biosensors also used in determining the nutritional content in food, and this can enhance the quality of food products. The safety of food products can be guaranteed as biosensor acts as a device to detect any adulteration in food that might harm the health of consumers. The applications of the biosensor in food sectors are shown clearly in Table 2.1.

Nanotechnology does not only exist within but also around food products, mainly as food packaging. Nanomaterials are being applied widely to food technology due to their ability to enhance the organoleptic properties and shelf life of food products. Nanomaterials have unique ability includes providing surface effect, small size effect, quantum size effect, and quantum tunneling effect, which based on the physicochemical properties of each nanomaterial. It is reported that nanoparticles such as zinc, calcium, and silver are natural potent antimicrobial; hence, these nanoparticles are incorporated with cinnamon or oregano oil to produce edible food packaging (Kumar, 2015). Besides, companies are using polymer nanocomposite such as silica nanocomposite in producing plastics due to its high barrier properties to prevent the penetration of oxygen and gas, thus extending the shelf life of food products. Other than that, food researchers have found that nanomicelles for encapsulation of nutraceuticals are possible to improve the bioavailability of nutraceuticals to be released into the membrane in the digestive system (Blasco & Picó, 2011).

Besides, nanotechnology, such as metal or metal oxide nanomaterials, possesses the ability to protect food against microbial. The mostly used nanoparticles in exterminating microbial are gold, silver, and zinc nanoparticles (Silvestre, Duraccio, & Cimmino, 2011) due to its intrinsic physicochemical properties allowing excess production of reactive oxygen species that lead to oxidative stress and causing damage on the microbial cell. Furthermore, it is reported that the production of metal ions outside the cell, at the cell surface, or within the cell has the probability of altering the cellular structure or function of the microbial cell (He & Hwang, 2016). Therefore, nanomaterials such as metal or metal oxide are suitable to be fabricated in the processing of food packaging and coating or exist as ingredients. Apart from that, a combination of nanosensors with the advancement of IT systems can help in food tracking to ensure food safety. In the food industry, traceability is the essential element that needs better attention to avoid expensive product recalls and prevent a food poisoning outbreak. Nowadays, food safety and quality indicators have been successfully done with the incorporation of nanomaterials, for example, poultry and meat freshness indicator via the visual quality label, microbiological food safety via deterioration products detection and the latest are radio frequency identification tagging

Table 2.1 Applications of the biosensor in food sectors.

Types of biosensor	Nanotechnology used	Analyte	Food sample	Limit of detection	Reference
Optical sensor	N/A	E. coli O157: H7	Milk, apple juice, ground beef	10^2–10^3 CFU/mL	Waswa, Irudayaraj, and DebRoy (2007)
	N/A	Gentamicin L-glutamate	Milk	10 ng/mL	Haasnoot and Verheijen (2001)
	N/A	Sulfonamide	Prepared soup, food stocks	5 µM	Md Muslim, Ahmad, Heng, and Saad (2012)
	N/A	Fluoroquinolone, β-lactam, tetracycline	Milk	0.5 ± 0.1– 34.2 ± 5.4 µg/L	Adrian et al. (2009)
	N/A	Melamine	Infant formula milk	<0.5 µg/mL	Fodey et al. (2011)
	N/A	Folic acid	Milk powder, infant formula, cereal	Not stated	Boström Caselunghe (2000)
	N/A	Bovine serum albumin	Milk	0.02 mg/g	Indyk, Gill, and Woollard (2015)
	N/A	Gluten	Food containing gluten products, biscuits, and gluten-free flou	4.77 ng/mL	Weng, Gaur, and Neethirajan (2016)
Electrochemical	N/A	Aflatoxin B1 (AF)	N/A	0.23 ng/mL	Srivastava et al. (2014)
	N/A	Biogenic amines	Salted anchovies	$5 \times$ mol/L	Draisci et al. (1998)
	Gold nanoparticles	E. coli O111	Pork	3 CFU/mL	Ma et al. (2014)
	N/A	Salmonella	Milk	305 CFU/mL	Luo et al. (2012)
	Gold nanoparticles	Hydrogen peroxide	Sterilized milk, apple juices, watermelon juice, coconut milk, mango juice	0.01 µM	Zhang et al. (2011)

Continued

Table 2.1 Applications of the biosensor in food sectors. *Continued*

Types of biosensor	Nanotechnology used	Analyte	Food sample	Limit of detection	Reference
	N/A	Parathion, carbaryl pesticides	Natural water, tomato, apple, orange	9.0–10.3 µg/L	Pedrosa, Caetano, Machado, and Bertotti (2008)
	N/A	Lysine	Ground farro	N/A	Marconi et al. (1996)
	Palladium-platinum (PdPt) bimetallic alloy nanoparticles	Tyrosine	Cheese, egg, yogurt	0.009 × mol/L	Varmira et al. (2018)
	Nanoporous gold electrode	Cholesterol	Margarine, butter, fish oil	0.5 mg/dL	Ahmadalinezhad and Chen (2011)

(RFIT) and nucleic acid engineered nanobio barcode (NAENB) (Sun-Waterhouse & Waterhouse, 2016).

Research and development of food industries should collaborate with food companies to set goals, which are to enhance the bioavailability of food, increase the nutritional content, improve the shelf life and to produce food with high quality and safety for the consumer's consumption. With the presence of nanotechnology and biosensors, consumers can tell the freshness of the food products inside the packaging materials that prevent consumers from having extensive sensory exposure to the food; consumers also can have food allergen detection that can prevent them from being exposed to allergy reaction during consumption. Nanotechnology shows more benefits in food development and processing processes. However, the incorporation of nanomaterials has become concerned with consumers due to some health issues.

Advantages and disadvantages of biosensor and nanotechnology in food sector

Biosensors and nanotechnology provide great benefits in the research world. However, some drawbacks needed to be overcome. The advantages of biosensors over conventional analytical techniques are they enable direct and real-time results. Besides, biosensors offer great benefits that include high specificity, sensitivity, small size, and cost-effectiveness (Damborský et al., 2016). Biosensors can be used in on-line control processes because biosensors can sense materials without damaging the system (Koyun et al., 2012). The biosensor is said to have a better limit of detection, high precision, high detectability, multi parameters detection, and compact design (Roda et al., 2016; Tereshchenko et al., 2016).

However, it is claimed that biosensors have a weak repeatability system, might have measurement error due to contamination factors that cause interference, temperature, and pH-dependent system. Biorecognition elements such as enzymes might be temperature and pH-dependent as specific temperature and pH might denature the enzyme (Azmi, Azman, Ibrahim, & Yunus, 2017). Biosensors must be replaced after positive prove causes by irreversible inhibition of many types of inhibitors (Pohanka, 2016). Apart from that, biosensor required another additional component to amplify the signal depends on the concentration of the analyte (Azmi et al., 2017).

Nanotechnology offers excellent advantages, including the incorporation of nanocomposite or nanosized filler into food packaging (Berekaa, 2015), which gives better barrier resistance, provide functional performance, and offers to sense of relevant information. Besides, polymer nanocomposites improved the flexibility and durability of the packaging (Omanovic-Miklicanin, Maksimovic, Vrcek, Mulaomerovic, & Doric, 2016). Nanotechnology applied widely in the food sector and even producing edible products with biodegradable nanomaterials, which also help in generating a better quality of food products. Through the bottom-up engineering process, nanomaterials are engineered and devised to detect chemical contaminations and pathogens, which can improve the quality and safety of food products (Duncan, 2011). Nanotechnology is commonly paired with biosensor due to its multiple molecular targets simultaneously, and the revolution of nanotechnology around electronic products, procedures, and applications might enhance the quality of the nanotechnology-upgraded products (Alok et al., 2013). Nanoencapsulation technology also allowed efficient drug accumulation at the site and sustained drug release for weeks besides isolating drugs from the surrounding environment (Hussain & Hussain, 2015).

The incorporation of nanomaterials in the food sector creates health concerns among consumers. It is claimed that nanoparticles can stimulate the production of free radicals that can cause cellular damage. Moreover, nanoparticles are reported, then it can cross blood–brain carriers and travel up to the nerve cells or even travel across the placenta and thus affecting the fetus due to its small size. The application of nanotechnology, such as carbon nanotubes, can release dangerous free radicals that harm human skin cells. The use of nanotechnology in food packaging as a potent antimicrobial leads to a significant concern as it also can negatively affect humans' cells that might put respiratory and digestive track at high risk (Sharon, 2016). Besides, nanoparticles, with its nanosize particles, increased risk to health as inhalation of those nanoparticles such as titanium dioxide nanoparticles might cause inhalation problems and fatal diseases such as lung damage. Minute particles can exist in the air; therefore, even just inhaling air containing nanoparticles for 60s can harm human health (Parveen, Banse, & Ledwani, 2016). Besides, nanotechnology requires substantial investment in research and development and is currently expensive as compared to other technology. Manufacturing of nanotechnology is also quite tricky as it required skilled human resources (Aithal & Aithal, 2016).

Impact of biosensor and nanotechnology

Never-ending scientific works of literature relating to biosensor have been published for the past few decades, and it is undeniable that biosensor caught the attention of researchers and not forgotten about the industries. The most significant contribution of the biosensor in the industry that can be seen nowadays is the point-of-care testing locations, even without the need to do analytical tests in the laboratory. The invention and revolution of biosensor into a device with excellent reliability, easy-to-use, and rugged instrumentation allow biosensor to assure the success rate of biosensor-based systems during the on-site testing (D'Orazio, 2011). The pioneers of the biosensor, Clark, and Lyons, open a new frontier in scientific research and thus leading to never-ending scientific literature related to biosensors nowadays. Besides, the field of biosensors has united researchers from different areas of science and engineering in teaming up and invent devices for the benefits of different areas, including healthcare, food industries, and the environment. Researchers from different fields have different skills and ideas, working and brainstorming together with other fields' researchers contribute to creating something that is out of the box. For example, a pregnancy test biosensor is available in the market in recent times, and this shows that biosensor does not confine to a research-based-niche, but also biosensor has been reached out to the customers worldwide (Bhalla et al., 2016).

Nanotechnology has been contributed to broad applications, including food processing, medical, agricultural, and environmental areas. Even though nanotechnology is well-known for its nanosized materials, it contributes to many factors in human lives such as faster, more functional and accurate medical diagnostic; nanoparticles in pharmaceutical also help in improving absorptions of the pharmaceutical products in the human body; nanoparticles also increase the efficiency of drug delivery to specific cells such as cancer cells; sunscreen made up from the nanoclays can absorb the UV light from reaching to the skin. Despite the fantastic contribution of nanotechnology in many different fields, the emerging technologies of nanotechnology have been viewed by the public as potential exposure to health risk issues. Besides, from the public point of view, exposure to nanoparticles causes an enormous impact on human safety and environmental pollutions. These issues have been concerning by society as the quantity and types of nanoparticles used in the industries have grown in number (Dreher, 2004).

Challenges and future prospective

Biosensors have been under development for about 50 years and had contributed to significant contributions in the academic field for the past 10 years. Nonetheless, other than pregnancy kit test and electrochemical glucose biosensors, very few biosensors have gained global retail-level commercial success. Bhalla et al. (2016) reported that these happened due to industries are having a hard time in translating the academic research into commercially viable prototypes; it is time-consuming to produce viable prototypes translated from the scientific literature; the existence of regulatory issues within the clinical field regarding nanotechnology paired with biosensors. To some extent, industries are reluctant to face risk as industries need to identify manufacturers and markets that are drawn into biosensors technology, taking count of the cost of manufacturing each component of the biosensors and the stability of the biosensor. Industries that are evolved around biosensors should acknowledge the hazard ethics associated with the development of biosensors. Biosensors have developed rapidly in the healthcare applications and show that the next generations might encounter new platforms of biosensors that are fast, easy-to-use, specific, and inexpensive. The alliance of that expertise might bring biosensors into a new level in the future with a better understanding of the principles of biosensors.

Innovations of nanotechnology invested massive investment in the research and development area; however, nanotechnology still yields minimal results. Fabrication of nanotechnology in nowadays technologies have severe facing opposition since nanoparticles might harm human health. Besides, recent findings found that artificially generated products from nanotechnology have taken over the functions of natural products such as rubber, cotton, various food grains, coffee, tea, and other products; these might cause an economic imbalance in particular developing countries (Aithal & Aithal, 2016). Furthermore, nanotechnology is a new kind of technology that will have far-reaching effects on society since the public has limited knowledge of nanotechnology. Companies also should consider nanotechnology as companies should consider the life cycle risk management and safety procedure to dispose of or recycle unwanted or nanowaste (Lamabam & Thangjam, 2018). Nanotechnology might be complicated for public acceptance due to its toxicity effect. Despite all the challenges, a glimpse of the future of nanotechnology can be seen in the medical field as there has been a growing interest in emerging a new field called nanomedicine. Patil, Mehta, and Guvva (2008) suggested that nanomedicine needs to overcome the challenges of nanotechnology and to take advantage of its small size for the applications in nanomedicine. Nanomedicine can increase the effectiveness of many types of therapies, produce more sophisticated and accurate diagnostic opportunities, and have preventive properties.

Conclusions

In general, biosensors and nanotechnology have been under much research and development for a few decades ago. Variety of applications of biosensors and nanotechnology that have been developed by researches from different fields of science, including primary and applied science. Both biosensor and nanotechnology have been applied daily in human lives without human realizing about those techniques. Both technologies aim to improve the quality of life of society in diverse areas such as in the field of food processing, agriculture, medicinal, and environmental. The biosensor companies must continue establishing these technologies to increase the emerging of biosensor and nanotechnology in the industrial market. Nanotechnology manufacturers should overcome the drawbacks of nanomaterials to reduce health and environmental impacts.

References

Adley, C. C. (2014). Past, present and future of sensors in food production. *Food*, *3*(3), 491–510.

Adrian, J., Pasche, S., Voirin, G., Adrian, J., Pinacho, D. G., Font, H., … Granier, B. (2009). Wavelength-interrogated optical biosensor for multi-analyte screening of sulfonamide, fluoroquinolone, β-lactam and tetracycline antibiotics in milk. *TrAC Trends in Analytical Chemistry*, *28*(6), 769–777.

Ahmadalinezhad, A., & Chen, A. (2011). High-performance electrochemical biosensor for the detection of total cholesterol. *Biosensors and Bioelectronics*, *26*(11), 4508–4513.

Aithal, P. S., & Aithal, S. (2016). Nanotechnology innovations and commercialization— Opportunities, challenges & reasons for delay. *International Journal of Engineering and Manufacturing (IJEM)*, *6*(6), 15–25.

Alfadul, S. M., & Elneshwy, A. A. (2010). Use of nanotechnology in food processing, packaging and safety–review. *African Journal of Food, Agriculture, Nutrition and Development*, *10*(6), 2719–2739.

Alok, A., Panat, S., Aggarwal, A., Upadhyay, N., Agarwal, N., & Kishore, M. (2013). Nanotechnology: A boon in oral cancer diagnosis and therapeutics. *SRM Journal of Research in Dental Sciences*, *4*(4), 154–160.

Ayesha, A. I. S. (2015). Biosensor: Concept, classification and applications. *Excel Journal of Engineering Technology and Management Science (An International Multidisciplinary Journal)*, *1*(6), 1–6.

Azmi, A., Azman, A. A., Ibrahim, S., & Yunus, M. A. M. (2017). Techniques in advancing the capabilities of various nitrate detection methods: A review. *International Journal on Smart Sensing & Intelligent Systems*, *10*(2), 223–261.

Berekaa, M. M. (2015). Nanotechnology in food industry; advances in food processing, packaging and food safety. *International Journal of Current Microbiology and Applied Sciences*, *4*(5), 345–357.

Bhalla, N., Jolly, P., Formisano, N., & Estrela, P. (2016). Introduction to biosensors. *Essays in Biochemistry*, *60*(1), 1–8.

Blasco, C., & Picó, Y. (2011). Determining nanomaterials in food. *TrAC Trends in Analytical Chemistry*, *30*(1), 84–99.

Boström Caselunghe, M. (2000). Biosensor-based determination of folic acid in fortified food. *Food Chemistry*, *70*(4), 523–532.

Carelli, D., Centonze, D., Palermo, C., Quinto, M., & Rotunno, T. (2007). An interference free amperometric biosensor for the detection of biogenic amines in food products. *Biosensors and Bioelectronics*, *23*(5), 640–647.

Chellaram, C., Murugaboopathi, G., John, A. A., Sivakumar, R., Ganesan, S., Krithika, S., & Priya, G. (2014). Significance of nanotechnology in food industry. *APCBEE Procedia*, *8*, 109–113.

Clark, L. C., Jr., & Lyons, C. (1962). Electrode systems for continuous monitoring in cardiovascular surgery. *Annals of the New York Academy of Sciences*, *102*(1), 29–45.

Damborský, P., Švitel, J., & Katrlík, J. (2016). Optical biosensors. *Essays in Biochemistry*, *60*(1), 91–100.

D'Orazio, P. (2011). Biosensors in clinical chemistry—2011 update. *Clinica Chimica Acta*, *412*(19–20), 1749–1761.

Draisci, R., Volpe, G., Lucentini, L., Cecilia, A., Federico, R., & Palleschi, G. (1998). Determination of biogenic amines with an electrochemical biosensor and its application to salted anchovies. *Food Chemistry*, *62*(2), 225–232.

Dreher, K. L. (2004). Health and environmental impact of nanotechnology: Toxicological assessment of manufactured nanoparticles. *Toxicological Sciences*, *77*(1), 3–5.

Duncan, T. V. (2011). Applications of nanotechnology in food packaging and food safety: Barrier materials, antimicrobials and sensors. *Journal of Colloid and Interface Science*, *363*(1), 1–24.

Ercole, C., Del Gallo, M., Mosiello, L., Baccella, S., & Lepidi, A. (2003). Escherichia coli detection in vegetable food by a potentiometric biosensor. *Sensors and Actuators B: Chemical*, *91*(1–3), 163–168.

Fanfair, D., Desai, S., & Kelty, C. (2007). The early history of nanotechnology. *Connexions*, *6*, 1–15.

Fodey, T. L., Thompson, C. S., Traynor, I. M., Haughey, S. A., Kennedy, D. G., & Crooks, S. R. H. (2011). Development of an optical biosensor based immunoassay to screen infant formula milk samples for adulteration with melamine. *Analytical Chemistry*, *83*(12), 5012–5016.

Haasnoot, W., & Verheijen, R. (2001). A direct (non-competitive) immunoassay for gentamicin residues with an optical biosensor. *Food and Agricultural Immunology*, *13*(2), 131–134.

He, X., & Hwang, H. -M. (2016). Nanotechnology in food science: Functionality, applicability, and safety assessment. *Journal of Food and Drug Analysis*, *24*(4), 671–681.

Hughes, W. S. (1922). The potential difference between glass and electrolytes in contact with the glass. *Journal of the American Chemical Society*, *44*, 2860–2867.

Hussain, K., & Hussain, T. (2015). Gold nanoparticles: A boon to drug delivery system. *South Indian Journal of Biological Sciences*, *1*(3), 128.

Indyk, H. E., Gill, B. D., & Woollard, D. C. (2015). An optical biosensor-based immunoassay for the determination of bovine serum albumin in milk and milk products. *International Dairy Journal*, *47*, 72–78.

Kalita, P., Singh, J., Kumar Singh, M., Solanki, P. R., Sumana, G., & Malhotra, B. D. (2012). Ring like self assembled Ni nanoparticles based biosensor for food toxin detection. *Applied Physics Letters*, *100*(9)093702.

Karunakaran, C., Rajkumar, R., & Bhargava, K. (2015). Introduction to biosensors. In *Biosensors and bioelectronics* (pp. 1–68). Elsevier.

Korotkaya, E. V. (2014). Biosensors: Design, classification, and applications in the food industry. *Foods and Raw Materials*, *2*(2), 161–171.

Koyun, A., Ahlatcolu, E., Koca, Y., & Kara, S. (2012). Biosensors and their principles. In *A roadmap of biomedical engineers and milestones* (pp. 117–142). IntechOpen.

Kumar, L. Y. (2015). Role and adverse effects of nanomaterials in food technology. *Journal of Toxicology and Health*, *2*(1), 2.

Lamabam, S. D., & Thangjam, R. (2018). Progress and challenges of nanotechnology in food engineering. In *Impact of nanoscience in the food industry* (pp. 87–112). Academic Press.

Luo, C., Lei, Y., Yan, L., Yu, T., Li, Q., Zhang, D., … Ju, H. (2012). A rapid and sensitive aptamer-based electrochemical biosensor for direct detection of Escherichia Coli O111. *Electroanalysis*, *24*(5), 1186–1191.

Ma, X., Jiang, Y., Jia, F., Yu, Y., Chen, J., & Wang, Z. (2014). An aptamer-based electrochemical biosensor for the detection of Salmonella. *Journal of Microbiological Methods*, *98*, 94–98.

Marconi, E., Panfili, G., Messia, M. C., Cubadda, R., Compagnone, D., & Palleschi, G. (1996). Fast analysis of lysine in food using protein microwave hydrolysis and an electrochemical biosensor. *Analytical Letters*, *29*(7), 1125–1137.

Md Muslim, N. Z., Ahmad, M., Heng, L. Y., & Saad, B. (2012). Optical biosensor test strip for the screening and direct determination of l-glutamate in food samples. *Sensors and Actuators B: Chemical*, *161*(1), 493–497.

Monošík, R., Streďanský, M., & Šturdík, E. (2012). Biosensors-classification, characterization and new trends. *Acta Chimica Slovaca*, *5*(1), 109–120.

Mungroo, N. A., & Neethirajan, S. (2014). Biosensors for the detection of antibiotics in poultry industry—A review. *Biosensors*, *4*(4), 472–493.

Neethirajan, S., Ragavan, V., Weng, X., & Chand, R. (2018). Biosensors for sustainable food engineering: Challenges and perspectives. *Biosensors*, *8*(1), 23.

Omanovic-Miklicanin, E., Maksimovic, M., Vrcek, I. V., Mulaomerovic, D., & Doric, A. (2016). Application of nanotechnology in food packaging. In *5th workshop: Specific methods for food safety and quality* (pp. 119–125).

Otles, S., & Yalcin, B. (2010). Nano-biosensors as new tool for detection of food quality and safety. *LogForum, 6*(4), 7.

Parveen, K., Banse, V., & Ledwani, L. (2016, April). Green synthesis of nanoparticles: Their advantages and disadvantages. *AIP conference proceedings* (p. 020048). Vol. 1724. (p. 020048). AIP Publishing LLC no. 1.

Patil, M., Mehta, D. S., & Guvva, S. (2008). Future impact of nanotechnology on medicine and dentistry. *Journal of Indian Society of Periodontology, 12*(2), 34.

Pedrosa, V., Caetano, J., Machado, S., & Bertotti, M. (2008). Determination of parathion and carbaryl pesticides in water and food samples using a self assembled monolayer/acetylcholinesterase electrochemical biosensor. *Sensors, 8*(8), 4600–4610.

Pilolli, R., Monaci, L., & Visconti, A. (2013). Advances in biosensor development based on integrating nanotechnology and applied to food-allergen management. *TrAC Trends in Analytical Chemistry, 47*, 12–26.

Pohanka, M. (2016). Electrochemical biosensors based on acetylcholinesterase and butyrylcholinesterase. A review. *International Journal of Electrochemical Science, 11*, 7440–7452.

Rashidi, L., & Khosravi-Darani, K. (2011). The applications of nanotechnology in food industry. *Critical Reviews in Food Science and Nutrition, 51*(8), 723–730.

Roda, A., Mirasoli, M., Michelini, E., Di Fusco, M., Zangheri, M., Cevenini, L., … Simoni, P. (2016). Progress in chemical luminescence-based biosensors: A critical review. *Biosensors and Bioelectronics, 76*, 164–179.

Sharon, M. (2016). Are we ignoring the considerations for the dark-side of nanotechnology. *Journal of Nanomedicine Research, 3*(2)00051.

Silvestre, C., Duraccio, D., & Cimmino, S. (2011). Food packaging based on polymer nanomaterials. *Progress in Polymer Science, 36*(12), 1766–1782.

Sozer, N., & Kokini, J. L. (2009). Nanotechnology and its applications in the food sector. *Trends in Biotechnology, 27*(2), 82–89.

Srivastava, S., Ali, M. A., Umrao, S., Parashar, U. K., Srivastava, A., Sumana, G., … Hayase, S. (2014). Graphene oxide-based biosensor for food toxin detection. *Applied Biochemistry and Biotechnology, 174*(3), 960–970.

Sun-Waterhouse, D., & Waterhouse, G. I. N. (2016). Recent advances in the application of nanomaterials and nanotechnology in food research. *Novel Approaches of Nanotechnology in Food, 1*, 21–66.

Tereshchenko, A., Bechelany, M., Viter, R., Khranovskyy, V., Smyntyna, V., Starodub, N., & Yakimova, R. (2016). Optical biosensors based on ZnO nanostructures: Advantages and perspectives. A review. *Sensors and Actuators B: Chemical, 229*, 664–677.

Theis, T., Parr, D., Binks, P., Ying, J., & Drexler, K. E. (2006). Nanotechnology. *Nature Nanotechnology, 1*(1), 8–10.

Tolochko, N. K. (2009). History of nanotechnology. In *Encyclopedia of life support systems (EOLSS)* (pp. 1–6). Nanoscience and Nanotechnologies.

Varmira, K., Mohammadi, G., Mahmoudi, M., Khodarahmi, R., Rashidi, K., Hedayati, M., … Jalalvand, A. R. (2018). Fabrication of a novel enzymatic electrochemical biosensor for determination of tyrosine in some food samples. *Talanta, 183*, 1–10.

Waswa, J., Irudayaraj, J., & DebRoy, C. (2007). Direct detection of E. Coli O157:H7 in selected food systems by a surface plasmon resonance biosensor. *LWT - Food Science and Technology, 40*(2), 187–192.

Weng, X., Gaur, G., & Neethirajan, S. (2016). Rapid detection of food allergens by microfluidics ELISA-based optical sensor. *Biosensors, 6*(2), 24.

Yman, I. M., Eriksson, A., Johansson, M. A., & Hellens, K. E. (2006). Food allergen detection with biosensor immunoassays. *Journal of AOAC International, 89*(3), 856–861.

Zhang, B., Cui, Y., Chen, H., Liu, B., Chen, G., & Tang, D. (2011). A new electrochemical biosensor for determination of hydrogen peroxide in food based on well-dispersive gold nanoparticles on graphene oxide. *Electroanalysis, 23*(8), 1821–1829.

Detection of foodborne organisms: In the perspective of biosensors

3

Introduction

Foodborne disease is specified as any illness caused by the ingestion of water or food spoiled by pathogenic microorganisms such as bacteria and viruses, pesticide residues, or toxins (Zhao, Lin, Wang, & Oh, 2014). In general, the food industry is responsible for the presence of pathogenic microorganisms in food products where there will be a terrible effect of failure to detect a pathogen. Although legislation has been established and control measures are being taken to improve the nutritional quality of food as well as to prevent contamination, progress is uneven, and foodborne pathogen outbreaks are still prevalent in many countries. The World Health Organization (WHO) estimated that worldwide intake of contaminated food and water accounted for 1.8 million deaths per year (Shen et al., 2014). Foodborne diseases caused by nonanimal food, resulting in outbreaks, hospitalizations, and even deaths, were also reported to have increased from 2008 through 2011. In 2011, 48 million cases were recorded in the US, with 128,000 hospitalizations and few deaths due to foodborne diseases. Most of these cases are *Salmonella, Campylobacter,* viruses, and several bacterial toxins (EFSA, 2012).

In 2007, the US Food and Drug Administration (FDA) introduced an inclusive "Food Protection Plan" to emphasize the role of pathogenic microorganisms as a potential vehicle capable of causing intentional contamination. Contamination intentionally may have adverse health effects on humans and may lead to death, as well as economic losses. Besides, food products should not contain microorganisms or toxins or metabolites in quantities that pose an unacceptable risk to human health, as stated in the European Union (EU) legislation on microbiological criteria for food. Furthermore, Velusamy, Arshak, Korostynska, Oliwa, and Adley (2010) claimed that the potential for foodborne pathogen outbreaks also contributes to the sale and purchase of contaminated food across borders. Food safety monitoring and management systems have made every effort to improve food quality. The steps taken include improved pathogen detection methods, as the current conventional methods that are commonly used to detect the presence of pathogens in the food sample are highly dependent on identified microbiological, biochemical, or genetic identification. Those techniques can easily be affected by the time of the test, as well as an enrichment step is often needed to identify target microorganisms that often occur in small numbers in the food sample. The limitations of available conventional

Advanced Food Analysis Tools. https://doi.org/10.1016/B978-0-12-820591-4.00003-7

methods result in the development of a fast, sensitive, and on-site detection method, with biosensors being a promising technique that can meet both characteristics (Adley & Ryan, 2015).

Foodborne pathogens and diseases

Foodborne illness, which could be categorized as food poisoning, and food poisoning remains a public health concern as the incidence is likely to increase. The ingestion of microorganism infected foods may cause diseases. Consequently, the occurrence of foodborne pathogens in food is becoming a primary concern for consumers and food manufacturers. The commonly found foodborne pathogen in the food sample includes *Escherichia coli, Listeria monocytogenes, Salmonella typhimurium, Campylobacter jejuni, Vibrio vulnificus, Clostridium botulinum,* and *Staphylococcus aureus,* as shown in Table 3.1.

Table 3.1 Foodborne pathogens and their diseases.

Foodborne pathogens	Sources	Diseases	References
E. coli	Yogurt, cheese, salad, vegetables	Diarrhea, vomiting, hemolytic uremic syndrome	Ferens and Hovde (2011)
L. monocytogenes	Milk, meat, seafood	Meningitis, encephalitis, septicemia	Ajayeoba, Atanda, Obadina, Bankole, and Adelowo (2016), Van de Venter (2000)
S. typhimurium	Meat, eggs, fruits	Salmonellosis	Bari and Yeasmin (2018)
C. jejuni	Raw milk, raw poultry, untreated water	Campylobacteriosis	Whiley, van den Akker, Giglio, and Bentham (2013)
V. vulnificus	Raw or undercooked shellfish	Primary septicemia, gastroenteritis	Daniels (2011)
C. botulinum	Improperly processed home-canned foods, commercially canned foods, herb-infused oils	Foodborne botulism	Angelo et al. (2017)
S. aureus	Cooked meat, dairy products, egg products	Nausea, vomiting, diarrhea	Angelo et al. (2017)

Escherichia coli

E. coli is one of the foodborne pathogens that can produce toxins called verotoxins commonly found in apple juice, yogurt, cheese, and salad vegetables. This pathogen can enter the human body through fecal contamination of food and water, cross-contamination during food processing, and person-to-person contact (Ferens & Hovde, 2011). According to the Department of Public Health of California (2015), *E. coli* can lead to diarrhea, cramping, and vomiting. In the meantime, long-term complications will lead to hemolytic uremic syndrome (HUS), where red blood cells slowly damaged, resulting in renal failure.

Listeria monocytogenes

L. monocytogenes is a gram-positive bacterium that naturally exists in the environment, such as soil and water, which can be identified in a wide range of raw and processed foods, such as milk, meat, and seafood. *L. monocytogenes* may survive and multiply rapidly during storage, which may affect individuals with weak immune systems, such as pregnant women, babies, and senior citizens, resulting in meningitis, encephalitis, or septicemia. Abortion or premature birth may also occur when the infection occurs in pregnant women (Ajayeoba et al., 2016; Van de Venter, 2000).

Salmonella typhimurium

S. typhimurium grows in animals such as livestock, poultry, sheep, and horses and is found in foods, including meat, eggs, and fruit. These pathogens are difficult to eliminate due to the development of a strain resistant to commonly used antibiotics and can cause individual infections by consuming contaminated foods from animal origin. *S. typhimurium* may cause a disease known as Salmonellosis, which is reported annually in 4500 cases of the most common gastrointestinal infections in the United States in California. Symptoms may include nausea, cramping, and fever (Bari & Yeasmin, 2018).

Campylobacter jejuni

C. jejuni can be found in raw or undercooked poultry and unchlorinated water. Sporadic disease caused by *C. jejuni* is often associated with the consumption of mishandled poultry products, such as raw milk. A commonly found disease caused by *C. jejuni* infections is known as campylobacteriosis and may result in a syndrome of Guillain-Barré. After several weeks of infection, the syndrome may cause weakness and paralysis. Initially, campylobacteriosis symptoms include only diarrhea, abdominal cramping, and fever. As a result, individuals with an illness often recover completely (Whiley et al., 2013).

Vibrio vulnificus

V. vulnificus is a type of naturally occurring bacteria that can be found in coastal waters and can survive in warm water. Consumption of raw or undercooked shellfish, especially oysters contaminated with this pathogen, may lead to primary septicemia and death if the infection spreads to the blood. *V. vulnificus* can cause gastroenteritis in which the symptoms will occur 12 h to 21 days after exposure and are often self-limiting in healthy adults. Besides, persons with chronic liver disease or chronic alcoholism are most susceptible to *V. vulnificus* infection (Daniels, 2011).

Clostridium botulinum

C. botulinum occurs naturally in the environment and can cause three different types of botulism in infants, including foodborne botulism, wound botulism, and botulism. Foodborne botulism is caused by food consumption containing the toxin, while wound botulism is caused by toxin formation in the infected wound. Consumption of the spores of *C. botulinum* by infants will result in infant botulism. There is a wide variety of foods usually associated with foodborne botulism, including poorly processed home-made canned foods like green beans and maize, commercially canned foods, and herbal oils. Symptoms of foodborne botulism, including blurred and double vision, usually start within 18 to 36 h of toxin exposure. While symptoms can be reversed within several days of botulinum antitoxin therapy, severe cases may also lead to paralysis of the respiratory muscles (WHO, 2018).

Staphylococcus aureus

S. aureus can be found in nature, humans, and animals. *S. aureus* is associated with a wide range of foods, in particular foods that require extensive handling during preparation, such as cooked meat products, egg products, and dairy products. Room temperature will provide the optimum condition for the pathogen to grow and multiply, producing harmful and heat-stable toxins on food. The toxin cannot be removed from the food, and when ingested in large quantities will cause illness. Symptoms of *S. aureus* infection include nausea, vomiting, and diarrhea, with temporary changes in blood pressure and heart rate (Channaiah, 2015).

Biosensors in the detection of foodborne organisms
Application of biosensors in the detection of foodborne pathogen
Bioreceptor
Antibody

Immunosensors are widely used to identify microbial agents in food for rapid and high-sensitivity reactions. The detection is based on a phenotype and does not involve the extraction of genetic information from a bioagent (Skládal et al.,

2013). The theory is based on the immobilization of antibodies, known as immunorecognition elements on the surface of the electrode. Immunoglobulin G (IgG) is commonly used in the development of immunosensors as antibodies to detect foodborne organisms because it quickly forms a covalent bond as antibodies are immobilized on the working electrode (Hart, Crew, Crouch, Honeychurch, & Pemberton, 2004). Various materials, including bare metal and carbon electrodes, and also noble metal electrodes, can be used to construct an electrode. Although bare metal and carbon electrodes may adsorb proteins due to the slow spontaneous release of proteins, the layers are not strong enough. Noble metal electrodes, which may consist of versions of gold, platinum, or screen printers, must be chemically activated by deposition of thiol-based self-assembled monolayers (SAM). Thiol-based SAM is used because one end of the usually linear thiol molecule (amino, carboxy, and hydroxyl groups) allows a capable antibody group to be added to (Skládal et al., 2013). Immunoglobulins will link directly to proteins A and G, forming an oriented linkage. The primary immobilized antibody will then capture the target microorganisms in the sample. The surface-bound immunocomplex obtained must be explicitly labeled using an enzyme-linked secondary antibody after the washing step. Skládal et al. (2013) classified immunosensor into three different types of sandwich assay, direct assay, and cell viability assay.

In the sandwich assay, the primary antibody captures the target microorganism and is labeled using the secondary antibody-enzyme conjugate or also known as the tracer. The added enzyme substrate will then be converted into an electrochemically active product measured at the electrode. The various sensing format is used in the sandwich assay as the double antibody system can improve the specificity of the procedure. Besides, the enzyme label will amplify a useful signal resulting in high sensitivity and robustness (Skládal, 1997). This independent sandwich test inspired by enzyme-linked immunosorbent assay (ELISA) provides benefits in terms of robustness and reliability, which successfully tested on real samples. The sensitivity of an assay that can be enhanced and also protects the sensing surface against fouling with biomolecules by using magnetic particles as for target pre-concentration and sample matrix portion washing. However, this test is the most complex as it involves incubation and washing (Che, Li, Slavik, & Paul, 2000).

Meanwhile, for the direct assay, the captured microbe will block the access of the correct redox probe to the electrode. The composition of the immunocomplex on the electrode surface can, therefore, be measured directly using the electrochemical method of the correct redox-active probe. For example, a decrease in redox ferrocyanide signals indicates a positive response. The downside of a direct assay is that nonspecifically collected microbes may also contribute to the measured signal (Skládal et al., 2013). The direct assay is widely used due to the simplicity of the working protocol. Nonetheless, some disadvantages may be experienced because more sophisticated methods are required to achieve a low detection limit as this test is label-free. The amplification techniques will make the test less reliable, and the procedures are more sensitive and strongly influenced by the sample matrix (Baldrich, Vigués, Mas, & Muñoz, 2008). According to Skládal et al. (2013), measurements may also be made based on the viability of the cells captured and the intracellular activity of the correct reporting enzyme, such as β-galactosidase, will be measured. When the microbe is located on the electrode, the enzyme activity will be improved by the use of an active inductor. The activity is then determined using a suitable substrate to supply the electroactive substance, e.g., phenyl-β-D-galactoside.

Kozitsina et al. (2017) produced a low-cost, simple-to-use of biosensor immunosensor based Fe_3O_4-SiO_2-NH_2 nanoparticles for the rapid detection of *Staphylococcus aureus* in foods. Steps involved the incubation of bacteria with excess magnetite nanoparticles, the magnetic separation of free nanoparticles followed by the formation of labeled immunocomplexes on the electrode surface, and the measurement of electrochemical reactions induced by magnetite nanoparticles in the immunocomplex. Under optimum condition, the detection limit was 8.7 CFU/mL linear, with a range from 10 to 105 CFU/mL. Besides, Güner, Çevik, Şenel, and Alpsoy (2017) demonstrated the use of a sandwich assay immunosensor based on the hybridization of PPy/AuNP/MWCNT/Chi composite onto pencil graphite electrode to detect the presence of *Escherichia coli* in food. An anti-*E. coli* monoclonal antibody was developed to modify the hybrid bionano composite platform. The study showed that the detection limit was 30 CFU/mL and concentrations ranging from 30 to 3×10^7 CFU/mL with higher selectivity of gram-negative (M. Xu, Wang, & Li, 2016) successfully developed a minimal-cost, scientifically valid, convenient-to-operate, and preserve immunosensor for the detection of *E. coli* in samples of ground beef. The detection limits of bacteria in foods were found 2.0510(3) CFU g (−1) and 1.0410 (3) CFU mL (−1). This immunosensor only needed a bare electrode to calculate the impedance changes, and no electrode surfing was needed and showed great potential for rapid, on-site detection of pathogenic bacteria in food.

Biomimetic

The biomimetic biosensor can be described as an artificial or synthetic sensor, designed to imitate a natural biosensor feature. Aptasensor is one of the biomimetic biosensors which commonly used in the food industry (Perumal & Hashim, 2014). Tombelli, Minunni, and Mascini (2005) defined aptasensor as a type of biosensor made up of aptamers that are single-stranded DNA or RNA ligands selected from random sequences. The function of aptamers is to bind to a non-nucleic acid target with a highly specific binding effect (Jayasena, 1999). Aptamers are selected through a process known as the systematic evolution of exponential enrichment ligands (SELEX), which involves numerous cycles consisting of three different steps: (1) incubation of the target in vitro synthesized DNA or RNA library, (2) separation of the target bound and unbound nucleic acid, and (3) use of target bound sequences as a template for subsequent PCR amplification (Teng et al., 2016). In recent years, the aptamer-based biosensor has gained interest as the affinity of aptamers to target organisms is comparable or perhaps higher than the monoclonal antibodies previously used.

Besides, aptamers come in small quantities, chemically stable, and low cost but some disadvantages need to be addressed. This is due to aptamers inherent in the properties of nucleic acids, such as structural pleomorphic and chemical simplicity, which may result in reduced assay efficiency and higher cost of production (Perumal & Hashim, 2014). Fluorescent aptasensor is one of the examples of aptamer-based biosensors that used the excitation of the valence electron from the ground to the excited singlet state by absorbing light with sufficient energy. A low-energy photon will be released as the electron returns to its initial ground state (Chung, Kang, Jurng, Jung, & Kim, 2015). Xu et al. (2015) demonstrated the use of fluorescent aptasensors coupled with nanobead-based immunomagnetic separation and quantum dots (QDs) as fluorescence reporters for simultaneous detection of foodborne pathogens including *E. coli*, *S. aureus*, *L. monocytogenes,* and *S. typhimurium* in ground beef. At the same time, streptavidin-coated 25 nm MNBs combined with four corresponding biotin-coated antibodies were used for capturing and magnetically separating pathogens. The detection limits recorded were 87, 100, 47, and 160 CFU/mL for *E. coli*, *S. aureus*, *L. monocytogenes,* and *S. typhimurium*, respectively.

Housaindokht et al. (2018) developed a label-free aptasensor to detect *E. coli* O157: H7 by using a single-wall carbon nanotube modified screen-printed electrode. Based on an analysis, it was known that the MB/Apt/SWNT/SPE layer provided an excellent current response for the detection of *E. coli* O157: H7 and interactions were observed using an electrochemical methylene blue (MB) probe. The proposed aptamer-based biosensor was able to detect the pathogen in the concentration range of 1.7×10^1–1.1×10^7 CFU/mL with a limit of detection of 1.7×10^1 CFU/mL. The aptasensor is a promising analytical technique as it is rapid, cost-effective, and straightforward with high sensitivity of detection. It was also proven that the developed aptasensor could be used in a real sample such as tap water.

Cell

The identification of a foodborne pathogen by cellular structures or cell-based bioreceptors may depend on the whole-cell or portion of the cell capable of performing a specific bond with the target organism. In cell-based biosensors (CBBs), two transduction phases and an entire cell are required to act as a molecular recognition element. The primary function of the cells is to act as the primary transducer and to convert the detected analyte into a cellular response, while the second transducer is to convert the cell signal into an electronic signal that can be processed and evaluated (Velusamy et al., 2010). Banerjee and Bhunia (2009) proposed three prototypes of a B lymphocyte Ped-2E9 CBB prototypes for the simultaneous identification of foodborne pathogens found in food and beverages, including L. *monocytogenes,* enterotoxigenic *Bacillus,* and *Serratia*. Type I collagen was mixed with Ped-2E9 cells in a three-dimensional scaffold cell culture to make the analyte-induced response becoming more physiologically relevant. The study was successfully detected using all three prototypes and proves that CBB is a promising technique for detecting *L. monocytogens* and *B. cereus* at a low initial concentration of 102–104 CFU/g.

CBB provides many advantages in foodborne pathogen identification, including exposure to a wide range of biochemical stimuli because the cells comprise multiple biochemical pathways that have evolved highly. Given the benefits, we also need to tackle limitations. Cells require a specific environment to function normally and subject to biological variability; for instance, cells may duplicate during the assay, resulting in sensor response variations. CBB also has a shelf-life drawback, as cell preservation requires a lot of effort (Ye, Guo, & Sun, 2019). However, the disadvantages encountered may be overcome by developing a genetically engineered cell-based biosensor (GECBB).

Enzyme

According to Yunus (2019), an enzyme-based biosensor is an analytical device that uses enzymes in either the biorecognition process, the transducing element, or both. The enzyme-based biosensor can be classified into two primary groups, the enzyme bioreceptor, and the enzyme transducer. In the first group, the enzyme acts as a bioreceptor with a specific mode of action, usually associated with oxidation (Kumar and Neelam, 2016). The transducer transforms the signals to generate a computable response, such as potential, electrical current, or heat shift. In general, binding capacity and catalytic activity will decide the option of the enzyme. The primary advantage of this approach is that enzymes can catalyze a wide range of reactions as well as identify different types of analytes. The enzyme-based transducer can be further divided into three main categories of optical, electrochemical, and calorimetric transducers (Yunus, 2019).

Enzymes serve as transducers in optical biosensors based on enzymes and catalyze the reaction to turn analytes into products that can be oxidized at a working electrode and retained at a particular potential. Ohk and Bhunia (2013) demonstrated the use of the enzyme-based fiber optic biosensor to detect the presence of *E. coli* O157 successfully: H7 with a detection limit as small as 103 CFU/mL in ground beef. The working principle of an enzyme-based amperometric biosensor is based on an enzyme structure that catalyzes the transformation of electrochemical non-active analytes into products that are susceptible to oxidation by the working electrode (Yunus, 2019). Previous studies conducted by (Yang, Ruan, & Li, 2001) demonstrated the use of horseradish peroxidase and tyrosinase bio-enzyme electrochemical biosensor coupled with an immunomagnetic separation to successfully detect the presence of *S. typhimurium* in chicken and ground beef. The detection limit was as low as 103 CFU/mL with a total assay time of 2.5 h.

Enzymes can also be integrated into biosensors based on colorimeters requiring the immobilization of biomolecules on temperature sensors. The working theory of this biosensor is based on the calorimetric principle and temperature changes due to the response of the biorecognition factor to the target analytes (Yunus, 2019). The temperature change is greatly influenced by the molar enthalpy and the number of molecules present in the phase, according to Xie, Ramanathan, and Danielsson (1999). The temperature shift is calculated using an enzyme thermistor fitted with an enzyme and a temperature sensor. Hossain et al. (2012) established an enzyme-based calorimetric biosensor to detect the presence of *E. coli* O157: H7 with a low detection limit of 5 CFU/mL.

DNA

A DNA-based biosensor consists of several discreetly positioned pathogen-specific detector sequences that are immobilized to build a solid support microarray. The target DNA to be analyzed will generally be amplified using consensus primers that target a genomic region consisting of pathogen-specific sequences and hybridized to the array. However, the selection of a common gene fragment must meet several criteria, such as that the gene should contain the conserved regions common to the target organism. Besides, the gene must contain sufficient sequencing diversity to allow species to be detected (Wong et al., 2000). The variability of ribosomal DNA genes is essential for the identification of a wide range of taxonomic levels, while the conservation of the region makes the gene suitable for the detection of different foodborne pathogen species (Wang, Beggs, Robertson, & Cerniglia, 2002). A previous study conducted by Bang et al. (2013) demonstrated the use of DNA microarray to detect L. *monocytogenes* in milk. The microarray image obtained in the study showed that DNA microarray probes were hybridized with milk extracted DNA, either in the presence of L. *monocytogens* or not. Nevertheless, positive signals or the fluorescing spots were only observed when genomic DNA with L. *monocytogenes* was hybridized.

Phage

The use of bacteriophages as elements of biorecognition to detect the presence of a foodborne pathogen in the sample has become an emerging trend. According to Velusamy et al. (2010), bacteriophages can be defined as viruses that may bind to specific receptors on the bacterial surface to inject genetic material inside the bacteria. The identification of bacterial receptors will be made through the bacteriophage protein tail spike. Bacteriophage based biosensor is a promising technique for pathogen detection in a food sample as the technique is highly specific. Niyomdecha et al. (2018) demonstrated the successful use of M13 bacteriophage in a capacitive flow injection system to detect *Salmonella* spp. The immobilization of the *Salmonella*-specific M13 bacteriophage on the polytyramine gold surface by the use of glutaraldehyde as a crosslinker occurred via the amino acid groups on the phage. In contrast, the alkaline solution was used to sever the binding of the sensing surface and the analyte. When testing the method on a real sample such as raw chicken meat, a detection limit of 200 CFU/mL was reached with a total assay time of 40 min, with high recovery rates of between 100% and 111%.

Transducer
Electrochemical biosensor

An electrochemical biosensor can be described by a chemical reaction involving immobilized biomolecules and target analytes, resulting in observable electrical properties such as electrical current or potential through the creation or consumption of ions (Zhang, Ju, & Wang, 2011). Generally, electrochemical biosensors are highly favorable as the process has high sensitivity and low-cost selectivity and can be used in turbid media (Palchetti & Mascini, 2008). Electrochemical biosensors are classified according to the type of transducer used. Various types of electrochemical biosensors are used to detect foodborne pathogens, including amperometric, potentiometric, impedimetric, and conductometric biosensors (Lazcka, Del Campo, & Muñoz, 2007). Three electrode cells are involved in the measurement of electrochemical biosensors, the working electrode, the reference electrode, and the auxiliary electrode. The working electrode described as an electrode that will undergo significant changes in its potential when the analyte concentration differentiates. The reference electrode, meanwhile, remains unchanged during the entire analysis (Ahmed, Rushworth, Hirst, & Millner, 2014).

Amperometric biosensors measure the quantity of currently produced at a constant potential between the operating electrode and the reference electrode (2011). The amperometric biosensor also requires a voltage source and a meter for both current and voltage (Mutlu, 2016). The process of detection is carried out by the use of a specific marker enzyme, specifically oxidoreductase produced during metabolic processes in the microorganism. Amperometric biosensors are typically used to detect coliform in a water sample based on the enzyme β-D-glucuronide, glucuronosohydrolase, and β-D-galactosidase released by the metabolic product (Arora, Sindhu, Dilbaghi, & Chaudhury, 2011). Another example of the application of amperometric biosensor illustrated by Abdalhai et al. (2014) simultaneously detected the gene of *E. coli* O157: H7 and the nuc gene of *S. aureus*. The working theory of these genosensors was based on the binding of target DNA (tDNA) to nanoparticle tracers such as lead sulfite and cadmium sulfite, which serve as a signal reporter and amplifier. The detective test was used as a parallel sequence to the other end of the tDNA. Theoretically, the signal will increase as the logarithmic concentration of tDNA increases because there was a linear relationship between the stripping signals of the nanoparticle tracers and the concentration of tDNAs.

Potentiometric biosensor involves measuring the potential based on specific interactions with ions present in the solution using ion-selective electrodes. In general, the method measures the difference in electrical potential between the working electrode and the reference electrode. The most widely used potentiometric biosensor in the food industry is a light-addressed potentiometric sensor (LAPS) due to its convenience and high sensitivity (2011). The LAPS can be constructed using a semiconductor chip coated with a silicon dioxide insulating layer placed in contact with the sample solution. Linking interactions at the surface of the insulating layer will directly influence the potential generated by the different load distributions that occur at the insulating layer/solution interface and the semiconductor/isolator interface. Zelada-Guillén, Sebastián-Avila, Blondeau, Riu, and Rius (2012) proposed a real-time potentiometric biosensor using a single-wall carbon nanotube chemically linked to an aptamer system to detect the presence of *S. aureus* in pig-skin. The detection limits differ significantly depending on the type of bond at which the detection limit when the aptamer was covalently bound to nanotubes was 8×10^2 cells/mL while 10^7 cells/mL when the aptamer was bound non-covalently.

The impedimetric biosensor includes unlimited measurement of the target molecule, the ability to analyze a large number of samples simultaneously, and short detection time. However, several challenges need to be overcome, such as high detection limits, nonspecific binding, and variable reproducibility. The impedimetric biosensor, also known as the capacitive biosensor, measures the change in conductivity of the medium caused by microbial growth or microbial metabolism of inert substrates converted into electrically charged ion compounds (Sharma et al., 2013). There are two types of impedimetric biosensors, depending on the presence or absence of specific elements of biorecognition. In the presence of specific biorecognition elements, the impedance changes that occur due to the binding of the bioreceptor target to the electrode surface. Meanwhile, the second type of measurement is based on metabolites produced by bacterial cells during growth.

The theory of a conductometric electrochemical biosensor is based on the relationship between conductivity and the biorecognition technique. Change in the concentration of ion species is associated with reactions that occur in the conductometric biosensor, resulting in a change in conductivity or current flow. In general, the conductometric biosensor consists of two metal electrodes, namely cathode and anode, which are separated by a distance. As the electrolyte dissociates into its ion components in a liquid, the liquid will become a conductive medium. When an AC voltage is applied across the electrodes to generate a current flow, migration of ions occurs and is influenced by the orderly, oppositely directed movement of ions in which negatively charged ions move toward anodes while positively charged ions move toward cathodes (Adley & Ryan, 2015). Changes in ion composition and conductivity between metal electrodes are measured during the detection of foodborne pathogens (Velusamy et al., 2010). Pal, Ying, Alocilja, and Downes (2008) demonstrated the use of a direct transfer conductometric biosensor for the identification of *B. cereus* in strawberries, spinach, tomatoes, and cooked foods such as corn and rice. The sensitivity of the biosensor was tested by the use of nontarget bacteria, *B. megaterium,* and *E. coli,* in pure culture. In the studies, antibodies serve as a biological sensing factor and polyaniline nanowires have been used as transducers. Although this method is widely used, Adley and Ryan (2015) also stated that there is a significant drawback to the fact that the ion species produced from the reaction must contribute to a significant change in the overall ion strength to obtain significant and reliable measurements. Nonetheless, this will result in intrusion due to the potential variation of the ion concentration of the sample. Therefore, it is believed that the efficiency of this technique is generally lower than that of other types of electrochemical biosensors.

Mass-sensitive biosensors

A mass-sensitive biosensor is commonly used for sensitive detection applications and can be divided into two main types, piezoelectric and magnetoelectric. The piezoelectric biosensor can be classified as bulk wave (BW) or quartz crystal microbalance (QCM) and surface acoustic wave (SAW) (Yasmin, Ahmed, & Cho, 2016). The piezoelectric biosensor is based on a transduction system that depends on the use of piezoelectric crystals which can be made to vibrate at a particular electrical frequency. Chemical binding can lead to increased mass and changes in crystal oscillation frequency when the antibody-coated sensor surface is placed in a solution that contains the target species. The resulting adjustment can be electrically measured and then used to calculate the extra crystal mass. This method is cost-effective and straightforward despite the generally lower application compared to optical and electrochemical biosensors (Velusamy et al., 2010).

Piezoelectric immunosensor is equipped with an antibody that acts as an element of biorecognition. The specificity of the entire immunosensor will vary greatly depending on the specificity of the antibody. In principle, a piezoelectric immunosensor is accurate if the antibody used is similar, and the electrode will not be sensitive to unspecific reactions with interfering compounds with the other sensitive parts of the piezoelectric content. The opposite reaction is also possible in which an antibody is detected using the immunosensor that may contain an immobilized antigen (Pohanka, 2018).

Su and Li (2005) demonstrated the application of a QCM immunosensor to detect the presence of *S. typhimurium* in chicken meat and at the same time calculate the resonance frequency and motion resistance. It can be seen that meanwhile, the changes in QCM resonant frequency and motion resistance were significant, the difference in static power, motion capacity, and motion inductance was negligible based on the study of high-frequency impedance. During the test with real samples, the analysis indicated that the resonant frequency and motion resistance was directly proportional to the cell concentration of 105 to 108 and 106 to 108 cells/mL, respectively. When using anti-*Salmonella*-magnetic beads, the detection limit was minimized to 102 cells/mL, but there was no significant relationship between the concentrationss of cells that were resistant to motion.

It can be summed up that piezoelectric immunosensors are ideal for analyzing high molecular weight as the frequency of oscillation decreases further. Nonetheless, this analytical approach is limited since it will be a bit difficult to directly identify a low molecular weight analyte by antibodies that have been immobilized on the surface of a piezoelectric immunosensor. Although microorganisms are a good analyte that can be analyzed directly by this biosensor, there are still several disadvantages, such as the microbial cell not functioning as an ideal mass point (Campbell, Uknalis, Tu, & Mutharasan, 2007; Maraldo & Mutharasan, 2007). Furthermore, the modification of the oscillations would require only part of the membrane in contact with the receptor captured by the immobilized antibody.

Therefore, efforts were made to overcome the limitation by incorporating antibodies-covered nanoparticles against analytes which can increase the mass on the biosensor surface as well as crosslinking the target organism into a firm layer. An assay in which the analyte is captured in a sandwich between an antibody immobilized and bound to nanoparticles on the surface of the crystal. Salam, Uludag, and Tothill (2013) successfully demonstrated the QCM immunosensor, which is coated with a gold nanoparticles antibody method to detect *S. typhymurium* in chicken meat. The method provided a low detection limit ranging from 10 to 20 CFU/mL.

Apart from the piezoelectric type of a mass-sensitive biosensor, phage-based magnetoelastic biosensors are also widely used to detect the presence of *Salmonella* in a food sample. This transduction platform detects signals through either magnetic, acoustic, or optical techniques. Magnetoelastic (ME) biosensors provide advantages in terms of wireless interrogation as magnetic fields are used, miniaturization capability, and simultaneous detection of different targets in a multiplexed fashion (Grimes, Roy, Rani, & Cai, 2011). Changes in frequency of resonance in the magnetoelastic sensor due to mass increase were measured to detect the binding of *S. typhimurium* to the phage. The filamentous phage specific for the target organism was physically adsorbed to the sensor surface. In this study, the detection limit was 103 CFU/mL (Lakshmanan et al., 2007).

Huang et al. (2009) explained the use of multiple magnetoelastic sensors to simultaneously detect two different pathogens, which were *S. typhimurium* and spores of *B. anthracis*. The proposed biosensor was developed with a reference sensor as control, a *Salmonella*-specific sensor, and a sensor coated with *B. anthracis* spore-specific filamentous phages. From the study, it was proven that only sensors coated with phages specific for the respective pathogens would produce measurable signals after continuous exposure to different pathogenic agents. In the real sample, the Salmonella-specific magnetoelastic biosensor was used for the direct detection of *S. typhimurium* on the surface of fresh tomatoes (Li et al., 2010). Phage-coated sensors and a phage-free control sensor were placed directly on the surfaces of tomatoes in a moist environment for 30 min after the samples were spiked with pathogens at different concentrations and air-coated. It can be concluded that there was a significant difference between the phage-coated sensor and the control sensor in terms of generated responses by tomato surfaces that had been spiked with *Salmonella* suspensions with concentrations as low as 5×10^2 CFU/mL. Chai et al. (2012) applied the same principle to successfully detect the presence of *S. typhimurium* on eggshells with a detection limit of 1.4×10^2 CFU/cm^2 within 30 min. A previous study conducted by Mutharasan and Campbell (2014) demonstrated the use of a sensor flow cell to obtain a piezoelectric-excited millimeter-size cantilever (PEMC) sensor. The sensor consisted of a portion of the reservoir that formed a sensing surface of the PEMC sensor and a portion or more of the fluid that can be in liquid or gas form and exposed to the environment. The ability of the PEMC sensor to detect the target organism or analyte in the medium can, therefore, be maximized under flow conditions compared to stable conditions. Theoretically, the flow of the medium stimulates the binding of analytes to the surface of the PEMC sensor, resulting in the detection of a small concentration of analytes.

Optical biosensor

Optical biosensors are widely applied to detect the presence of foodborne pathogens in food samples due to sensitivity and selectivity. Optical biosensors can be classified into multiple groups, including infrared, Raman, chemiluminescent, fluorescence, and phosphorous. It is also recognized that all subgroups need an effective spectrometer to test the spectrochemical properties of the target analyte. Chiefly, surface plasmon resonance (SPR) is the most commonly used technique in the food industry (Velusamy et al., 2010).

SPR is a label-free method that involves sending first polarized light rays through a thin film made of two transparent media with distinct refractive indexes. As a result, some of the photons will be absorbed by the conductive film while the remaining non-absorbed light is reflected at a specific angle known as the SPR angle due to the difference in refractive indexes. A change in the refractive index will occur due to the binding of affinity partners, such as antigen or antibody, and can be detected using SPR biosensors. SPR-based biosensors provide benefits in terms of speed as they are label-free technology, sensitivity, and selectivity through the incorporation of nanoparticles. Recently, molecular recognition elements (MREs) are immobilized on the metal surface to improve the sensitivity and selectivity of SPR biosensors. Nonetheless, some limitations need to be addressed since the approach needs costly and complicated pretreatment, such as biosensor surface coating of the antibodies (Mungroo & Neethirajan, 2016).

Vaisocherová-Lísalová et al. (2016) demonstrated the use of SPR-based biosensor on ultra-low fouling, and functionalizable poly(carboxybetaine acrylamide) (pCBAA) brushes for simultaneous detection of *Salmonella* sp. and *E. coli* O157: H7 in hamburger and cucumber samples which required three steps. The first step is the incubation of a sensor with raw food samples, which will lead to the capture of bacteria through the immobilization of antibodies to pCBAA coating. Then, binding of secondary biotinylated antibody (Ab$_2$) to previously captured bacteria will take place, followed by the binding of streptavidin-coated gold nanoparticles to the biotinylated Ab$_2$ to enhance the sensitivity of the proposed biosensor. In this study, it was proven that pCBAA provides better surface resistance in terms of fouling from complex food samples compared to standard OEG-based alkanethiol self-assembled monolayers.

The fiber optic biosensors are a method based on the reflective properties of light for the simultaneous identification of analytes. The fiber optic biosensors with their respective refractive indexes are made of core, cladding, and jacket. Core and cladding are generally required for light transmission. The optical fibers can be divided into two categories, which are the grating for Fiber Bragg and the construction-based long-term grating. Optical-based biosensor provides many advantages including high sensitivity with minimal light loss and low detection limits (Martins et al., 2013). However, this method also has limitations such as the short lifetime of incident light reagents, and slow response time due to analyte diffusion (Nyachuba, 2010).

Kaushik, Tiwari, Pal, and Sinha (2019) illustrated the use of molybdenum disulfide based fiber optic biosensor nanosheets using the immunosensor SPR to detect the presence of *E.coli* in the food sample. Monoclonal antibodies to *E.coli* were immobilized by hydrophobic interactions on the molybdenum disulfide surface. *S. typhimurium* and *S. aureus* were used to investigate the nonspecificity and cross-reactivity of the proposed immunosensor. It has been established from the analysis that the technique has a low detection limit of 94 CFU/mL when checked on an actual sample, which is orange juice. It can also be assumed that this label-free immunosensor gives better efficiency and greater sensitivity compared with the traditional SPR fiber optic biosensor.

Surface-Enhanced Raman Spectroscopy (SERS) is a technique of surface spectroscopy that magnifies Raman's signals, which generates information about chemical structures when they are subject to molecules. In SERS, the excitation laser resonates with a metal substrate's surface plasmon, which is typically gold or silver in the form of a roughened metal film, colloids, or colloidal solution that has been immobilized on the surface. As the analyte gets closer to the metal, the energy resulting from the plasmon resonance will be coupled into analyte bonds, resulting in a significant increase in the Raman signal (Mungroo & Neethirajan, 2016). In ideal conditions, the identification of a foodborne pathogen is achieved using the target organism's natural vibrational fingerprint (Zourob, Elwary, & Turner, 2008; Le Ru & Etchegoin, 2008).

A previous study conducted by Sundaram, Park, Kwon, and Lawrence (2013) indicated the use of a silver nanoparticle biopolymer with silver nitrate, polyvinyl alcohol (PVA) solution, and trisodium citrate deposited on a mica sheet to be used as a SERS substrate. The sample is containing *S. typhimurium, E. coli, S. aureus,* and *L. innocua* placed individually on the substrate before being exposed to 785 nm HeNe laser excitation. The results showed significant differences between $1200 \, cm^{-1}$ and $1700 \, cm^{-1}$ in nucleic acid and amino acid structure detail and between $400 \, cm^{-1}$ and $700 \, cm^{-1}$ in the fingerprint area. Hence, it can be concluded that SERS is a promising technique in the determination of foodborne pathogens. Chen, Huang, Cai, Wang, and Lin (2018) developed an optical biosensor in combination with immunomagnetic separation, urease catalysis, and pH indication to quickly identify the presence of *L. monocytogenes* in lettuce samples. Magnetic nanobeads conjugated with monoclonal antibodies using streptavidin-biotin binding were used to effectively separate *Listeria* cells from the background. Gold nanoparticles have been modified with urease and polyclonal antibodies (PAbs) by electrostatic adsorption to react with previously labeled bacteria to form MNB-Mab-*Listeria*-PAb-AuNP-urease complexes. The primary function of urease is to catalyze urea hydrolysis to produce ammonium carbonate and result in an increase in the urea solution's pH. The study also demonstrated that optical biosensor is a promising technique for microbiological detection due to its simplicity, sensitivity, and cost-effectiveness.

Current status and future perspectives of biosensor

The biosensor has been used for pathogen detection in recent years to address the limitations of traditional analytical techniques regarding the detection time. Although biosensors such as electrochemical and optical-based biosensors may overcome the limitations of conventional techniques, some drawbacks remain, particularly in terms of sensitivity and cost. Optical biosensors are better than electrochemical biosensors in terms of sensitivity, but high costs and more complicated procedures are required. Electrochemical biosensors, on the other hand, provide a more straightforward protocol, but better performance is needed in the detection of foodborne pathogens. Nonetheless, DNA-based and immunosensors offer excellent results in terms of precision and durability, but both biosensor-based techniques are not capable of distinguishing between living and dying microbial cells.

In general, there are insufficient numbers of foodborne pathogens in the middle of millions of other bacteria. Hence, detecting the target organism is a challenge, resulting in a higher chance for the pathogen to get lost during detection. Foodborne pathogens are present at a deficient concentration in the sample. Therefore, a method that is sufficient for in-situ real-time monitoring must also be created. In this case, the use of a biosensor allows the rapid detection of a foodborne pathogen so that the uncontaminated food can be released in hours or even minutes compared to several days when conventional techniques are used. Several critical steps will be taken to determine the performance of biosensors, such as sample preparation, enrichment, and selection. Besides, an appropriate and specific separation technique to extract the target cell from the sample matrix must be chosen to enhance the sensitivity and specificity of the biosensor being developed. The isolation will also reduce sensory identification of inhibitory compounds, microflora, and physical interferences.

More attention has recently been paid to the development of biosensors using nanoparticles. Nanoparticles can improve the precision, responsiveness, and detection limits of femtomolar detection. Detection of foodborne pathogens in food is expected to be completed in minutes using nanomaterial-based biosensors. Nanoparticles should, therefore, be used in the development of biosensors. Theoretically, foodborne pathogens present in food may grow and multiply, resulting in toxin production during food processing. More studies should, therefore, be conducted to develop a biosensor that can be used to detect the presence of foodborne pathogens during the processing phase.

Conclusions

Foodborne pathogens are any species that are found in food and may cause illness when ingested. Foodborne pathogens are becoming a significant concern in the food industry as ingestion can lead to serious health problems. A rapid detection system using biosensors is, therefore, established to mitigate contamination caused by a foodborne pathogen. As described earlier, biosensors can be divided into two classes that are bioreceptor dependent and transducer-based detection. Bioreceptor-based detection methods, including DNA, enzyme, biomimetic, phage, cell, and antibody, are discussed in this chapter as molecules provide high sensitivity and selectivity during detection. Transducer-based detection, which is an optical, electrochemical, and mass-sensitive biosensor, is also presented. While biosensor is a promising technique for foodborne detection, more research should be done to develop a faster and more cost-effective biosensor (Table 3.2).

Table 3.2 Summary of biosensors available for the detection of foodborne pathogens.

Microorganism	Method	Limit of detection	Food sample	References
E. coli	Immunosensor	30 CFU/mL	Ground beef	Güner et al. (2017), Xu et al. (2016)
E. coli, S. aureus, L. monocytogenes, S. typhimurium	Biomimetic sensor	87 CFU/mL, 100 CFU/mL, 47 CFU/mL, 160 CFU/mL	Ground beef	Xu et al. (2015)
E. coli O157: H7	Biomimetic sensor	1.7×101 CFU/mL	Water	Housaindokht et al. (2018)
E. coli S. aureus	Amperometric electrochemical biosensor	Amperometric electrochemical biosensor	Water	Abdalhai et al. (2014), Arora et al. (2011)
S. aureus	Potentiometric electrochemical biosensor	8×10^2 cells/mL	Pigskin	Zelada-Guillén et al. (2012)
S. typhimurium	Quartz crystal microbalance immunosensor	10^2 cells/mL	Chicken meat	Su and Li (2005)
S. typhimurium	Phage-based magnetoelastic biosensor	5×10^2 CFU/mL	Fresh tomatoes	Li et al. (2010)
S. typhimurium	Phage-based magnetoelastic biosensor	1.4×10^2 CFU/cm2	Eggshells	Chai et al. (2012)
S. typhimurium	Quartz crystal microbalance immunosensor	10–20 CFU/mL	Chicken meat	Salam et al. (2013)
B. cereus	Conductometric-based biosensor	35.3 CFU/mL	Lettuce	Pal et al. (2008)
B. cereus	Conductometric-based biosensor	88.4 CFU/mL	Tomatoes	Pal et al. (2008)
E. coli O157:H7 *Salmonella* sp.	SPR-based optical biosensor	57 CFU/mL, 7.4×10^3 CFU/mL	Hamburger	Vaisocherová-Lísalová et al. (2016)
E. coli O157:H7 *Salmonella* sp.	SPR-based optical biosensor	17 CFU/mL, 11.7×10^3 CFU/mL	Cucumber	Vaisocherová-Lísalová et al. (2016)
E. coli	Fiber optic biosensor	94 CFU/mL	Orange juice	Kaushik et al. (2019)
E. coli	Optical biosensor	1×10^2 CFU/mL	Lettuce	Chen et al. (2018)
E. coli O157: H7	Enzyme-based fiberoptic biosensor	10^3 CFU/mL	Ground beef	Ohk and Bhunia (2013)
S. typhimurium	Enzyme-based electrochemical biosensor	10^3 CFU/mL	Ground beef	Yang et al. (2001)

References

Abdalhai, M. H., Maximiano Fernandes, A., Bashari, M., Ji, J., He, Q., & Sun, X. (2014). Rapid and sensitive detection of foodborne pathogenic bacteria (*Staphylococcus aureus*) using an electrochemical DNA genomic biosensor and its application in fresh beef. *Journal of Agricultural and Food Chemistry*, *62*(52), 12659–12667. https://doi.org/10.1021/jf503914f.

Adley, C. C., & Ryan, M. P. (2015). Conductometric biosensors for high throughput screening of pathogens in food. In *High throughput screening for food safety assessment* (pp. 315–326). Woodhead Publishing. https://doi.org/10.1016/B978-0-85709-801-6.00014-9.

Ahmed, A., Rushworth, J. V., Hirst, N. A., & Millner, P. A. (2014). Biosensors for whole-cell bacterial detection. *Clinical Microbiology Reviews*, *27*(3), 631–646. https://doi.org/10.1128/CMR.00120-13.

Ajayeoba, T. A., Atanda, O. O., Obadina, A. O., Bankole, M. O., & Adelowo, O. O. (2016). The incidence and distribution of Listeria monocytogenes in ready-to-eat vegetables in South-Western Nigeria. *Food Science & Nutrition*, *4*(1), 59–66. https://doi.org/10.1002/fsn3.263.

Angelo, K. M., Conrad, A. R., Saupe, A., Dragoo, H., West, N., Sorenson, A., Barnes, A., Doyle, M., Beal, J., Jackson, K. A., & Stroika, S. (2017). Multistate outbreak of Listeria monocytogenes infections linked to whole apples used in commercially produced, pre-packaged caramel apples: United States, 2014–2015. *Epidemiology & Infection*, *145*(5), 848–856.

Arora, P., Sindhu, A., Dilbaghi, N., & Chaudhury, A. (2011). Biosensors as innovative tools for the detection of food borne pathogens. *Biosensors and Bioelectronics*, *28*(1), 1–12. https://doi.org/10.1016/j.bios.2011.06.002.

Baldrich, E., Vigués, N., Mas, J., & Muñoz, F. X. (2008). Sensing bacteria but treating them well: Determination of optimal incubation and storage conditions. *Analytical Biochemistry*, *383*(1), 68–75. https://doi.org/10.1016/j.ab.2008.08.005.

Banerjee, P., & Bhunia, A. K. (2009). Mammalian cell-based biosensors for pathogens and toxins. *Trends in Biotechnology*, *27*(3), 179–188. https://doi.org/10.1016/j.tibtech.2008.11.006.

Bang, J., Beuchat, L. R., Song, H., Gu, M. B., Chang, H. I., Kim, H. S., & Ryu, J. H. (2013). Development of a random genomic DNA microarray for the detection and identification of Listeria monocytogenes in milk. *International Journal of Food Microbiology*, *161*(2), 134–141. https://doi.org/10.1016/j.ijfoodmicro.2012.11.023.

Bari, M. L., & Yeasmin, S. (2018). Foodborne diseases and responsible agents. In *Food safety and preservation* (pp. 195–229). Academic Press. https://doi.org/10.1016/B978-0-12-814956-0.00008-1.

Campbell, G. A., Uknalis, J., Tu, S. I., & Mutharasan, R. (2007). Detect of Escherichia coli O157: H7 in ground beef samples using piezoelectric excited millimeter-sized cantilever (PEMC) sensors. *Biosensors and Bioelectronics*, *22*(7), 1296–1302. https://doi.org/10.1016/j.bios.2006.05.028.

Channaiah, L. (2015). Staphylococcus aureus food poisoning: Food safety risks and prevention strategies. Quality Assurance & Food Safety [veebileht]. Available from: https:/www.qualityassurancemag.com/article/aib0815-staphylococcus-aureus-food-safetyrisks/ (Accessed 16 March 2019).

Chai, Y., Li, S., Horikawa, S., Park, M. K., Vodyanoy, V., & Chin, B. A. (2012). Rapid and sensitive detection of Salmonella typhimurium on eggshells by using wireless biosensors. *Journal of Food Protection*, *75*(4), 631–636. https://doi.org/10.4315/0362-028X.JFP-11-339.

Chen, Q., Huang, F., Cai, G., Wang, M., & Lin, J. (2018). An optical biosensor using immunomagnetic separation, urease catalysis and pH indication for rapid and sensitive detection of Listeria monocytogenes. *Sensors and Actuators B: Chemical*, *258*, 447–453. https://doi.org/10.1016/j.snb.2017.11.087.

Che, Y. H., Li, Y., Slavik, M., & Paul, D. (2000). Rapid detection of Salmonella typhimurium in chicken carcass wash water using an immunoelectrochemical method. *Journal of Food Protection*, *63*(8), 1043–1048. https://doi.org/10.4315/0362-028X-63.8.1043.

Chung, J., Kang, J. S., Jurng, J. S., Jung, J. H., & Kim, B. C. (2015). Fast and continuous microorganism detection using aptamer-conjugated fluorescent nanoparticles on an optofluidic platform. *Biosensors and Bioelectronics*, *67*, 303–308. https://doi.org/10.1016/j.bios.2014.08.039.

Daniels, N. A. (2011). Vibrio vulnificus oysters: pearls and perils. *Clinical Infectious Diseases*, *52*(6), 788–792. https://doi.org/10.1093/cid/ciq251.

EFSA (2012). The European Union summary report on trends and sources of zoonoses, zoonotic agents and food-borne outbreaks in the European Union in 2010. *The EFSA Journal*, *10*, 2597.

Ferens, W. A., & Hovde, C. J. (2011). Escherichia coli O157: H7: animal reservoir and sources of human infection. *Foodborne Pathogens and Disease*, *8*(4), 465–487. https://doi.org/10.1089/fpd.2010.0673.

Grimes, C. A., Roy, S. C., Rani, S., & Cai, Q. (2011). Theory, instrumentation and applications of magnetoelastic resonance sensors: A review. *Sensors*, *11*(3), 2809–2844. https://doi.org/10.3390/s110302809.

Güner, A., Çevik, E., Şenel, M., & Alpsoy, L. (2017). An electrochemical immunosensor for sensitive detection of Escherichia coli O157: H7 by using chitosan, MWCNT, polypyrrole with gold nanoparticles hybrid sensing platform. *Food Chemistry*, *229*, 358–365. https://doi.org/10.1016/j.foodchem.2017.02.083.

Hart, J. P., Crew, A., Crouch, E., Honeychurch, K. C., & Pemberton, R. M. (2004). Some recent designs and developments of screen-printed carbon electrochemical sensors/biosensors for biomedical, environmental, and industrial analyses. *Analytical Letters*, *37*(5), 789–830. https://doi.org/10.1081/AL-120030682.

Hossain, S. Z., Ozimok, C., Sicard, C., Aguirre, S. D., Ali, M. M., Li, Y., & Brennan, J. D. (2012). Multiplexed paper test strip for quantitative bacterial detection. *Analytical and Bioanalytical Chemistry*, *403*(6), 1567–1576. https://doi.org/10.1007/s00216-012-5975-x.

Housaindokht, M. R., Verdian, A., Sheikhzadeh, E., Pordeli, P., Rouhbakhsh Zaeri, Z., Janati Fard, F., Nosrati, M., Mashreghi, M., Haghparast, A., Nakhaei Pour, A., & Esmaeili, A. A. (2018). A sensitive electrochemical aptasensor based on single wall carbon nanotube modified screen printed electrode for detection of Escherichia coli O157:H7. *Advanced Materials Letters*, *9*, 369–374. https://doi.org/10.5185/amlett.2018.1701.

Huang, S., Yang, H., Lakshmanan, R. S., Johnson, M. L., Wan, J., Chen, I. H., Wikle Iii, H. C., Petrenko, V. A., Barbaree, J. M., & Chin, B. A. (2009). Sequential detection of Salmonella typhimurium and Bacillus anthracis spores using magnetoelastic biosensors. *Biosensors and Bioelectronics*, *24*(6), 1730–1736. https://doi.org/10.1016/j.bios.2008.09.006.

Jayasena, S. D. (1999). *Aptamers: An emerging class of molecules that rival antibodies in diagnostics.* https://doi.org/10.1093/clinchem/45.9.1628.

Kaushik, S., Tiwari, U. K., Pal, S. S., & Sinha, R. K. (2019). Rapid detection of Escherichia coli using fiber optic surface plasmon resonance immunosensor based on biofunctionalized molybdenum disulfide (MoS2) nanosheets. *Biosensors and Bioelectronics, 126,* 501–509. https://doi.org/10.1016/j.bios.2018.11.006.

Kozitsina, A., Svalova, T., Malysheva, N., Glazyrina, Y., Matern, A., & Rusinov, V. (2017). Determination of Staphylococcus aureus B-1266 by an enzyme-free electrochemical immunosensor incorporating magnetite nanoparticles. *Analytical Letters, 50*(6), 924–935. https://doi.org/10.1080/00032719.2016.1204312.

Kumar, H., & Neelam, R. (2016). Enzyme-based electrochemical biosensors for food safety: A review. *Nanobiosensors in Disease Diagnosis, 5,* 29–39. https://doi.org/10.2147/NDD.S64847.

Lakshmanan, R. S., Guntupalli, R., Hu, J., Kim, D. J., Petrenko, V. A., Barbaree, J. M., & Chin, B. A. (2007). Phage immobilized magnetoelastic sensor for the detection of Salmonella typhimurium. *Journal of Microbiological Methods, 71*(1), 55–60. https://doi.org/10.1016/j.mimet.2007.07.012.

Lazcka, O., Del Campo, F. J., & Muñoz, F. X. (2007). Pathogen detection: A perspective of traditional methods and biosensors. *Biosensors and Bioelectronics, 22*(7), 1205–1217. https://doi.org/10.1016/j.bios.2006.06.036.

Li, S., Li, Y., Chen, H., Horikawa, S., Shen, W., Simonian, A., & Chin, B. A. (2010). Direct detection of Salmonella typhimurium on fresh produce using phage-based magnetoelastic biosensors. *Biosensors and Bioelectronics, 26*(4), 1313–1319. https://doi.org/10.1016/j.bios.2010.07.029.

Maraldo, D., & Mutharasan, R. (2007). 10-Minute assay for detecting Escherichia coli O157: H7 in ground beef samples using piezoelectric-excited millimeter-size cantilever sensors. *Journal of Food Protection, 70*(7), 1670–1677. https://doi.org/10.4315/0362-028X-70.7.1670.

Martins, T. D., Ribeiro, A. C. C., de Camargo, H. S., da Costa Filho, P. A., Cavalcante, H. P M., & Dias, D. L. (2013). New insights on optical biosensors: Techniques, construction and application. *State of the Art in Biosensors—General Aspects,* 112–139.

Mungroo, N. A., & Neethirajan, S. (2016). Optical biosensors for the detection of food borne pathogens. *Institution of Engineering and Technology,* 181–208. https://doi.org/10.1049/PBHE001E (Chapter 10).

Mutharasan, R., & Campbell, G. A. (2014). In MutluM. (Ed.), *U.S. Patent No. 8,778,446. Washington, DC: U.S. Patent and Trademark Office.* Biosensors in food processing, safety, and quality control. CRC Press (2016).

Niyomdecha, S., Limbut, W., Numnuam, A., Kanatharana, P., Charlermroj, R., Karoonuthaisiri, N., & Thavarungkul, P. (2018). Phage-based capacitive biosensor for Salmonella detection. *Talanta, 188,* 658–664. https://doi.org/10.1016/j.talanta.2018.06.033.

Nyachuba, D. G. (2010). Foodborne illness: Is it on the rise? *Nutrition Reviews, 68*(5), 257–269. https://doi.org/10.1111/j.1753-4887.2010.00286.x.

Ohk, S. H., & Bhunia, A. K. (2013). Multiplex fiber optic biosensor for detection of Listeria monocytogenes, Escherichia coli O157: H7 and Salmonella enterica from ready-to-eat meat samples. *Food Microbiology, 33*(2), 166–171. https://doi.org/10.1016/j.fm.2012.09.013.

Pal, S., Ying, W., Alocilja, E. C., & Downes, F. P. (2008). Sensitivity and specificity performance of a direct-charge transfer biosensor for detecting Bacillus cereus in selected food matrices. *Biosystems Engineering*, *99*(4), 461–468. https://doi.org/10.1016/j.biosystemseng.2007.11.015.

Palchetti, I., & Mascini, M. (2008). Electroanalytical biosensors and their potential for food pathogen and toxin detection. *Analytical and Bioanalytical Chemistry*, *391*(2), 455–471. https://doi.org/10.1007/s00216-008-1876-4.

Perumal, V., & Hashim, U. (2014). Advances in biosensors: Principle, architecture and applications. *Journal of Applied Biomedicine*, *12*, 1–15. https://doi.org/10.1016/j.jab.2013.02.001.

Pohanka, M. (2018). Overview of piezoelectric biosensors, immunosensors and DNA sensors and their applications. *Materials*. *11*(3), https://doi.org/10.3390/ma11030448.

Le Ru, E., & Etchegoin, P. (2008). *Principles of surface-enhanced Raman spectroscopy: And related plasmonic effects*. Elsevier.

Salam, F., Uludag, Y., & Tothill, I. E. (2013). Real-time and sensitive detection of Salmonella typhimurium using an automated quartz crystal microbalance (QCM) instrument with nanoparticles amplification. *Talanta*, *115*, 761–767. https://doi.org/10.1016/j.talanta.2013.06.034.

Sharma, H., Agarwal, M., Goswami, M., Sharma, A., Roy, S. K., Rai, R., & Murugan, M. S. (2013). Biosensors: Tool for food borne pathogen detection. *Veterinary World*, *6* (12), 968–973. https://doi.org/10.14202/vetworld.2013.968-973.

Shen, Z., Hou, N., Jin, M., Qiu, Z., Wang, J., Zhang, B., … Li, J. (2014). A novel enzyme-linked immunosorbent assay for detection of Escherichia coli O157: H7 using immunomagnetic and beacon gold nanoparticles. *Gut Pathogens*, *6*(1).

Skládal, P. (1997). Advances in electrochemical immunosensors. *Electroanalysis*, *9*(10), 737–745. https://doi.org/10.1002/elan.1140091002.

Skládal, P., Kovář, D., Krajíček, V., Krajíček, P., Přibyl, J., & Švábenská, E. (2013). Electrochemical immunosensors for detection of microorganisms. *International Journal of Electrochemical Science*, *8*(2), 1635–1649. Retrieved fromhttp:/www.electrochemsci.org/papers/vol8/80201573.pdf.

Su, X. L., & Li, Y. (2005). A QCM immunosensor for Salmonella detection with simultaneous measurements of resonant frequency and motional resistance. *Biosensors and Bioelectronics*, *21*(6), 840–848. https://doi.org/10.1016/j.bios.2005.01.021.

Sundaram, J., Park, B., Kwon, Y., & Lawrence, K. C. (2013). Surface enhanced Raman scattering (SERS) with biopolymer encapsulated silver nanosubstrates for rapid detection of foodborne pathogens. *International Journal of Food Microbiology*, *167*(1), 67–73. https://doi.org/10.1016/j.ijfoodmicro.2013.05.013.

Teng, J., Yuan, F., Ye, Y., Zheng, L., Yao, L., Xue, F., … Li, B. (2016). Aptamer-based technologies in foodborne pathogen detection. *Frontiers in Microbiology*. *7*, https://doi.org/10.3389/fmicb.2016.01426.

Tombelli, S., Minunni, M., & Mascini, M. (2005). Piezoelectric biosensors: Strategies for coupling nucleic acids to piezoelectric devices. *Methods*, *37*(1), 48–56. https://doi.org/10.1016/j.ymeth.2005.05.005.

Vaisocherová-Lísalová, H., Víšová, I., Ermini, M. L., Špringer, T., Song, X. C., Mrázek, J., … Homola, J. (2016). Low-fouling surface plasmon resonance biosensor for multi-step detection of foodborne bacterial pathogens in complex food samples. *Biosensors and Bioelectronics*, *80*, 84–90. https://doi.org/10.1016/j.bios.2016.01.040.

Van de Venter, T. (2000). Emerging food-borne diseases: A global responsibility. *Food Nutrition and Agriculture, 26,* 4–13.

Velusamy, V., Arshak, K., Korostynska, O., Oliwa, K., & Adley, C. (2010). An overview of foodborne pathogen detection: In the perspective of biosensors. *Biotechnology Advances, 28*(2), 232–254. https://doi.org/10.1016/j.biotechadv.2009.12.004.

Wang, R. F., Beggs, M. L., Robertson, L. H., & Cerniglia, C. E. (2002). Design and evaluation of oligonucleotide-microarray method for the detection of human intestinal bacteria in fecal samples. *FEMS Microbiology Letters, 213*(2), 175–182. https://doi.org/10.1016/S0378-1097(02)00802-9.

Whiley, H., van den Akker, B., Giglio, S., & Bentham, R. (2013). The role of environmental reservoirs in human campylobacteriosis. *International Journal of Environmental Research and Public Health, 10*(11), 5886–5907. https://doi.org/10.3390/ijerph10115886.

WHO (2018). https://www.who.int/news-room/fact-sheets/detail/botulism.

Wong, H. C., Liu, S. H., Ku, L. W., Lee, I. Y., Wang, T. K., Lee, Y. S., … Shih, D. Y. C. (2000). Characterization of Vibrio parahaemolyticus isolates obtained from foodborne illness outbreaks during 1992 through 1995 in Taiwan. *Journal of Food Protection, 63*(7), 900–906. https://doi.org/10.4315/0362-028X-63.7.900.

Xie, B., Ramanathan, K., & Danielsson, B. (1999). Principles of enzyme thermistor systems: Applications to biomedical and other measurements. *Advances in Biochemical Engineering/Biotechnology, 64,* 1–33.

Xu, L., Callaway, Z. T., Wang, R., Wang, H., Slavik, M. F., Wang, A., & Li, Y. (2015). A fluorescent aptasensor coupled with nanobead-based immunomagnetic separation for simultaneous detection of four foodborne pathogenic bacteria. *Transactions of the ASABE, 58*(3), 891–906. https://doi.org/10.13031/trans.58.11089.

Xu, M., Wang, R., & Li, Y. (2016). Rapid detection of Escherichia coli O157:H7 and Salmonella typhimurium in foods using an electrochemical immunosensor based on screen-printed interdigitated microelectrode and immunomagnetic separation. *Talanta, 148,* 200–208. https://doi.org/10.1016/j.talanta.2015.10.082.

Yang, L., Ruan, C., & Li, Y. (2001). Rapid detection of Salmonella typhimurium in food samples using a bienzyme electrochemical biosensor with flow injection. *Journal of Rapid Methods and Automation in Microbiology, 9*(4), 229–240. https://doi.org/10.1111/j.1745-4581.2001.tb00249.x.

Yasmin, J., Ahmed, M. R., & Cho, B. K. (2016). Biosensors and their applications in food safety: A review. *Journal of Biosystems Engineering, 41*(3), 240–254.

Ye, Y., Guo, H., & Sun, X. (2019). Recent progress on cell-based biosensors for analysis of food safety and quality control. *Biosensors and Bioelectronics, 126,* 389–404. https://doi.org/10.1016/j.bios.2018.10.039.

Yunus, G. (2019). *Biosensors: An enzyme-based biophysical technique for the detection of foodborne pathogens. In Enzymes in food biotechnology*: (pp. 723–738). Academic Press. https://doi.org/10.1016/B978-0-12-813280-7.00042-6.

Zelada-Guillén, G. A., Sebastián-Avila, J. L., Blondeau, P., Riu, J., & Rius, F. X. (2012). Label-free detection of Staphylococcus aureus in skin using real-time potentiometric biosensors based on carbon nanotubes and aptamers. *Biosensors and Bioelectronics, 31*(1), 226–232. https://doi.org/10.1016/j.bios.2011.10.021.

Zhang, X., Ju, H., & Wang, J. (Eds.), (2011). *Electrochemical sensors, biosensors and their biomedical applications.* Academic Press.

Zhao, X., Lin, C. W., Wang, J., & Oh, D. H. (2014). Advances in rapid detection methods for foodborne pathogens. *Journal of Microbiology and Biotechnology, 24*(3), 297–312. https://doi.org/10.4014/jmb.1310.10013.

Zourob, M., Elwary, S., & Turner, A. P. (Eds.), (2008). *Principles of bacterial detection: Biosensors, recognition receptors and microsystems.* Springer Science & Business Media.

Novel biosensors for detection of the parasite in food

4

Introduction

Foodborne parasites (FBPs) are often referred to as overlooked disease and not received the same level of concern as other foodborne biological and chemical hazards, even though they have posed a high burden of human disease, especially in the area with inadequate sanitary facilities and have caused numerous outbreaks. In 2011, the outbreak was the largest affecting 80 people who had consumed raw marinated fish at Lake Bolsena, and the outbreak in 2010 was caused by raw tench filets serving at the restaurant due to lower costs and higher demand during the summer season (Cacciò, Chalmers, Dorny, & Robertson, 2018). However, parasites are living beings who reside permanently or temporarily in or on other living organisms (hosts) for feed, growth, and reproduction purposes, which cause human disease and are transmitted through various routes, including waterborne, soil, food, animal-to-human as well as human-to-human contact. FBPs are expected to have a significant impact on public safety in the future due to the growing demand for meat and fresh food worldwide.

Symptoms of foodborne parasitic infections vary widely depending on the type of parasite and the strain of infection. Protozoa is the most common cause of diarrhea and other gastrointestinal symptoms. They are less common, but some parasites may cause serious illness in the elderly, pregnant women, immunocompromised, and other persons with lower immune systems, which may have serious consequences for the immunocompetent. Since FBPs have become a global food safety concern, there are many approaches to improving the identification and management of FBPs, such as sanitation and hygiene, cooking and heat treatment, freezing, other physical processes, picking, smoking and fermentation, and filtration, chlorination, and disinfection.

Biosensors are popular in a variety of fields, including medicine, food production, environmental safety, and foodborne pathogens. There are three important elements for identifying a parasite in the biosensor that is a live capture molecule, a mechanism for translating trap molecule-target interactions into signs, and a framework for the output of information. Yunus (2018) emphasized on developing new biosensor methods that can identify foodborne pathogens in a limited time with sensitivity and selectivity relative to the old methods that can potentially be used as stand-alone devices for on-site pathogen detection. Moreover, recent advances in nanomaterial-based sensors provide a number of technical innovations in the

Advanced Food Analysis Tools. https://doi.org/10.1016/B978-0-12-820591-4.00004-9

identification of foodborne pathogens by attaching or reacting biological components to target organisms and gradually converting them into observable signals, enabling rapid identification of food pollutants, and ensuring early preventive food protection (Inbaraj & Chen, 2016). The key advantages of biosensors are rapid real-time detection, portability, sensitivity, user-friendly, ease of use, and simultaneous pathogen detection for field and laboratory investigations. This chapter offers current approaches and views for integrating modern sensing technologies to identify the parasite in food.

Biosensor

Biosensors are analytical instruments that transform biological reactions to electrical signals and are deemed promising because of their specific properties such as high sensitivity, ease of miniaturization, and rapid response. Biosensor and nanotechnology progress has recently increased as leading research in several forms of industrial or educational industries and provides opportunities to boost the potential generation of biosensor innovations that will improve the mechanical, electrochemical, optical, and magnetic features of biosensors with high-performance biosensor arrays. Nanotechnology-enabled goods are rapidly commonplace and one of the most promising technological developments that have contributed to significant advances in the modern diet and food sciences. Biosensors and nanotechnologies are increasingly emerging in current areas such as food, forestry, biomedical, medicinal, and pharmaceutical sciences, catalysis, and environmental regeneration. Since biosensor has high sensitivity and reliability, which is improved by the usage of nanomaterials that have rendered it possible to incorporate in the field of parasitology. Recent advances in biosensor development over the last few years have paved the way for potential researchers to improve these biosensory aspects further and optimize them for the identification of dangerous diseases triggered by parasites.

Classification of parasites

Parasites look like roundworms, gross-looking tapeworms, fleas, or blood-borne diseases (malaria and schistosomiasis) ranging from several centimeters to many meters in length. Their size is very small compared to their food sources, which can protect them from predators, and they often consume other living things. Parasites are species that receive food from other living organisms; therefore, a "good" or well-adapted parasite will not destroy its host, as it relies on the host to provide food consistently over a long period of time. In the meantime, according to Doyle (2013), those parasites live only in one animal species. Nevertheless, other parasites, especially worms, invest their sexually reproductive lives in a primary or definite host and emerge as larvae in an intermediate host of different organisms during another part of their lives.

The protozoan parasite is a completely different class of eukaryotic organisms that can cause disease in living organisms. Robertson (2018) discovered that the majority of parasitic infections are asymptomatic, induce acute short-lived, as well as remain in the body causing chronic effects. This situation can be considered confined to tropical countries, primarily in areas with minimal sanitary facilities where the communities are typically eating raw and undercooked food. Generally, the transmission occurs through various sampling techniques, preparation routines, detection targets used, as well as through a variety of routes and vehicles, including soil, water, food, and human-animal contact (Ortega & Sterling, 2018; Rozycki et al., 2020).

Parasites tend to be attributed to multiple factors, including parasitic infections, which do not appear to be serious diseases but affect their hosts chronically and gradually. A host is described as an organism that harbors the parasite, provides food and shelter, comparatively more substantial in size, and maybe a definitive host, intermediate host, reservoir host, paratenic hosts, and accidental hosts. Robertson (2018) explains another reason in 2018 as it relates to poverty, here populations live in areas with a lack of primary infrastructure, water system, hygiene, and accommodation and they are the most vulnerable to parasite infections and are unable to combat these diseases. However, the worldwide prevalence of human parasite disease has been reported at 407 million cases per year, which approximately 22% infections, and nearly 52,000 fatalities are predicted caused by foodborne (Gargouri et al., 2015; Rozycki et al., 2020).

Fig. 4.1 describes three classes of parasitic worms that are tapeworms (cestodes), flukes (trematodes), and roundworms (nematodes) and some protozoans. Such selected parasites are very different from each other, not only in terms of taxonomy but also anatomy, symptoms, and life cycle. In the meantime, few commonalities are of zoonotic potential where it is important for those whose route of transmission to humans is through the ingestion of an animal already infected by itself.

The protozoans, a tiny unicellular eukaryotic species belonging to the Protista kingdom, have nuclei and cellular organs enclosed by a membrane. Their size is between 5 and 1000 μm which only can be seen under a microscope, as well as possess a simpler and more primitive structure than the species in the animal kingdom. Protozoan has flagella or cilia, which allows them to travel and get nutrients. According to Cavalier-Smith (2010) and Hampl et al. (2012), protozoans are a diverse assemblage containing a variety of different lineages covering almost all major eukaryote clades (alveolates, stramenopiles, amoebozoans, opisthokonts, rhizarians, and excavates) which are capable of sexual reproduction and typically reproduce asexually by binary or multiple fission. Besides, protozoan is mainly aquatic, living in moist conditions, freshwater (including the soil), brackish, and marine environments (Thorp, Rogers, & Covich, 2015). Protozoans often are found in sources of fresh water that have been polluted with waste, thus food which is washed with such infected water allows the parasite to immobilize onto the contact and cause infection. Some protozoa can survive in only one animal species, whereas, human pathogens can exist in humans and animals. Therefore, five of the most common parasites are *Toxoplasma*, *Cryptosporidium*, *Cyclospora*, *Entamoeba*, and *Giardia*.

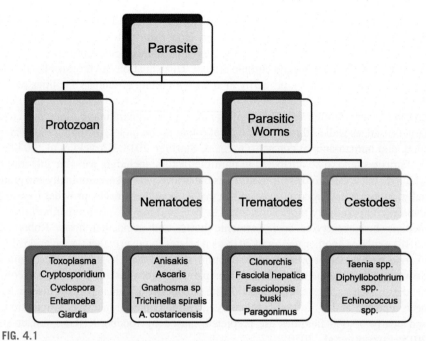

FIG. 4.1

Type of parasite in various of food.

Parasitic worms cestodes, or tapeworms, are flat, tape-like worms, just a few millimeters in size that can reside in the human gastrointestinal tract, comprising both male and female reproductive organs, and they do not have a digestive tract and consists of strobila (the major part of worm) including segments and proglottids (formed in the neck of the worms). Besides, the tapeworms absorb their nutrients from the host intestine directly through the outer surface of the tegument (Cobo, 2014; Saari, Näreaho, & Nikander, 2018). Typically, pork (*Taenia solium*) and beef (Taenia. saginata) tapeworm eggs are found on waste-treated fruits or vegetables, and in meat or fish muscles that may mature in the human intestine to adults. Doyle, 2013 clarified that the impact of consuming *T. solium* on humans can cause severe complications when larvae hatching from the eggs burrow out of the intestine and spread to the lungs, muscles, brain, and other parts of the body where they encyst. Generally, dogs and humans serve as their hosts, but humans are the only definitive host for *T. solium* (pork tapeworm) and *T. saginata* (beef tapeworm) while *Taenia asiatica* is mostly found in pigs in certain countries of Southeast Asia (Vietnam, Indonesia, and Taiwan). Therefore, the typical cestodes worms are *Taenia* spp., *Diphyllobothrium* spp., and *Echinococcus* spp.

Nematodes or roundworms are microscopic, nonsegmented, typically 0.5–2.0 mm in length, worm-like, cross-sectionally cylindrical, and have a complete dietary tract and body cavity. It also has a well-developed nervous system, excretory system and musculature, as well as living in freshwater, soil, and marine ecosystems. In addition, the nematodes have a complete digestive system with an anterior mouth which is fitted for complex structures (lips, sensory organs, and chitinous teeth or plates) for eating or attaching to the host and a posterior anus (Levsen, Lunestad, & Berland, 2008; Saari et al., 2018). Nematodes consist of *Trichinella, Ascaris, Anisakis, Angiostrongylus, Gnathostoma,* and can be located in various food matrices, where Ascaris can be identified in polluted water or vegetables. At the same time, Angiostrongylus found in snails and on leafy vegetables, and others live as cysts in meat or fish muscles (Doyle, 2013). However, nematodes often inhabit the intestinal tract, and their larvae can be found in the respiratory tract and respiratory exudate.

Trematodes are flatworms or flukes with female and male reproductive organs of the same individual, with the incomplete digestive tract. It has more than one intermediate host, long-lived parasites, flat and leaf-like with a bilaterally symmetrical body. There are four specific trematodes of relevance to human infestation, namely Clonorchis, *Fasciola hepatica, Fasciolopsis buski*, and Paragonimus (Wanger et al., 2017). According to Doyle (2013), *Fasciola* and *Fasciolopsis* are present in aquatic crops or foods washed in polluted water while *Paragonimus* contained in wild boar and others are encyst in fish or crabs (Clonorchis); however, flukes may also be identified in a variety of human organs (intestine, lungs, and liver).

The life cycle is the process of emergence, creation, and replication of a parasite that proceeds in one or more different hosts based on the species of parasites. For instance, the life cycle of a parasite may be direct reinfection, completion of the life cycle in one host, one intermediate host, and two intermediate hosts. These differences represent alternate approaches for dealing with environmental vagaries and their eventual hosts (Nielsen & Reinemeyer, 2018). Some have a simplistic life cycle where all phases of growth are achieved in a single host, while in other cases, certain parasites have a complex life cycle containing more than one host animal. Complex life cycles offer advantages to parasites that have a longer life span, greater fecundity, but often reflect the sequence of unforeseeable events that many adaptations have evolved.

Effect of the parasite in food to human

Individuals may acquire animal-dependent zoonotic infections, including contact with an infected arthropod vector or an infected animal, ingestion of food or water contaminated with parasites, ingestion of tissue from an infected animal, or ingestion of environmental friendly food. Parasites are species which remove metabolic substances from their host organisms to complete their life cycle, and parasites may also be primary sources and vectors of infectious disease. Parasites are species that extract metabolism from their host organisms to complete their life cycle and parasites can also be the primary epidemic disease sources and vectors.

In humans, intestinal protozoan parasites typically cause moderate to serious diarrhea, while malnourished kids, aged, and immunocompromised persons experience extreme and persistent gastrointestinal symptoms may be life-threatening (Doyle, 2013). Besides, infection with the tapeworm *T. saginata* induces taeniosis where most human infections with *T. saginata* are asymptomatic (showing no symptoms). However, mild abdominal symptoms may occur, including pain, lack of appetite, weight loss, nausea, and proglottids, triggering pruritis due to the inferior sensitivity of the meat inspection and the environmental spread of eggs from sewage. Gottstein, Pozio, and Nöckler (2009) defined trichinellosis (syn. Trichinosis) as a global disease triggered by the ingestion of undercooked meat containing viable nematode larvae, *Trichinella* spp. Pork is the most common source of human infection, but meat from other sources such as horses, wild boars, bears, walruses, and badgers has also induced outbreaks. Infection with this parasite may cause severe disease in humans, including diarrhea, fever, periorbital edema, and myalgia, as well as other possible complications such as myocarditis, thromboembolic disease, and encephalitis.

Anyone may be diagnosed with *T. gondii*, and the outcomes depend on both individual and infective strain, where most infections in generally healthy people are asymptomatic or cause flu-like symptoms. During pregnancy, primary infection with *T. gondii* may trigger miscarriage or the birth of a congenitally infected child with severe health issues, whereas acute or chronic *T. gondii* infection is dangerous for people who have weakened immune systems, and life-threatening complications may develop such as encephalitis (Rozycki et al., 2020). In most cases, infections are asymptomatic, although they may have catastrophic effects for the immunocompromised and unborn children who become infected during pregnancy. Nevertheless, most of the time, the pregnant woman hardly notices being infected because *Toxoplasma* can cross the placenta and infect the fetus. The most severe result of such infection in children is weakened vision or blindness after birth, and more severe consequences are hydrocephalus, convulsions, and calcium deposits in the brain whereas adults may also develop signs of retinitis and swollen lymph nodes following exposure to contaminated meat or water (Carboni & Tully, 2009). Also, *Cyclospora* induces prolonged watery diarrhea, nausea, and vomiting that can be debilitating, especially in infants and the immunocompromised (Dorny, Praet, Deckers, & Gabriel, 2009).

Control of parasite

Parasite prevention is complicated due to the presence of zoonotic reservoir (mainly dogs and cats) and the firmly rooted customs of eating raw, undercooked, or freshly pickled crabs or crayfish in endemic areas. Control of the parasites can be accomplished by prevention and some simple technique (sanitation and proper cooking of foods), where it is useful and helpful in combating all the parasites in food. Besides, other approaches, as seen in Fig. 4.2, might be useful in controlling the parasites.

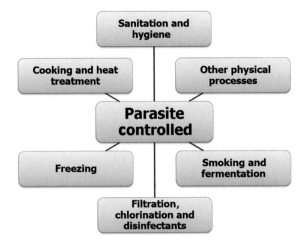

FIG. 4.2

Methods on control the parasites.

Sanitation and hygiene

Sanitation and hygiene are some of the simple approaches that can be used to monitor the parasite in food as it is a function to interrupt the life cycle of parasites and reducing the likelihood of a fecal-oral transmission route. For example, proper disposal of human and animal wastes to prevent from food and drinking water contamination is an excellent and easy technique to deter certain parasitic infections that are spread through the fecal-oral route. However, in many developing countries, this waste serves as fertilizer for crops, and the composting of this substance may destroy parasite eggs and could also regulate the increasing of flies, cockroaches, and other insects in the dispersal of infective stages of parasites to foods. Besides, washing raw vegetables and fruits can remove cysts, oocysts, and eggs of parasites, but it is difficult to clean certain leafy vegetables and berries properly. Thus, frequent handwashing, use of clean utensils, and measures to avoid cross-contamination during food processing are also necessary in order to prevent any parasite contamination (Doyle, 2013; Thompson, 2015).

Cooking and heat treatment

In cooking and heat treatment, it is apparent that all the infective phases of pathogens are destroyed by adequate cooking of food and boiling drinking water. However, microwave cooking (2450 MHz, 700 W) may not consistently destroy all parasites in meat and fish because the heating is uneven and cooler spots may permit survival but consumers are encouraged to cook pork and any wild game meat that may be contaminated with trichinae at an internal temperature of 160 °F (71 °C). For *Anisakis*, heating at ≥60°C core temperature of fishery products for at least 1 min is necessary to destroy the larvae, hence the fish fillets of 3 cm thickness should be heated for 10 min to exceed and maintain 60°C in the core (EFSA, 2010) while cooking the fish for 10 min at 60°C or 7 min at 70°C would also destroy the *Anisakis*. Robertson et al. (2019) and Gajadhar (2015) highlight many types of heat treatment research as the most effective tool for controlling and preventing contamination of food by the parasite, as well as emphasizing that heating duration is required to be uniformly spread across meat or any food product.

Freezing

Freezing is another thermal technique that can be successful in controlling certain parasites. Raw or fresh food (fish and some meats) need to be frozen over many days in order to inactivate or destroy the parasites, for example, fish should be frozen at −30°C over ≥15 h using industrial blast freezer or − 20°C for ≥7 days in a domestic freezer to destroy *Anisakis*. Meanwhile, cold meat freezing at 5°F (−17°C) for 20 days, 10°F (−23.3°C) for 10 days, or 20°F (−29°C) for 6 days is the safest way to kill trichinae in pork, although that might not be effective for trichinae in wild game meat. Unexpectedly, the infective trichinae have been found in polar bears and grizzly bears meat frozen for 24 months (Cédric et al., 2019; Doyle, 2013).

Filtration, chlorination, and disinfectants

Besides, filtration systems can remove protozoan cysts and oocysts from water, while disinfection is a crucial move to defend consumers from foodborne infectious diseases triggered by parasites, and it can eliminate the organisms, including bacteria, virus, and parasites (Mian, Hu, Hewage, Rodriguez, & Sadiq, 2018). In addition, chlorination methods are able to kill bacteria and certain parasites from water. Nevertheless, cysts and oocysts are immune to chlorine when soaking vegetables in bleach solution, vinegar, potassium permanganate solution, or saturated cooking salt that killed specific nematode and trematode parasites from contagious larvae, as well as ammonium hydroxide solution, which killed 94% of Ascaris eggs after 3 h, but other disinfectants were less efficient.

Other physical processes

Other physical processes by irradiation can eliminate parasites in particular raw foods and by reducing doses of irradiation capable of destroying larvae and inhibiting infectivity. However, higher doses are needed to kill all the trichinae in meat, although irradiation doses have been recorded to kill trematode cysts in fish. High hydrostatic pressure has been documented to be a theoretically useful nonthermal tool for destroying *Anisakis*. At the same time, ultraviolet light will disinfect water containing *Giardia* cysts, and ozone destroys protozoan parasites in the water, and ultrasound treatment inactivates *Cryptosporidium* oocysts in water (Doyle, 2013). Food irradiation is utilized in food manufacturing to further guarantee food health by utilizing ionizing radiation that uses electricity, X-rays, and gamma rays to kill microorganisms (bacteria, viruses, or insects) in food. In 2013, Marcus clarified that irradiation has the potential to slow ripening, boost rehydration, increase juice yield, and prevent sprouting, which helps preserve foods and keeps them at their peak. Therefore, food irradiation technology is allowed in nearly 60 countries, but its usage is restricted to a few, mainly in Asia and North America (Prakash & de Jesús Ornelas-Paz, 2019).

Pickling, smoking, and fermentation

Pickling is a process of soaking food in a salt, acid, or alcohol solution that may be used in a number of foods that resist and kill bacteria, parasites, and other microorganisms (Iordache et al., 2017). In contrast, pickling pork kills the larvae of tapeworms (cysticerci). Hot smoking processes kill *Anisakis* but those parasites survive cold smoking. According to Verni et al. (2019), fermentation became one of the oldest forms of preservation, but it is still capable of enhancing the sensory and nutritional quality of food, altering its structural characteristics, and extending its shelf-life.

Detection of the parasite in food based on biosensors

Biosensor technology has been given significant attention because of its high precision, high sensitivity, and cheapness. From previous analysis by Kumar, Dilbaghi, Barnela, Bhanjana, and Kumar (2012), they explained the use of biosensors in the food industry to detect numerous pathogens, allergens, residues of pesticides, natural pollutants, and other toxic materials. Some of these parasites may be spread by contact with water, soil, or from person-to-person. Parasitic diseases affect many people across the world, leading to crippling diseases and death. Parasite detection approaches need to be rapid and cheap, particularly in resource-limited settings.

Previously, Jain, Costa Melo, Dolabella, and Liu (2019) reported that biosensors and nanotechnology-based parasites such as *Cryptosporidium*, *Giardia*, *Entamoeba*, and *Toxoplasma* could be used to detect the cysts and oocyst of the parasites in the environment. Besides, Webb et al. (2016) designed many modular biosensors based on *Escherichia coli* and *Bacillus subtilis* that integrate an interchangeable motif for protease recognition into their designs. This whole-cell biosensor evolved to identify the presence and activity of elastase, an enzyme released through the *Schistosoma mansoni* cercarial larvae stage. Additionally, Ullah, Qadeer, Rashid, Rashid, and Cheng (2019) established nucleic acid-based biosensors for the identification of biomarkers of nucleic acid, which can theoretically be used to diagnose helminth infection.

Gavriilidou & Bridle (2018) proposed the lectin immobilization using an 11-mercaptoundecanoic acid protocol accompanied by EDC-sulfo-NHS (carbodiimide-*N*-hydroxysulfosuccinimide crosslinker) to detect pathogenic protozoa such as *Cryptosporidium*. Additionally, Lin, Luo, Zhou, Wan, and Wu (2018) reported that immunosorbent enzyme-linked assay (ELISA) and immunoelectrotransfer blot enzyme (EITB) are relevant approaches for identifying *T. solium*, which is not only infected but also infected pigs. Nazari-Vanani et al. (2018) produced a sensor that used toluidine blue as a hybridization marker and a *Leishmania infantum*-specific capture sequence of DNA immobilized as an electrochemical transducer to identify a synthetic L. *infantum* on a high surface gold nanostructure. Also, Hou, Cai, Zheng, and Lin (2019) successfully developed a microfluidic biosensor using magnetic nanoparticles that incorporated with catalases for the detection of *Salmonella typhimurium*.

Meat

Meat is flesh or other edible animal parts, including tendons and ligaments, as well as muscles, used for foods containing full protein and all the amino acids required for living things. *Sarcocystis* species are the most frequently observed parasitic organisms in animals commonly found in muscle tissue of beef cattle. *Sarcocystis* species are also found in minced meat, meatballs, cured meat, and beef sausages. The parasite generally produces toxins and causes food poisoning by zoonotic parasites transmitted through beef consumption (Kamber, Arslan, Gülbaz, Tasçi, & Akça, 2018). Vidic, Manzano, Chang, and Jaffrezic-Renault (2017) proposed biosensing mechanisms for the identification and diagnosis of pathogens in livestock and poultry-based on DNA receptors, glycan, aptamers, antibodies, and ELISA. Toubanaki, Athanasiou, and Karagouni (2016) implemented lateral flow biosensor by merely detecting the PCR product using a lateral nucleic acid flow integrated with functionalized gold nanoparticles studied with leishmaniasis of high specificity, caused by *Leishmania* parasites in dog meat. In previous research, Luka et al. (2019) developed simultaneously microfluidic biosensors based on impedance for the identification of *Salmonella* serotypes in the ready-to-eat (RTE) turkey matrix.

Xu, Wang, and Li (2016) developed an electrochemical biosensor in food to rapidly detect pathogenic bacteria, *E. coli* and *S. typhimurium*, based on immunomagnetic separation, enzyme labeling, and electrochemical impedance spectroscopy (EIS) techniques. They integrated bifunctional nanocomposites based on electrochemical apta-biosensors using modified SP-IDMEs using polymeric nanocomposites (PMNCs), GOx-polydopamine (PDA), and Prussian blue (PB). Additionally, Alves et al. (2019) established a novel electrochemical immunosensor based on the immobilization of a predicted peptide (PepB$_3$) obtained from *T. gondii* membrane protein and poly modified graphite electrode (3-hydroxybenzoic acid) for the detection of mouse serum anti-*T. gondii* immunoglobulins.

Fish and shellfish

All living things may have parasites, particularly the raw one, like fish. *Anisakis* is a group of widely spread nematodes whose presence in foodborne infections caused by the ingestion of raw or undercooked seafood has acquired high social relevance. *Anisakis simplex* has been identified as a significant cause of disease in humans and as a source of foodborne allergens (Herrero, Vieites, & Espiñeira, 2011; Lopez & Pardo, 2010). Previous researchers developed a method of electromagnetic detection of parasites in the fish muscle. The use of electrical properties of the fish muscle and related parasites simplified the identification problem by moving it from complicated pattern recognition to simple current identification (Choudhury & Bublitz, 1994; Smith & Hemmingsen, 2003). Yang et al. (2013) established a promising application of UV fluorescent imagery as an efficient and flexible technique for *Anisakis* larvae identification in fishery products. From the previous study by Srisuphanunt, Saksirisampant, and Karanis (2009), they used the immunofluorescence antibody method to detect the oocysts of the *Cryptosporidium* spp. in the green mussels' population of Samut Prakan. Recently, Mutro, Georgette, Manuel, Peter, and Patrick (2020) mentioned new rapid and nanotechnology-based methods for enhanced detection in clinical and field settings that can be used to detect *Schistosoma* infection rapidly. Besides, Chinnappan et al. (2020) evolved an aptamer biosensor for the identification of significant shrimp allergens tropomyosin (TM) using graphene oxide (GO) as a screening platform for the minimal aptamer sequence needed for high-affinity target binding. *Kudoa thyrsites* is a parasite located inside fibers of the fish muscle. From the previous research by Lee, Lee, Kim, and Cho (2017), they applied a portable microscopic imaging tool to get information and detect the parasite in raw fish slices.

Fresh produce (fruits and vegetables)

Fresh produce can be explained as fruits and vegetables, which are not been appropriately processed yet. Several types of research had been conducted to analyze the role of raw vegetables in intestinal parasite transmission. The ingestion of raw vegetables and fruits are among how intestinal parasite species are transmitted to humans. *Cryptosporidium parvum* is a parasite of the zoonotic protozoan causing cryptosporidial enteritis. *Cryptosporidium* is spread to hosts via polluted water and food intake but also by direct contact with contaminated soil or infected hosts (Hong et al., 2014). The infectious phases of protozoan and helminth parasites were identified on a wide range of fresh produce globally and led to numerous epidemics and diseases. Earlier, Campbell and Mutharasan (2008) used a piezoelectric-excited millimeter cantilever biosensor for identification of *Cryptosporidium parvum* oocyst in drinking water, which was manufactured and functionalized with immunoglobulin M (IgM). Likewise, Iqbal et al. (2015) were focused on acquiring DNA aptamers that attach to the *Cryptosporidium parvum* oocyst wall and using aptamers to determine the presence of this parasite in pineapples and mango. As for sensing this parasite, the use of a gold nanoparticle-modified screen-printed carbon electrode employed a simple electrochemical sensor. Fresh produce may be contaminated with parasites from farm to consumer at any of the various stages, including the use of untreated water, application of animal or human waste to crops, or contact with contaminated farm workers or food handlers (Dixon, 2015).

Previous studies have shown that the use of lectin-magnetic separation with corresponding microscopic or molecular detection can separate *T. gondii* oocysts from concentrate water samples (Harito, Campbell, Tysnes, Dubey, & Robertson, 2017). Besides, Iqbal, Liu, Dixon, Zargar, and Sattar (2019) previously developed a DNA-aptamer-based aptasensor, coupled with magnetic beads, to detect and classify *Cryptosporidium* oocysts for tracking recreational and drinking water sources. The electrochemical aptasensor was used as a secondary ligand to attach the streptavidin-coated magnetic beads incorporated in a probe via screen-printed carbon electrodes modified in gold nanoparticles. Recently, Lalle, Possenti, Dubey, and Pozio (2018) developed a sensitive and reliable method for the identification of *T. gondii* oocysts in RTE baby lettuce based on a Loop-Mediated Isothermal Amplification-Lateral-Flow Dipstick (LAMP-LFD) assay. Additionally, Luka et al. (2019) published a label-free interdigitated capacitive biosensor for the analysis of *Cryptosporidium* oocysts in water samples. *Cryptosporidium* monoclonal antibodies (IgG3) were covalently immobilized as the capture probes on interdigital gold electrodes, and bovine serum albumin was used to prevent nonspecific adsorption.

Dairy product

Dairy products or milk products are a form of food that is made from, or that contains, mammalian milk. Dairy foods like yogurt, butter, and cheese might contain parasites if they do not undergo a proper process. In addition, animals typically often live with parasites without any apparent symptoms of illness. Raw milk is milk from any animal not pasteurized and may contain harmful germs, such as bacteria, viruses, and disease-causing parasites. *Campylobacter jejuni* is a frequent contaminant found in dairy products and is remarkably hard to separate from complex food matrix. Núñez-Carmona, Abbatangelo, and Sberveglieri (2019) recently implemented a metal oxide gas sensor to identify the presence and volatile organic compounds of *C. jejuni* in the raw milk. Besides, Núñez-Carmona et al. (2019) proposed the nanostructured metal oxide semiconductor sensors for the identification of *C. jejuni* in milk samples. Additionally, Dehghani, Hosseini, Mohammadnejad, and Ganjali (2019) discovered a novel colorimetric sensor-based aptamer for tracing *C. jejuni* DNA presence in milk samples. About 12 cytosine nucleotides were used as a scaffold for the stabilization of gold/platinum nanoclusters. Previously, Singh, Flampouri, and Dempsey (2019) established an electrochemical immunoassay to identify *Ostertagia ostertagi*, a gastrointestinal parasite nematode in infected samples. The proposed sensor exhibits fast screening techniques in a lightweight, portable format, leading to the quest for effective treatment and prevention of parasitic *O. ostertagi* diseases in cattle. Epifluorescence microscopy use of fluorescent dye to detect and visualize helminth eggs and protozoan oocysts identified in domestic animals (Marques et al., 2018). A summary of the types of parasites and methods of detection is presented in Table 4.1.

Table 4.1 Types of parasites and methods of detection.

Types of parasite	Method of detection	Limit of detection	Host	References
Eimeria	DNA receptors, glycan, aptamers, antibodies, and enzyme-linked immunosorbent assays (ELISA)	0.09 ng/mL	Beef	Vidic et al. (2017)
Leishmania	Lateral flow biosensor	100 fmol	Meat (dog)	Toubanaki et al. (2016)
Salmonella	Impedance-based microfluidic biosensor	100 CFU/mL	Meat (turkey matrix)	Liu et al. (2019)
Anisakis larvae	UV fluorescent imaging	N/S	Fish	Yang et al. (2013)
Cryptosporidium	Immunofluorescence antibody method (IFA)	N/S	Shellfish (green mussel)	Srisuphanunt et al. (2009)
Tropomyosin	Aptamer biosensor-based graphene oxide (GO) as a platform	3.3 SD/s	Shellfish (shrimp)	Chinnappan et al. (2020).
Kudoa thyrsites	A portable microscopic	N/S	Fish	Lee et al. (2017)
Toxoplasma gondii	Lectin-magnetic separation (LMS)	N/S	Water	Harito et al. (2017)
Ostertagia ostertagi	Electrochemical ELISA	N/S	Dairy product (cattle)	Singh et al. (2019).
Escherichia coli and Salmonella typhimurium	Electrochemical biosensor based on the techniques of immunomagnetic separation and electrochemical impedance spectroscopy (EIS) techniques	$2.05 \times 103\,\text{CFU}\,\text{g}^{-1}$ and $1.04 \times 103\,\text{CFU}\,\text{mL}^{-1}$	N/S	Xu et al. (2016).
Elastase (Schistosoma mansoni)	Whole-cell-based biosensors	N/S	N/S	Webb et al. (2016)
Helminth	Nucleic acid-based biosensors	1.8×10–$20\,\text{mol}\,\text{L}^{-1}$	N/S	Ullah et al. (2019)

Continued

Table 4.1 Types of parasites and methods of detection—*cont'd*

Types of parasite	Method of detection	Limit of detection	Host	References
Cryptosporidium	Lectin immobilization using a protocol of 11-mercaptoundecanoic acid by EDC-sulfo-NHS	60 cells/mL	N/S	Gavriilidou and Bridle (2018)
Taenia solium	Enzyme-linked immunosorbent assay (ELISA) and enzyme immunoelectrotransfer blot (EITB)	N/S	Pig	Lin et al. (2018)
Leishmania	Electrochemical transducer-based gold nanostructure	0.2 mol L^{-1}	N/S	Nazari-Vanani et al. (2018)
Salmonella typhimurium	Microfluidic biosensor using magnetic nanoparticles (MNPs)	100 CFU/mL	N/S	Hou et al. (2019)
Toxoplasma gondii	Electrochemical immunosensor based on immobilization of an in silico predicted peptide (PepB3)	N/S	Mouse serum	Alves et al. (2019)
Cryptosporidium oocysts	Label-free interdigitated-based capacitive biosensor	40 cells/mm^2	Water	Luka et al. (2019)
Campylobacter jejuni	Metal oxide (MOX) gas sensors	104 CFU/mL	Raw milk	Núñez-Carmona et al. (2019)
Campylobacter jejuni	Nanostructured metal oxide semiconductor (MOS) sensors	105 CFU/mL	Milk	Núñez-Carmona et al. (2019)
Campylobacter jejuni	Colorimetric DNA sensor	20 pM	Milk	Dehghani et al. (2019)
Helminth	Epifluorescence microscopy (fluorescent dye)	N/S	N/S	Marques et al. (2018)
Cryptosporidium oocysts	DNA-aptamer based aptasensor, coupled with magnetic beads	50 oocysts	pineapples and mango	Iqbal et al. (2019)
Cryptosporidium oocysts	DNA aptamers use of a gold nanoparticle-modified screen-printed carbon electrode	100 oocysts	Fresh fruit	Iqbal et al. (2015)
Toxoplasma gondii	Loop-mediated isothermal amplification-lateral-flow dipstick (LAMP-LFD) assay	100 fg	lettuce	Lalle et al. (2018)
Cryptosporidium oocysts	Label-free interdigitated-based capacitive biosensor	40 cells/mm^2	Water	Luka et al. (2019)
Cryptosporidium parvum	Piezoelectric-excited millimeter cantilever (PEMC)	N/S	Drinking water	Campbell and Mutharasan (2008)

Conclusion

For the prevention and elimination of infectious and parasitic diseases caused by the parasites in the food, successful and rapid diagnosis is essential. Biosensors are a possible driving force in resource-limited settings with increasing biomedical demands for on-site diagnostics. The recent interest in biosensor research and the progress made from published data with the prototypes suggest that the technology may have a significant effect on parasite-causing diseases. Biosensors offer the opportunity of a convenient, responsive, and cheap technology platform for parasite diseases, which can quickly identify parasites and predict successful treatment compared to traditional methods. In addition, nowadays, nano and biosensor innovations are being to improvise the diagnostic dimension. Biosensors that have been established in the research showed excellent specificity, reproducibility, and flexibility and are expected to find wide-ranging applications in the identification of foodborne pathogens.

Developing and applying systematic and validated techniques of identification for these identified FBPs will improve our awareness of their foodborne transmission routes, strengthen risk assessment, and help determine and validate critical points of control. The critical aspects of identification assays included sample preparation, parasite separation from background material, and either visualization of the parasite itself, which microscopy is often required, or identification of antigens, DNA, or other unique markers. More likely, the merging of proteomics and nanotechnology would include unique immune sensors and immune-assays to detect infection-related biomarkers. In this regard, the invention of portable point-of-care diagnostic tools to identify circulating exosomes as biomarkers, therapeutic targets, and signals of parasitic origin molecules is a feasible and significant aim in parasitology study. Integrating data from identified parasite molecules and changes observed in host immune and metabolic responses to the infection may provide extensive sensory data for accurate diagnostic and monitoring tools at the molecular level. Future approaches should concentrate on designing techniques suitable for standardization, providing for validation, and ensuring that they are available to analytical laboratories with minimal costs and time-to-outcomes.

References

Alves, L. M., Barros, H. L., Flauzino, J. M., Guedes, P. H., Pereira, J. M., Fujiwara, R. T., & Brito-Madurro, A. G. (2019). A novel peptide-based sensor platform for detection of antitoxoplasma gondii immunoglobulins. *Journal of Pharmaceutical and Biomedical Analysis, 175*, 112778–112785.

Cacciò, S. M., Chalmers, R. M., Dorny, P., & Robertson, L. J. (2018). *Foodborne parasites: Outbreaks and outbreak investigations. A meeting report from the European network for foodborne parasites (euro-FBP). Food and waterborne parasitology.* Italy: Elsevier Inc. https://doi.org/10.1016/j.fawpar.2018.01.001.

Campbell, G. A., & Mutharasan, R. (2008). Near real-time detection of Cryptosporidium parvum oocyst by IgM-functionalized piezoelectric-excited millimeter-sized cantilever biosensor. *Biosensors and Bioelectronics, 23*(7), 1039–1045. https://doi.org/10.1016/j.bios.2007.10.017.

Carboni, D., & Tully, T. N. (2009). Marsupials. In *Manual of exotic pet practice* (pp. 299–325). Canada: Elsevier Inc. https://doi.org/10.1016/B978-141600119-5.50014-7.

Cavalier-Smith, T. (2010). Kingdoms protozoa and chromista and the eozoan root of the eukaryotic tree. *Biology Letters, 6*(3), 342–345. https://doi.org/10.1098/rsbl.2009.0948.

Cédric, G., Frits, F., Silivia, M., Anamaria, C. P., Utaaker, K. S., Anet, R. J., ... Robertson, L. J. (2019). Inactivation of parasite transmission stages: Efficacy of treatments on foods of non-animal origin. *Trends in Food Science and Technology, 91*, 114–128.

Chinnappan, R., Rahamn, A. A., AlZabn, R., Kamath, S., Lopata, A. L., Abu-Salah, K. M., & Zourob, M. (2020). Aptameric biosensor for the sensitive detection of major shrimp allergen, tropomyosin. *Food Chemistry. 314*, https://doi.org/10.1016/j.foodchem.2019.126133.

Choudhury, G. S., & Bublitz, C. G. (1994). Electromagnetic method for detection of parasites in fish. *Journal of Aquatic Food Product Technology, 3*(1), 1–4. https://doi.org/10.1300/J030v03n01_06.

Cobo, F. (2014). *Imported infectious diseases: The impact in developed countries. Imported infectious diseases: The impact in developed countries*: (pp. 1–277). Spain: Elsevier Inc. https://doi.org/10.1016/C2013-0-18223-2.

Dehghani, Z., Hosseini, M., Mohammadnejad, J., & Ganjali, M. R. (2019). New colorimetric DNA sensor for detection of campylobacter jejuni in milk sample based on peroxidase-like activity of gold/platinium nanocluster. *ChemistrySelect, 4*(40), 11687–11692. https://doi.org/10.1002/slct.201901815.

Dixon, B. R. (2015). Transmission dynamics of foodborne parasites on fresh produce. In *Foodborne parasites in the food supply web* (pp. 317–353). Woodhead Publishing.

Dorny, P., Praet, N., Deckers, N., & Gabriel, S. (2009). Emerging food-borne parasites. *Veterinary Parasitology, 163*(3), 196–206. https://doi.org/10.1016/j.vetpar.2009.05.026.

Doyle, M. E. (2013). *Foodborne parasites: A review of the scientific literature*. Food Research Institute.

EFSA (2010). Opinion of the scientific panel on biological hazards on "Risk assessment of parasites in fishery products" *EFSA J, 8*(4), 1543.

Gajadhar, A. (2015). *Foodborne parasites in the food supply web: Occurrence and control. Foodborne parasites in the food supply web: Occurrence and control*: (pp. 1–454). Canada: Elsevier Inc. Retrieved from http://www.sciencedirect.com/science/book/9781782423324.

Gargouri, N., Fürst, T., Budke, C. M., Carabin, H., Kirk, M. D., Angulo, F. J., ... Sripa, B. (2015). World Health Organization estimates of the global and regional disease burden of 11 foodborne parasitic diseases, 2010: A data synthesis. *PLoS Medicine. 12*(12) https://doi.org/10.1371/journal.pmed.1001920.

Gavriilidou, D., & Bridle, H. (2018). High capture efficiency of lectin surfaces for Cryptosporidium parvum biosensors. *Biochemical Engineering Journal, 135*, 79–82. https://doi.org/10.1016/j.bej.2018.04.001.

Gottstein, B., Pozio, E., & Nöckler, K. (2009). Epidemiology, diagnosis, treatment, and control of trichinellosis. *Clinical Microbiology Reviews, 22*(1), 127–145. https://doi.org/10.1128/CMR.00026-08.

Hampl, V., Heiss, A., Hoppenrath, M., Lara, J., Gall, L., Lynn, D., ... Dunthorn, M. (2012). The revised classification of the eukaryotes. *Journal of Eukaryotic Microbiology, 59*, 429–493.

Harito, J. B., Campbell, A. T., Tysnes, K. R., Dubey, J. P., & Robertson, L. J. (2017). Lectin-magnetic separation (LMS) for isolation of Toxoplasma gondii oocysts from concentrated water samples prior to detection by microscopy or qPCR. *Water Research, 114,* 228–236. https://doi.org/10.1016/j.watres.2017.02.044.

Herrero, B., Vieites, J. M., & Espiñeira, M. (2011). Detection of anisakids in fish and seafood products by real-time PCR. *Food Control, 22*(6), 933–939. https://doi.org/10.1016/j.foodcont.2010.11.028.

Hong, S., Kim, K., Yoon, S., Park, W. Y., Sim, S., & Yu, J. R. (2014). Detection of Cryptosporidium Parvum in environmental soil and vegetables. *Journal of Korean Medical Science, 29*(10), 1367–1371. https://doi.org/10.3346/jkms.2014.29.10.1367.

Hou, Y., Cai, G., Zheng, L., & Lin, J. (2019). A microfluidic signal-off biosensor for rapid and sensitive detection of Salmonella using magnetic separation and enzymatic catalysis. *Food Control, 103,* 186–193. https://doi.org/10.1016/j.foodcont.2019.04.008.

Inbaraj, B. S., & Chen, B. H. (2016). Nanomaterial-based sensors for detection of foodborne bacterial pathogens and toxins as well as pork adulteration in meat products. *Journal of Food and Drug Analysis,* 15–28. https://doi.org/10.1016/j.jfda.2015.05.001.

Iordache, F., Gheorghe, I., Lazar, V., Curutiu, C., Ditu, L. M., Grumezescu, A. M., & Holban, A. M. (2017). Nanostructurated materials for prolonged and safe food preservation. In *Food preservation* (pp. 305–335). Academic Press.

Iqbal, A., Labib, M., Muharemagic, D., Sattar, S., Dixon, B. R., & Berezovski, M. V. (2015). Detection of Cryptosporidium parvum oocysts on fresh produce using DNA aptamers. *PLoS One. 10*(9), https://doi.org/10.1371/journal.pone.0137455.

Iqbal, A., Liu, J., Dixon, B., Zargar, B., & Sattar, S. A. (2019). Development and application of DNA-aptamer-coupled magnetic beads and aptasensors for the detection of cryptosporidium parvum oocysts in drinking and recreational water resources. *Canadian Journal of Microbiology, 65*(11), 851–857. https://doi.org/10.1139/cjm-2019-0153.

Jain, S., Costa Melo, T. G., Dolabella, S. S., & Liu, J. (2019). Current and emerging tools for detecting protozoan cysts and oocysts in water. *TrAC, Trends in Analytical Chemistry. 121,* https://doi.org/10.1016/j.trac.2019.115695.

Kamber, U., Arslan, M. ö., Gülbaz, G., Tasçi, G. T., & Akça, A. (2018). Identification of Sarcocystis spp. by polymerase chain reaction and microscopic examination in various beef products (minced meat, meatballs, fermented sausage). *Turkish Journal of Veterinary and Animal Sciences, 42*(1), 1–6. https://doi.org/10.3906/vet-1705-84.

Kumar, S., Dilbaghi, N., Barnela, M., Bhanjana, G., & Kumar, R. (2012). Biosensors as novel platforms for detection of food pathogens and allergens. *BioNanoScience, 2*(4), 196–217. https://doi.org/10.1007/s12668-012-0057-2.

Lalle, M., Possenti, A., Dubey, J. P., & Pozio, E. (2018). Loop-mediated isothermal amplification-lateral-flow dipstick (LAMP-LFD) to detect Toxoplasma gondii oocyst in ready-to-eat salad. *Food Microbiology, 70,* 137–142. https://doi.org/10.1016/j.fm.2017.10.001.

Lee, J., Lee, H., Kim, M. S., & Cho, B. (2017). Rapid detection of parasite in muscle fibers of fishes using a portable microscope imaging technique (conference presentation). *Sensing for agriculture and food quality and safety IX.* Vol. 10217. International Society for Optics and Photonics.

Levsen, A., Lunestad, B. T., & Berland, B. (2008). Parasites in farmed fish and fishery products. In *Improving farmed fish quality and safety* (pp. 428–445). Norway: Elsevier Inc. https://doi.org/10.1533/9781845694920.2.428.

Lin, X., Luo, H., Zhou, Y., Wan, N., & Wu, J. (2018). *A rapid serologic diagnosis sensor for Taenia Soliubm Cysticercosis.* AMA Publisher.

Liu, J., Jasim, I., Shen, Z., Zhao, L., Dweik, M., Zhang, S., & Almasri, M. (2019). A microfluidic based biosensor for rapid detection of *Salmonella* in food products. *PLoS ONE*, *14* (5), 1–18. https://doi.org/10.1371/journal.pone.0216873.

Lopez, I., & Pardo, M. A. (2010). Evaluation of a real-time polymerase chain reaction (PCR) assay for detection of anisakis simplex parasite as a food-borne allergen source in seafood products. *Journal of Agricultural and Food Chemistry*, *58*(3), 1469–1477. https://doi.org/10.1021/jf903492f.

Luka, G., Samiei, E., Dehghani, S., Johnson, T., Najjaran, H., & Hoorfar, M. (2019). Label-free capacitive biosensor for detection of Cryptosporidium. *Sensors (Switzerland)*. *19*(2) https://doi.org/10.3390/s19020258.

Marques, S. M. T., Barros, H. L. B., Glasenapp, R., & Stefani, V. (2018). Evaluation of benzazolic fluorescent dye for the detection of parasites diagnosed by simple flotation. *PUBVET*, *12*(4), 1–5.

Mian, H. R., Hu, G., Hewage, K., Rodriguez, M. J., & Sadiq, R. (2018). Prioritization of unregulated disinfection by-products in drinking water distribution systems for human health risk mitigation: A critical review. *Water Research*, *147*, 112–131. https://doi.org/10.1016/j.watres.2018.09.054.

Mutro, N. M., Georgette, S. -B., Manuel, B., Peter, O., & Patrick, H. (2020). Schistosomiasis: From established diagnostic assays to emerging micro/nanotechnology-based rapid field testing for clinical management and epidemiology. *Precision Nanomedicine*, 439–458. https://doi.org/10.33218/prnano3(1).191205.1.

Nazari-Vanani, R., Sattarahmady, N., Yadegari, H., Delshadi, N., Hatam, G. R., & Heli, H. (2018). Electrochemical quantitation of Leishmania infantum based on detection of its kDNA genome and transduction of non-spherical gold nanoparticles. *Analytica Chimica Acta*, *1041*, 40–49. https://doi.org/10.1016/j.aca.2018.08.036.

Nielsen, M. K., & Reinemeyer, C. R. (2018). *Handbook of equine parasite control. Handbook of equine parasite control*: (pp. 1–229). United States: Wiley. https://doi.org/10.1002/9781119382829.

Núñez-Carmona, E., Abbatangelo, M., & Sberveglieri, V. (2019). Innovative sensor approach to follow campylobacter jejuni development. *Biosensors*. *9*(1), https://doi.org/10.3390/bios9010008.

Ortega, Y. R., & Sterling, C. R. (Eds.), (2018). In *Foodborne parasites: Vol. 2*. Springer, https://doi.org/10.1007/978-3-319-67664-7.

Prakash, A., & de Jesús Ornelas-Paz, J. (2019). Irradiation of fruits and vegetables. In *Postharvest technology of perishable horticultural commodities* (pp. 563–589). Woodhead Publishing.

Robertson, L. J. (2018). Parasites in food: From a neglected position to an emerging issue. *Advances in food and nutrition research* (pp. 71–113). Vol. 86 Norway: Academic Press Inc. https://doi.org/10.1016/bs.afnr.2018.04.003.

Robertson, L., Gerard, C., Cozma-Petruţ, A., Vieira-Pinto, M., Jambrak, A. R., Rowan, N., ... Rodriguez-Lazaro, D. (2019). Inactivation of parasite transmission stages: Efficacy of treatments on food of animal origin. *Trends in Food Science and Technology*, *83*, 114–128. https://doi.org/10.1016/j.tifs.2018.11.009.

Rozycki, M., Bilska-Zajac, E., Schares, G., Mayer-Scholl, A., Trevisan, C., Tysnes, K., ... Mladineo, I. (2020). Parasite detection in food: Current status and future needs for validation. *Trends in Food Science and Technology*, *99*, 337–350. https://doi.org/10.1016/j.tifs.2020.03.011.

Saari, S., Näreaho, A., & Nikander, S. (2018). *Canine parasites and parasitic diseases. Canine parasites and parasitic diseases*: (pp. 1–287). Elsevier. Undefined, https://doi.org/10.1016/C20160052865.

Singh, B., Flampouri, E., & Dempsey, E. (2019). Electrochemical enzyme-linked immunosorbent assay (e-ELISA) for parasitic nematode: Ostertagia ostertagi (brown stomach worm) infections in dairy cattle. *Analyst, 144*(19), 5748–5754. https://doi.org/10.1039/c9an00982e.

Smith, J. W., & Hemmingsen, W. (2003). Atlantic cod *Gadus morhua* L.: Visceral organ topography and the asymetrical distribution of larval ascaridoid nematodes in the musculature. *Ophelia, 57*(3), 137–144. https://doi.org/10.1080/00785236.2003.10409510.

Srisuphanunt, M., Saksirisampant, W., & Karanis, P. (2009). Detection of cryptosporidium oocysts in green mussels (perna viridis) from shell-fish markets of Thailand. *Parasite, 16*(3), 235–239. https://doi.org/10.1051/parasite/2009163235.

Thompson, R. C. A. (2015). Foodborne, enteric, non apicomplexan unicellular parasites. In *Foodborne parasites in the food supply web: Occurrence and control* (pp. 149–164). Australia: Elsevier Inc. https://doi.org/10.1016/B978-1-78242-332-4.00007-2.

Thorp, J. H., Rogers, D. C., & Covich, A. P. (2015). Introduction to "Crustacea" *Thorp and Covich's freshwater invertebrates: Ecology and general biology* (pp. 671–686). (4th ed.). Vol. 1(pp. 671–686). United States: Elsevier Inc. https://doi.org/10.1016/B978-0-12-385026-3.00027-9.

Toubanaki, D. K., Athanasiou, E., & Karagouni, E. (2016). Gold nanoparticle-based lateral flow biosensor for rapid visual detection of Leishmania-specific DNA amplification products. *Journal of Microbiological Methods, 127*, 51–58. https://doi.org/10.1016/j.mimet.2016.05.027.

Ullah, H., Qadeer, A., Rashid, M., Rashid, M. I., & Cheng, G. (2019). Recent advances in nucleic acid-based methods for detection of helminth infections and the perspective of biosensors for future development. *Parasitology.* https://doi.org/10.1017/S0031182019001665.

Verni, M., Coda, R., & Rizzello, C. G. (2019). The use of faba bean flour to improve the nutritional and functional features of cereal-based foods: perspectives and future strategies. In *Flour and breads and their fortification in health and disease prevention* (pp. 465–475). Academic Press.

Vidic, J., Manzano, M., Chang, C. M., & Jaffrezic-Renault, N. (2017). Advanced biosensors for detection of pathogens related to livestock and poultry. *Veterinary Research. 48*(1) https://doi.org/10.1186/s13567-017-0418-5.

Wanger, A., Chavez, V., Huang, R. S. P., Wahed, A., Actor, J. K., & Dasgupta, A. (2017). *Microbiology and molecular diagnosis in pathology: A comprehensive review for board preparation, certification and clinical practice:* (pp. 1–300). United States: Elsevier Inc. Retrieved from, http://www.sciencedirect.com/science/book/9780128053515.

Webb, A. J., Kelwick, R., Doenhoff, M. J., Kylilis, N., MacDonald, J. T., Wen, K. Y., & Freemont, P. S. (2016). A protease-based biosensor for the detection of schistosome cercariae. *Scientific Reports, 6*(1), 1–14. https://doi.org/10.1038/srep24725.

Xu, M., Wang, R., & Li, Y. (2016). Rapid detection of Escherichia coli O157:H7 and Salmonella Typhimurium in foods using an electrochemical immunosensor based on screen-printed interdigitated microelectrode and immunomagnetic separation. *Talanta, 148*, 200–208. https://doi.org/10.1016/j.talanta.2015.10.082.

Yang, X., Rui, N., Hong, L., Cui, D., Sui, J., & Cao, L. (2013). Detection of anisakid larvae in cod fillets by uv fluorescent imaging based on principal component analysis and gray value analysis. *Journal of Food Protection, 76*(7), 1288–1292. https://doi.org/10.4315/0362-028X.JFP-12-471.

Yunus, G. (2018). Biosensors: An enzyme-based biophysical technique for the detection of foodborne pathogens. In *Enzymes in food biotechnology: Production, applications, and future prospects* (pp. 723–738). Saudi Arabia: Elsevier. https://doi.org/10.1016/B978-0-12-813280-7.00042-6.

Classification and application of nanomaterials for foodborne pathogens analysis

Introduction

Nowadays, the demand for customer-free food increases as the awareness of public health grows. Foodborne pathogens are commonly caused by pathogens, including *Escherichia coli*, *Salmonella enterica*, *Campylobacter jejuni*, *Listeria monocytogenes*, *Bacillus cereus*, and *Shigella* (Muniandy et al., 2019). Salmonellosis and campylobacteriosis are the most frequently reported as foodborne pathogens in the world. WHO (2015) recorded an overall median percentage of foodborne diseases, and deaths are due to *Campylobacter* spp. (16% and 5%) and *Salmonella spp.* (13% and 14%) were higher compared to other pathogens. *S. enterica* and *C. jejuni* that found in the gut content or skin of birds and might be carried inside the meat as vehicle transmission exits (Furukawa et al., 2016). Pathogen surveillance has a major impact on public health, which is important to prevent and monitor the presence of foodborne pathogens in food products. Hence, various techniques have been developed to monitor and maintain the quality and safety of food products since high market on poultry consumption (King, Osmond-McLeod, & Duffy, 2018). The development of advanced nanotechnology-based nanomaterials has demonstrated a full range of applications that shows rapid and stable for the identification of foodborne pathogens. Alternatively, reliable interfaces focusing on functional nanomaterials and bioactive molecules such as nanoparticles, metal oxides, carbon-based nanomaterials, polymer-conductive, and heme proteins have been thoroughly studied for the advancement of nanotechnology (Potonik, 2010)

Nanomaterials

In this era, the technology-based biosensor is well recognized as the fast detection of diverse types of the target analyte. Nonetheless, there are still a few difficulties that need to overcome related to the specificity, sensitivity, and detection period. Thus, the inclusion of nanomaterials in biosensors provides an alternative strategy due to the unique optical, hydraulic, catalytic, electrical, and thermal properties of nanomaterials which originate from the surface area and quantum coefficient (Alhamoud

Advanced Food Analysis Tools. https://doi.org/10.1016/B978-0-12-820591-4.00005-0

et al., 2019; Lv et al., 2018). Nanomaterials are classified into nine major groups, which are metal-based nanomaterials, ceramic nanomaterials, semiconductor-based nanomaterials (quantum dots), carbon-based/organic nanomaterials, organic-inorganic hybrid nanomaterials, silica-based nanomaterials, polymeric nanomaterials and nanoconjugates, biological nanomaterials, and self-assembled/biologically directed materials. The classification is based on their shape, size, composition, surface charge, aggregation, and chemical nature (Ball, Patil, & Soni, 2019).

Carbon-based nanomaterials

Carbon nanomaterials comprising carbon nanotubes (CNTs), graphene (Gr), carbon nanofibers (CNFs), graphene quantum dots, and fullerene have been used frequently in a variety of applications due to their magnificent properties (Li, Wang, Li, Feng, & Feng, 2019)

Carbon nanotubes (CNTs)

Recently, CNTs offer desirable and promising materials due to high electrical conductivity, biocompatibility, high mechanical strength, high surface-to-volume ratio, and chemical stability, which make them good candidates for applications in analytical science, biomedical sciences, and energy equipment (Zhang, Zhang, & Wei, 2017). CNTs are known as one-dimensional (1D) carbon nanomaterials that rolled-up sheets of graphene, which divided into single-walled CNTs (SWCNTs) and multiwalled CNTs (MWCNTs) (Lawal, 2016; Zeng, Zhu, Du, & Lin, 2016). It is referred to as the hollow cylindrical tubes formed by "rolled" up single or multiple graphene sheets, which consists of the sp^2 hybridized carbon atoms in crystal honeycomb lattice structure (Ramnani, Saucedo, & Mulchandani, 2016). The feature of CNTs is the transduction of physicochemical interactions that involve a large surface area that is efficient in identifying small amounts of target analytes (Yang, Chen, Ren, Zhang, & Yang, 2015). In electrochemical biosensors, the modification of the CNT surface is broadly utilized to immobilize the working electrode on a solid support surface to improve sensing performance. Besides, CNTs have also been blended with optical biosensors due to their function as a quencher for different types of fluorophores, resulting in a less framework and show constant signal-to-noise ratio (Xue, Zhang, et al., 2019).

SWCNTs are formed when a single graphene sheet is smoothly wrapped in a cylinder tube with a diameter of approximately 0.4–2 nm and a length of 1–100 μm. The size depends on the synthesizing method (Klumpp, Kostarelos, Prato, & Bianco, 2006; Ramnani et al., 2016). The structure can also be removed by several arrangements, such as an armchair, zigzag and chiral tubes (Danailov, Keblinski, Nayak, & Ajayan, 2002) that are useful for bioconjunction and adequate drug loading capacity due to the presence of ultra-high surface area. MWCNTs formed when multiple graphene sheets were rolled into a cylinder tube with two categories; (i) parchment-like structure and (ii) concentric structure. MWCNTs also comprise an outer and inner diameter of 2–100 nm and 1–3 nm, respectively. The outer nanotube has a larger diameter than the inner nanotube with a length of one to several microns

(Madani, Naderi, Dissanayake, Tan, & Seifalian, 2011; Vaibhav et al., 2014). The structure is less flexible and more defective as a dislocated electron cloud along the generated wall, which is essential for the interaction of adjacent cylindrical layers in MWCNTs (Xia, Guduru, & Curtin, 2007). The parchment-like structure formed by enveloping multiple times a single graphene sheet, while the concentric structure formed by the Russian Doll model, which includes extra nanotube inside the CNT (Eatemadi et al., 2014). The multilayer nature of MWCNTs protects internal CNTs from chemical interactions with external substances, so that their tensile strength is high, which is not present in SWCNTs (Vander Wal, Berger, & Ticich, 2003).

Generally, CNTs have higher tensile strength compare to steel and copper due to their carbon-carbon sp^2 bonding that enables them to twist, bend, buckle, and kink without damage and return to their original shape when exposed to a tremendous axial compressive force. However, there is an elasticity limit when nanotube deformation occurs when the limit is exceeded (Hone, 2004; Eatemadi et al., 2014). Wong, Sheehan, and Lieber (1997) stated that the mechanical properties of MWCNTs were smaller compared to silicon carbide nanotubes. Besides, Yu, Files, Arepalli, and Ruoff (2000) found that SWCNT's mechanical properties in the ropes as load-bearing elements support the theoretical prediction that SWCNT's will have high Young's modulus and break strength values. For thermal conductivity, SWCNTs have a high thermal conductivity of 6600 $Wm^{-1}K^{-1}$ along their long axis of nanotube at room temperature, while MWCNTs recorded 3000 $Wm^{-1}K^{-1}$ using a suspended microdevice (Berber, Kwon, & Tománek, 2000; Kim, Shi, Majumdar, & McEuen, 2001). The thermal conductivity of MWCNTs increases as the number of atomic walls present in MWCNTs decreases due to its interaction of phonons and electrons between MWCNTs (Fujii et al., 2005). Thus, the high thermal conductivity of CNTs is useful to the application of microelectromechanical systems and nanoelectromechanical systems designs. Subsequently, the electrical transport mechanism through the CNTs useful in nanoscale electronic devices application, for example, CNT field-effect transistors and diodes. CNTs are capable of discharging powerful electrical waves under specific conditions that have both metallic and semiconductor properties, depending on their chiral indices. Chirality in CNTs is referred to as the degree of twisted graphene sheet that will determine conductivity in nanotubes (Kaushik & Majumder, 2015). The multilayer nature of MWCNT's internal-wall interaction affects its electrical conductivity, which has been observed for nonuniform distribution of current through individual nanotubes (Kaushik & Majumder, 2015).

Graphene (Gr)

Graphene (Gr) has been identified as a two-dimensional (2D) crystal honeycomb lattice monolayer of carbon atoms with more energetic mechanical and thermal features as well as electrical conductivity compared to CNTs (Lan, Yao, Ping, & Ying, 2017). Each presence of carbon atoms in graphene is covalently bound to three other carbon atoms with an sp^2 hybridization mechanism. The sp^2 hybridized carbon atomic layers are held together by weak Van der Waals forces with a length of 0.142 nm

(Warner, Schaffel, Rummeli, & Bachmatiuk, 2012). The honeycomb lattice structure is the basic building block for other carbon allotropes such as graphite, CNT, and fullerene. The three-dimensional (3D) graphite consists of graphene layer stacking. Rolled-up graphene cylinders are forming 1D CNTs. Furthermore, zero-dimension fullerence (C60) is a molecule consisting of graphene wrapped (Neto, Guinea, Peres, Novoselov, & Geim, 2009). Gr and its derivatives are referred to as graphene oxide (GO), and reduced GO (rGO) are extraordinarily biocompatible and well-received nanomaterials for biosensor advancements. Gr is useful in electrochemical and optical biosensors as it has a higher surface-to-volume ratio and a greater π stacking interaction between the hexagonal Gr honeycomb lattice and the biomolecular cyclic carbon structures. As such, they are commonly used as alternatives to improve the adsorbability of biomolecules (Sun et al., 2019). Besides, Gr acts as a fluorescent emission and serves as an energy-acceptor (quencher) for optical fluorescent biosensors. It exhibits useful nanomaterials in fluorescent biosensors, as it plays the roles of both energy acceptors and donors. However, adsorption and Gr and GO desorption efficiencies are higher than CNTs, resulting in a higher ratio of signal-to-background detection (Alibolandi, Hadizadeh, Vajhedin, Abnous, & Ramezani, 2015; Liu, Dong, & Chen, 2012). A distinctive feature of Gr is its nanomaterial composition to enhance the biosensing properties, particularly nanoparticles from metal oxides (Mohammadian & Faridbod, 2018).

Moreover, Gr exhibited several properties in the electronic, chemical, mechanical, thermal, and optical aspects. It has high the electronic properties of the graphene are strongly dependent on the presence of the graphene layer. Single-layer graphene and bilayer graphene are the only single type of electrons and holes present as zero-gap semiconductors. Their conduction and valence bands began to overlap and to be touched at the points of Dirac. The linear dispersion showed by the graphene at this point, and its state of electronic density is zero. Several charge carriers appearing to be massless will have an impact on the inherent mobility of the carrier. Hence, in the application of electronics, graphene is developed as suitable materials with its sensitivity to both electron-donating and electron-removing molecules (Warner et al., 2012). Additionally, the chemical aspect of pure graphene sheets is generally not reactive to other issues. Chen, Shu, Li, Xu, and Hu (2018) stated that graphene is a relatively chemical inert that can withstand hydrogen peroxide and prevent oxidation of metals. The functionalization cycle is performed to reactivate the reactive graphene by adding reactive species such as hydroxyl, bromine, carboxyl, and amino to covalently bind to the graphene surface (H. He & Gao, 2010).

Sharma, Baik, Perera, and Strano (2010) reported that single-layer graphene is more reactive compared to bi- or multilayer graphene through determining the related disorder (D) peak in Raman spectroscopy. Apart from that, the chemical bond strength of graphene mainly attributes to its physical and mechanical properties. According to Zhao and Aluru (2010), the chemical bond of C-C in sp^2 hybrid carbon materials, such as graphene, is stable compared to other materials. Lee, Wei, Kysar, and Hone (2008) also reported that graphene is the most robust nano-identified material with 130 GPa tensile strength, where the single-layer graphene had 1 TPa Young modulus with a breaking strength 200 times higher than that of steel. Zhao and Aluru (2010) found that the mechanical properties of graphene sheets depend heavily on temperature and strain rate despite stimulation. As a result of this increase, the surrounding temperature will result in a decrease in fracture strength and fracture strain. Graphene is thus a lighter and more durable substance accessible to specific research areas (Zhu et al., 2010).

Heat conductivity in carbon materials is regulated by the transportation of phonons, which can be transported by diffusive conduction at high temperatures and ballistic conduction at low temperatures (Zhu et al., 2010). Owing to its relatively low carrier density of undoped graphene, the electronic contribution to thermal conductivity in graphene would be negligible. Mechanically cleaved graphene thermal conductivity is more significant than natural diamonds, multiple walls, and SWCNTs. Gr also presented high thermal properties that permitted the development of devices such as thermal biosensors (Balandin et al., 2008; Cai et al., 2010; Kim et al., 2001). The narrowband structure, zero bandgaps, and intense interaction with electromagnetic radiation between Dirac Fermions account for the optical properties in graphene. Inter-band and intra-band optical transitions enable graphene to be absorbed across a wide range of the spectrum. The optical graphene response from the visible to the near-infrared region is due to interband transitions, which is independent of the wavelength. Although graphene is absorbed in the far-infrared region, intra-band transitions are modeled (Fai, Lui, Misewich, & Heinz, 2008; Gierz et al., 2013). Gr also exhibits high fluorescence quenching capability for a number of dyes and quantum dots resulting from the transfer of energy or electrons from dyes to graphene (Chang, Tang, Wang, Jiang, & Li, 2010).

Carbon quantum dots (CQDs)

Carbon quantum dots (CQDs) or carbon dots (CDs) or carbon nanoparticles (CNPs) are evolving nanomaterials of small size (<10 nm), quasi-spherical morphology, with substantial benefits including chemical inertness, low toxicity, inexpensive, secure processing, high yield, adjustable fluorescence, photobleaching resistance, and good water solubility. Because of their chemical and electrochemical fluorescence, they are commonly used as electron acceptors or as electron donors in analytical sensors (Yao, Huang, Liu, & Kang, 2019).

Metal nanomaterials

Nobel metal nanomaterials have been widely used in the design of biosensors due to unique chemical, physical, and optoelectronic characteristics relevant to their shape, size, composition, and structure (Mahmoudpour et al., 2019). Several metal nanoparticles are popular in biosensors such as gold nanoparticles, silver nanoparticles, and platinum nanoparticles that display excellent biocompatibility with biomolecules, chemical stability, accessible to synthesis, and modify (Holzinger, Goff, & Cosnier, 2014; Malekzad, Sahandi Zangabad, Mirshekari, Karimi, & Hamblin, 2017). For example, the colorimetric sensor is widely incorporated with nanoparticles, particularly gold nanoparticles, since it has unique properties of surface plasmon resonance (SPR) along with elastic light-scattering properties resulting in a change in wavelength and color (Xue, Zhang, et al., 2019). The optical properties of metal nanoparticles are dependent on their particle size and distance (Bülbül, Hayat, & Andreescu, 2015). Several nanomaterials displayed unique enzyme properties, called "nanozymes," which that overcome the inherent limitations of natural enzymes that have been expected to suffer from various environmental factors. Furthermore, compared to natural enzymes, artificial enzymes have significant advantages, like improved design versatility, high efficiency, and specificity of the substrate, mainly their excellent stability—scientists struggling to establish successful mimetic enzymes based on colorimetric approaches for biosensing.

Numerous colorimetric sensors were developed by transforming a colorless substrate into a colored substance in the presence of hydrogen peroxide, based on the peroxidase-like activity of some nanozymes (Chen et al., 2018; Zhang, Tian, Huang, & Wu, 2020). For example, Ray, Biswas, Banerjee, and Biswas (2020) synthesized highly dispersed aggregation-free gold nanoparticles intercalated into the walls of mesoporous silica using nanozymes (thioether-functionalized silica) that demonstrated enhanced the peroxidase mimic performance for the determination of dopamine. Similarly, (Swaidan et al., 2020) synthesized CuS-BSA-Cu$_3$(PO4)$_2$ nanoparticles as organic-inorganic hybrid nanoscale materials via biomineralization for monitoring the presence of glucose and hydrogen peroxide. The artificial colorimetric probes nanozyme displayed excellent stability and biocompatibility. Furthermore, metal nanomaterials have also been regularly utilized for designing electrochemical biosensors because of their high electron transfer capability and because they provide more absorption sites to improve the immobilization cycle (Lan et al., 2017). Metal nanomaterial is conveniently placed on the electron surface to improve electron transfer and synergistic sensitization (Yu et al., 2013). Safoura, Hamideh, Hossein, and Soheila (2020) established an electrochemical biosensor for the detection of a particular sequence of DNA based on MWCNTs, chitosan, and gold nanoparticles modified glass carbon electrode. The proposed sensing provides simple, stable, high selectivity, and responsiveness for the future in electrochemical DNA biosensors.

Magnetic nanoparticles

Magnetic nanoparticles (magnetic beads) are one of the nanomaterials that are suitable for the isolation and detection of targeted pathogens from complex matrices, resulting in a highly efficient detection system (Liu et al., 2016). The modification of magnetic nanoparticles into nanometers (<100 μm to <100 nm) can improve the adsorptive region that can be directly incorporated into the transducer materials to attract target analytes after exposure to the external magnetic field (Lan et al., 2017; Majdinasab, Hayat, & Marty, 2018). This also provides a higher surface area for the detection of analytes resulting in improved signal response. Besides, nanoparticles can be combined with different recognition components, resulting in a reduction in background signals and an improvement in detection sensitivity in the biosensor system (Xu, Akakuru, Zheng, & Wu, 2019). Recently, Zou et al. (2019)

developed Fe_3O_4 nanoparticle cluster biosensor based on nuclear magnetic resonance with correctly recognized *Salmonella* at different sites in milk samples. Chattopadhyay, Sabharwal, Jain, Kaur, and Singh (2019) successfully capturing and separation of *S. typhimurium* on functionalized polymeric magnetic nanoparticles-based SERS immunosensor strategy. The proposed immunosensor demonstrated more sensitive and precise pathogen detection, which has a strong potential to be used to detect contamination in food sample analysis. Similarly, Guo et al. (2019) developed a portable biosensor-based magnetic nanoparticle immunoseparation, nanocluster signal amplification, and smartphone image analysis for detection of *S. typhimurium* in chickens. The sensor provides a simple, compact, and economic system for the detection of *S. typhimurium* in food and has the potential to be extended for the screening of foodborne pathogens by varying the antibodies.

Quantum dots (QDs)

Quantum dots (QDs) are described as relatively 3D spherical nanomaterials and semiconductor nanoscale colloidal particles with significant quantum effects from Bohr radii. The size of QDs is between 1-10 nm and originated from quantum confinement results in some unique optical and electronic properties (Stanisavljevic, Krizkova, Vaculovicova, Kizek, & Adam, 2015; Xue, Wang, Jeong, & Yan, 2019). QDS as new materials and commonly used in many areas due to their characteristics of tunable photoluminescent, high quantum performance, high absorption, excellent photobleaching resistance. The significant interest of QDs in the production of biosensors compared to traditional fluorescent materials is their size-tunable optical characteristics along with the emission spectrum that allows the identification of various analytes by using different sizes of QDs. Also, the brightness of QDs is enhanced, and photo-bleaching resistance is better compared to natural dyes, which dramatically increases the efficiency and consistency of the recognition process. Several QDs may be stimulated by a single wavelength owing to the broad absorption and narrow emission range. The modification is simple by employing various biorecognition elements to create QD-labeled probes. Moreover, QDs frequently applied as the chemiluminescent emitters and fluorescent labels to produce different forms of chemiluminescent and fluorescent biosensors. For example, Xue et al. (2020) designed an advancement of nanomaterials by combining quantum dots, immunomagnetic nanobeads, and manganese dioxide nanoflowers for simultaneous detection of *E. coli* and *S. typhimurium* in the chicken sample with satisfactory recovery values. The sensor has the potential to be combined with microfluidics for miniaturized, automated, and smart detection of various target pathogens.

Upconversion nanoparticles (UCNPs)

Recently, the advanced type of fluorescent nanomaterials has been implemented known as upconversion nanoparticles (UCNPs) with specific physicochemical features. The new nanoparticles can convert lower energy (near-infrared radiation) into higher energy (visible radiation) or fluorescent labeling in the construction of biosensors (Wang, Abbineni, Clevenger, Mao, & Xu, 2011). Also, UCNPs engaged in high sensitivity to photobleaching and photoblinking, a major Stokes shift, constant energy level, and long lifespan. UCNPs display high color purity, multicolor tunable, less toxicity, low background fluorescence, good emission bands, and chemical stability (Wu et al., 2015). UCNPs able couple with several recognition components and used as fluorescent probes in optical biosensors for pathogen detection.

Synthesis method
Graphene

Several methods for synthesizing graphene have been developed, such as mechanical exfoliation, chemical exfoliation, chemical synthesis, and thermal CVD. Mechanical exfoliation is a top-down technique applied in nanotechnology by producing longitudinal or transverse stress on the surface of the layered structural materials and by using a simple scotch tape or Atomic Force Microscopy (AFM) tip to slice a single or a few layers down onto a substrate (Choi & Lee, 2011). Different thicknesses of graphene sheets can be obtained by mechanical exfoliation by slice down layers from graphic materials onto SiO2 or Si substratum using scotch tape applied with mechanical force. The high-quality graphene was obtained easily by using mechanically exfoliated scotch-tape (Novoselov et al., 2004). However, the mechanical exfoliation method can produce high-quality graphene with the least defects, but it is limiting the production of graphene with thickness about 10nm. During deposition to a substrate, the pressure on the graphene layer may also be caused, and different forms of defects can occur, such as atomic defects (Choi et al., 2011). Defects may harm the electronic properties of graphene as a translational or rotational symmetry in a graphene break.

Chemical exfoliation is the process of isolating a few graphene layers that dispersed alkali metals in a solution interspersed with the graphite structure. The first chemical graphene is exfoliated by the use of potassium as an alkali metal intercalating agent that leads to the generation of hydrogen and help the separation of graphite layers for further purification (Viculis, Mack, & Kaner, 2003; Viculis, Mack, Mayer, Hahn, & Kaner, 2005). Alloy metals react more violently with graphite compared to potassium and allow graphene to be produced at low ambient temperatures. Boland et al. (2008) stated that graphite exfoliation is a mild sonication process in polar organic solvents such as N-methyl-pyrrolidone. Micron-sized single or small-layer graphene sheets are obtained, and this process enables scale-up production in nanotechnology equipment applications. Furthermore, Gr can also be chemically synthesized by reducing GO, an indirect top-down synthesis approach. This method involves graphite oxide synthesis by graphite oxidation followed by sonication to disperse the flakes and reduce them to graphene again (Choi & Lee, 2011). The graphite oxide is prepared in the (Stankovich et al., 2007) studies using the Hummers process, which involved acid treatment with potassium permanganate (KMnO4) and concentrated sulfuric acid (H2SO4) and is then chemically modified to form the water-dispersible graphite oxide. The polar oxygen functional groups formed through acid treatment, such as carbonyl and hydroxyl, make the graphite oxide hydrophilic (Paredes, Villar-Rodil, Martínez-Alonso, & Tascón, 2008). After mild sonication, the water-dispersible graphite oxide sheets were produced. Graphite oxide sheets can be reduced back to graphene by chemical reduction by adding reduction agents (Stankovich et al., 2007), heat treatment thermal reduction (Aksay et al., 2007) or electrochemical reduction involving immobilization of graphite oxide on the surface of the electrode (Zhou et al., 2009).

Chemical vapor deposition (CVD) is a chemical process for the synthesis of high-quality thin graphene films by the activation of gaseous reactants following a subsequent chemical reaction and the resulting decomposition of stable graphene over the substrate (Muñoz & Gómez-Aleixandre, 2013). The metal substrates used in CVD serve as a catalyst to help lower the energy barrier and ensure that the graphene deposition process is successful (Warner et al., 2012). There are two types of CVD, namely, thermal CVD and plasma CVD. The thermal CVD method refers to low carbon solubility in metal as the presence of weak interaction between graphene and transition metals such as copper (Cu). The high carbon solubility in metal is strong when graphene interaction with transition metals such as nickel (Ni) is strong (Pushpendra et al., 2013). The Cu transition metal is more favored than Ni because it is capable of increasing large areas on Cu foil using methane as a precursor and producing high quality, uniform, thick graphene film (Muñoz & Gómez-Aleixandre, 2013). The plasma-enhanced CVD approach is referred to as the thermal CVD process involving the creation of plasma in a vacuum chamber and contributes to the deposition of thin graphene film on the surface of the substrate (Choi & Lee, 2011). This method allows thin graphene film to be deposited at a lower temperature as opposed to thermal CVD and ideal for industrial production.

Gr can also be synthesized on a single crystalline silicon carbide (SiC) surface employing the epitaxial thermal growth. The process involved the Si atoms, which, when annealed at high temperatures, would desorb selectivity from a surface, while the carbon left behind will eventually form the graphene of few layers. For example, De Heer et al. (2004) obtained 1-3 mono-atomic graphene layers by processing ultrathin graphite on silicone-terminated (0001) 6H-SiC single-crystal surfaces. Graphene can also grow on 4H-SiC single-cristal faces with carbon-terminated (000-1) faces. Epitaxial graphene grown on the SiC surface showed a long period of consistency and revealed high mobility of more than 500cm2/Vs (Conrad et al., 2006). It is also a practical and flexible approach to the application of electronic devices.

Carbon nanotubes

There are many methods used to produce SWCNTs and MWCNTs, such as arc discharge, laser ablation, and CVD. Arc discharge process involved the use of nanotubes to synthesize high temperatures above 1700°C. There are two graphite electrodes mounted at low pressure between 50 and 10 mbar in a sealed chamber with inert gas, for example, helium or argon filled. Two electrodes are held apart for a short time, which is around 1 mm to 2 mm during arching with various potentials. High-temperature discharge vaporizes the surface of anode electrodes, and the thin rod-shaped electrode collects on the cathode. The nanotubes depositing on the cathode electrode can be collected after the de-pressurization and cooling cycle (Mathur, 2016). This technique enables a high yield of approximately 90% in the production of SWCNTs and MWCNTs with controllable dimensions of the nanotubes produced (Prasek et al., 2011). SWCNTs can be synthesized using precursor catalysts, but without them, MWCNTs cannot be synthesized (Pandey & Dahiya, 2016). High yields of SWCNTs with an average diameter of 1–4 nm are obtained by the use of Ni-Y-graphite mixtures (Eatemadi et al., 2014).

The laser ablation method is very similar to the arc discharge method, which used high-temperature precursors and catalyst precursors filled with inert gas. This method included a sealed quartz tube composed of a pure graphite block by using high-power laser vaporization and heated $1200 \pm °$ C in a furnace with an atmosphere of inert argon (Eatemadi et al., 2014). The use of powerful laser pulses will synthesize the MWCNTs and reduce the carbon target. Nevertheless, the synthesis of the SWCNTs includes the addition of catalysts such as iron, yttrium, sulfur nickel, and molybdenum. Besides, SWCNTs with a uniform diameter and self-assembly into ropes could be produced by dual pulsed laser vaporization. Two consecutive laser pulses are used in this process to reduce the volume of carbon accumulated as soot. The first laser pulse eliminates the carbon mixture followed by the separation of larger ablated particles by second laser pulses and has gradually developed into structures of nanotubes (Awasthi et al., 2006).

CVD method is useful for large-scale processing of CNTs that will decompose at elevated temperature, and hydrocarbon vapors move through a tubular reactor with the presence of transition metal catalysts (iron and nickel). The metal catalyst gradually sat on the substrate and formed into a nanotube structure (Mathur, 2016). The CVD methods involved two underlying mechanisms for the development of nanotubes. For the tip growth model, the catalytic particle site is at the top of the growing nanotube when the substrate-catalyst interaction is weak. However, the primary growth model that the catalytic particle remains on the growth substrate, and its interaction with substrate-catalyst is sustainable (Baker, 1989). The size of the catalyst particle is an account of the formation of SWCNTs and MWCNTs. SWCNTs will be formed when the catalyst particle is small in size, while a few ten nanometres will result in the formation of MWCNTs (Koziol, Boskovic, & Yahya, 2010).

Nanotechnology biosensors in the detection of foodborne pathogens

Aptamer-based nanosensors

Aptamers referred to the short sequences of oligonucleotides or peptides that are directly synthesized to bind with the target bacterial and are used as biosensor recognition components. Aptamers are synthesized by exponential enrichment (SELEX) in vitro artificial processes via the systematic evolution of the ligands

(Mustafa, Hassan, & Andreescu, 2017). Moreover, Lian, He, Wang, and Tong (2015) integrated an aptamer with Gr through the π-π stacking interaction-based piezoelectric sensor to identify *S. aureus*. The aptamers detach from the graphene surface and bind to the target *S. aureus* result in a change in oscillator frequency. Moreover, Abbaspour, Norouz-Sarvestani, Noori, and Soltani (2015) developed a combination of nanoparticle-based aptasensor with immunomagnetic separation and electrochemical detection using a dual aptamer method. The sensor consists of biotinylated primary aptamers attached to streptavidin-modified magnetic beads and secondary aptamers conjugated with silver nanoparticles for signal quantification. When a sample containing the target, bacteria are attached to aptamer-magnetic beads accompanied by attaching aptamer-AgNPs to the bacteria-carrying magnetic beads. The external magnetic field is then used to separate them, and the electrochemical signal is calculated using voltammetry with differential pulse stripping.

Immuno-based nanosensor

Immuno-based nanosensor uses similar concepts to traditional immunosorbent enzyme-linked (ELISA) assay. AuNPs nanosensing systems are designed to integrate with antibodies, and the identification of pathogens can be confirmed by plasmon resonance (SPR) or color changes when binding target bacteria. The SPR-based immunosensor for the detection of *E. coli* and Lactobacillus fermentium has developed, according to Baccar et al. (2010). Specific antibodies for both bacteria over AuNPs are immobilized using the 16-mercaptoundecanoic acid and carbodiimide coupling between the gold surface acid group and the amine residue. Li, Cao, Han, and Sim (2009) published a colorimetric AuNPs-based immunosensor assay to detect Giardia lamblia cysts with antibodies-functionalized NP probes. The bounded immunoprobes on the Giardia lamblia cysts surface result in changes in color. According to Sapna (2012), *Salmonella* is detected using a nanobiosenser that integrates CNTs. This procedure involved the covalent attachment of high CNT surface area with *Salmonella* monoclonal antibodies by using diimide-activated imitation as the method of binding and immobilization onto a glassy carbon electrode. The sensing mechanism for bacteria or pathogen detection is calculated as the dynamic formation of antigen-antibody by the changes in charge-transfer resistance and impedance.

Electrochemical biosensor

The electrochemical approach used is a distinctive feature of a biosensor with electrochemical functions. Besides the electrochemical process, the sample handling method and the sensor signal read-out format both provide differentiated characteristics of a pathogen recognition system based on a biosensor (Riu & Giussani, 2020). Various electrochemical methods can be performed using functionalized electrodes to enable pathogen detection. These methods differ in electrode configuration, applied signals, measured signals, mass transport regimes, binding information provided (Thévenot, Toth, Durst, & Wilson, 2001), and target size-selectivity (Amiri, Bezaatpour, Jafari, Boukherroub, & Szunerits, 2018). Electrochemical methods used for pathogen detection can be classified as potentiometric, amperometric, conductometric, impedimetric, or ion-charge/field-effect, which often signify the measured time-varying, quantitative signal (Thévenot et al., 2001).

Hai et al. (2017) applied potentiometry with a conductive polymer-based sensor to identify the presence of the human influenza A virus (H1N1) in a blood sample. Also, Singh, Hong, and Jang (2017) using a reduced GO-based electrode and chronoamperometry for the detection of H1N1. Iqbal et al. (2015) developed an electrochemical sensor-based AuNP-modified carbon electrodes for the detection of *C. parvum* in samples taken from the fruit. Bhardwaj, Devarakonda, Kumar, and Jang (2017) used DPV with a carbon-based electrode to detect *S. aureus*. Also, Mannoor et al. (2012) used a previously described conductometric biosensor to detect *S. aureus* and *Helicobacter pylori* on tooth enamel. Yoo et al. (2017) used a conductometric biosensor with CNT-based electrodes for the detection of *B. subtilis*. Hernández et al. (2014) used potentiometry to detect *S. aureus* with a carbon-rod electrode modified with reduced GO. Lee and Jun (2016) utilized wire-based electrodes for amperometric detection of *E. coli* and *S. aureus*. Boehm, Gottlieb, and Hua (2007) detected *E. coli* via potentiometry, utilizing a platinum wire as a working electrode. Similarly, He, Wu, Yin, and Zhang (2012) used FETs based on PEDOT: PSS organic electrochemical transistor electrodes for the detection of *E. coli* using Pt and Ag/AgCl gate electrodes. Meanwhile, Wu, Meyyappan, and Lai (2016) used a graphene-based FET to detect *E. coli* in nutrient broth diluted with phosphate-buffered saline solution with amperometry using an Ag/AgCl gate electrode. Moreover, Kim et al. (2012) successfully developed a light electrode-based sensor for the detection of DNA. Subramanian et al. (2012) developed CNTFET arrays to detect *E. coli*. In the field-effect transistors (FET)-type biosensor, graphene transferred onto a substrate, then the metal contacts are patterned by using electron beam lithography or photolithography (He, Zhang, et al., 2012). However, for CNTs-based FET fabrication, the metals electrodes are patterned onto a substrate, followed by bridging of the electrode gap with CNTs (S. N. Kim, Rusling, & Papadimitrakopoulos, 2007).

CNT-based gas sensors

Typically, the gas sensors have mainly used in the detection of the safeness and quality control of food products in the food industry. Incorporation of the carbon nanotechnology with a gas sensor has improved the efficiency of pathogen detection, which can be done in a short time and fast response. According to (Kong et al., 2000), there is a change in the conductivity of a single semiconducting SWCNT when exposed to ammonia. The resistance response of CNTs on adsorption of gas can be quantified by using field emit transistor (FET). The high surface area of CNTs enables the sensor to give a fast response, which less than 1 minute to complete the detection. Huang, Huang, Jang, Tsai, and Yeh (2005) again proven that nitrogen gas is detected by using a three-terminal device based on MWCNTs. There are two metal electrodes placed on the vertical alignment of MWCNTs film, which deposit on the substrate of Si/SiO$_2$ and the silicon substrate as the back gate. Also, Suehiro, Ikeda, Ohtsubo, and Imasaka (2009), a Bio-MEMS (microelectromechanical systems)-type device has developed for the detection of bacteria by using a CNT gas sensor coupled with a microheater. This method involved the heating of bacteria by microheater in the air and led to ammonia gas formation by the reaction of oxidation in bacterial organic components. The detection technique used in this method is dielectrophoretic impedance measurement (DEPM), which the positive dielectrophoretic force utilizes to trap the *E. coli*.

Conclusion and future perspectives

Nanomaterial-based sensors require binding or reaction of biological components with specific organisms and gradually converting them into measurable signals, thus allowing fast identification of food contaminants in food products. Indeed, carbon nanomaterials are a valuable tool for the diagnosis of foodborne pathogens due to the excellent mechanical, electrical, chemical, and desired properties of carbon nanomaterials described in previous sections. Carbon nanomaterials are integrated into detection systems that are ideal for rapid screening and detection. Nevertheless, there is still a challenge to make them an off-the-shelf tool that can be commercially available for regular and environmentally friendly use like interference in real-sample analysis, reproducibility, and nanomaterial toxicity. As the development in nanotechnology is currently possible, a simplified process for the manufacture and assembly in new sensors can be created. Nonetheless, the critical problems in pathogen sensor systems are reliability, repeatability, longevity, and ease of operation. Further focus and motivation must also be put on a better fundamental understanding of carbon nanomaterials and their practical application in the biosensor.

References

Abbaspour, A., Norouz-Sarvestani, F., Noori, A., & Soltani, N. (2015). Aptamer-conjugated silver nanoparticles for electrochemical dual-aptamer-based sandwich detection of Staphylococcus aureus. *Biosensors and Bioelectronics, 68*, 149–155. https://doi.org/10.1016/j.bios.2014.12.040.

Aksay, I. A., Li, J. L., Adamson, D. H., Schniepp, H. C., Abdala, A. A., Liu, J., ... Prud'homme, R. K. (2007). Single sheet functionalized graphene by oxidation and thermal expansion of graphite. *Chemistry of Materials, 19*(18), 4396–4404. https://doi.org/10.1021/cm0630800.

Alhamoud, Y., Yang, D., Fiati Kenston, S. S., Liu, G., Liu, L., Zhou, H., ... Zhao, J. (2019). Advances in biosensors for the detection of ochratoxin A: Bio-receptors, nanomaterials, and their applications. *Biosensors and Bioelectronics. 141*, https://doi.org/10.1016/j.bios.2019.111418.

Alibolandi, M., Hadizadeh, F., Vajhedin, F., Abnous, K., & Ramezani, M. (2015). Design and fabrication of an aptasensor for chloramphenicol based on energy transfer of CdTe quantum dots to graphene oxide sheet. *Materials Science and Engineering C*, *48*, 611–619. https://doi.org/10.1016/j.msec.2014.12.052.

Amiri, M., Bezaatpour, A., Jafari, H., Boukherroub, R., & Szunerits, S. (2018). Electrochemical methodologies for the detection of pathogens. *ACS Sensors*, *3*(6), 1069–1086. https://doi.org/10.1021/acssensors.8b00239.

Awasthi, K., Awasthi, S., Srivastava, A., Kamalakaran, R., Talapatra, S., Ajayan, P. M., & Srivastava, O. N. (2006). Synthesis and characterization of carbon nanotube-polyethylene oxide composites. *Nanotechnology*, *17*(21), 5417–5422. https://doi.org/10.1088/0957-4484/17/21/022.

Baccar, H., Mejri, M. B., Hafaiedh, I., Ktari, T., Aouni, M., & Abdelghani, A. (2010). Surface plasmon resonance immunosensor for bacteria detection. *Talanta*, *82*(2), 810–814. https://doi.org/10.1016/j.talanta.2010.05.060.

Baker, R. T. K. (1989). Catalytic growth of carbon filaments. *Carbon*, *27*(3), 315–323. https://doi.org/10.1016/0008-6223(89)90062-6.

Balandin, A. A., Ghosh, S., Bao, W., Calizo, I., Teweldebrhan, D., Miao, F., & Lau, C. N. (2008). Superior thermal conductivity of single-layer graphene. *Nano Letters*, *8*(3), 902–907. https://doi.org/10.1021/nl0731872.

Ball, A. S., Patil, S., & Soni, S. (2019). Introduction into nanotechnology and microbiology. *Methods in microbiology* (pp. 1–18). Vol. 46(pp. 1–18). Australia: Academic Press Inc. https://doi.org/10.1016/bs.mim.2019.04.003.

Berber, S., Kwon, Y. K., & Tománek, D. (2000). Unusually high thermal conductivity of carbon nanotubes. *Physical Review Letters*, *84*(20), 4613–4616. https://doi.org/10.1103/PhysRevLett.84.4613.

Bhardwaj, J., Devarakonda, S., Kumar, S., & Jang, J. (2017). Development of a paper-based electrochemical immunosensor using an antibody-single walled carbon nanotubes bioconjugate modified electrode for label-free detection of foodborne pathogens. *Sensors and Actuators, B: Chemical*, *253*, 115–123. https://doi.org/10.1016/j.snb.2017.06.108.

Boehm, D. A., Gottlieb, P. A., & Hua, S. Z. (2007). On-chip microfluidic biosensor for bacterial detection and identification. *Sensors and Actuators, B: Chemical*, *126*(2), 508–514. https://doi.org/10.1016/j.snb.2007.03.043.

Boland, J. J., Niraj, P., Duesberg, G., Krishnamurthy, S., Goodhue, R., Hutchison, J., … Gun'ko, Y. K. (2008). High-yield production of graphene by liquid-phase exfoliation of graphite. *Nature Nanotechnology*, *3*(9), 563–568. https://doi.org/10.1038/nnano.2008.215.

Bülbül, G., Hayat, A., & Andreescu, S. (2015). Portable nanoparticle-based sensors for food safety assessment. *Sensors (Switzerland)*, *15*(12), 30736–30758. https://doi.org/10.3390/s151229826.

Cai, W., Moore, A. L., Zhu, Y., Li, X., Chen, S., Shi, L., & Ruoff, R. S. (2010). Thermal transport in suspended and supported monolayer graphene grown by chemical vapor deposition. *Nano Letters*, *10*(5), 1645–1651. https://doi.org/10.1021/nl9041966.

Chang, H., Tang, L., Wang, Y., Jiang, J., & Li, J. (2010). Graphene fluorescence resonance energy transfer aptasensor for the thrombin detection. *Analytical Chemistry*, *82*(6), 2341–2346. https://doi.org/10.1021/ac9025384.

Chattopadhyay, S., Sabharwal, P. K., Jain, S., Kaur, A., & Singh, H. (2019). Functionalized polymeric magnetic nanoparticle assisted SERS immunosensor for the sensitive detection of S. typhimurium. *Analytica Chimica Acta*, *1067*, 98–106. https://doi.org/10.1016/j.aca.2019.03.050.

Chen, J., Shu, Y., Li, H., Xu, Q., & Hu, X. (2018). Nickel metal-organic framework 2D nanosheets with enhanced peroxidase nanozyme activity for colorimetric detection of H2O2. *Talanta*, *189*, 254–261. https://doi.org/10.1016/j.talanta.2018.06.075.

Choi, J. S., Kim, J. S., Byun, I. S., Lee, D. H., Lee, M. J., Park, B. H., Lee, C., Yoon, D., Cheong, H., Lee, K. H., & Son, Y. W. (2011). Friction anisotropy–driven domain imaging on exfoliated monolayer graphene. *Science*, *333*(6042), 607–610. https://doi.org/10.1126/science.1207110.

Choi, W., & Lee, J. W. (Eds.), (2011). *Graphene: synthesis and applications*. CRC Press.

Conrad, E. H., First, P. N., De Heer, W. A., Wu, X., Brown, N., Naud, C., … Marchenkov, A. N. (2006). Electronic confinement and coherence in patterned epitaxial graphene. *Science*, *312*(5777), 1191–1196. https://doi.org/10.1126/science.1125925.

Danailov, D., Keblinski, P., Nayak, S., & Ajayan, P. M. (2002). Bending properties of carbon nanotubes encapsulating solid nanowires. *Journal of Nanoscience and Nanotechnology*, *2*(5), 503–507. https://doi.org/10.1166/jnn.2002.132.

De Heer, W. A., Song, Z., Li, T., Li, X., Ogbazghi, A. Y., Feng, R., … First, P. N. (2004). Ultrathin epitaxial graphite: 2D electron gas properties and a route toward graphene-based nanoelectronics. *Journal of Physical Chemistry B*, *108*(52), 19912–19916. https://doi.org/10.1021/jp040650f.

Eatemadi, A., Daraee, H., Karimkhanloo, H., Kouhi, M., Zarghami, N., Akbarzadeh, A., … Joo, S. W. (2014). Carbon nanotubes: Properties, synthesis, purification, and medical applications. *Nanoscale Research Letters*, *9*(1), 1–13. https://doi.org/10.1186/1556-276X-9-393.

Fai, M. K., Sfeir, M. Y., Wu, Y., Lui, H., Misewich, J. A., & Heinz, T. F. (2008). Measurement of the optical conductivity of graphene. *Physical Review Letters*. https://doi.org/10.1103/physrevlett.101.196405.

Fujii, M., Zhang, X., Xie, H., Ago, H., Takahashi, K., Ikuta, T., … Shimizu, T. (2005). Measuring the thermal conductivity of a single carbon nanotube. *Physical Review Letters*. *95*(6) https://doi.org/10.1103/PhysRevLett.95.065502.

Furukawa, I., Ishihara, T., Teranishi, H., Saito, S., Yatsuyanagi, J., Wada, E., & Kobayashi (2016). Prevalence and characteristics of Salmonella and Campylobacter in retail poultry meat in Japan. *Japanese Journal of Infectious Diseases*, *70*(3), 239–247. https://doi.org/10.7883/yoken.JJID.2016.164.

Gierz, I., Petersen, J. C., Mitrano, M., Cacho, C., Turcu, I. C. E., Springate, E., … Cavalleri, A. (2013). Snapshots of non-equilibrium Dirac carrier distributions in graphene. *Nature Materials*, *12*(12), 1119–1124. https://doi.org/10.1038/nmat3757.

Guo, R., Wang, S., Huang, F., Chen, Q., Li, Y., Liao, M., & Lin, J. (2019). Rapid detection of Salmonella Typhimurium using magnetic nanoparticle immunoseparation, nanocluster signal amplification and smartphone image analysis. *Sensors and Actuators, B: Chemical*, *284*, 134–139. https://doi.org/10.1016/j.snb.2018.12.110.

Hai, W., Goda, T., Takeuchi, H., Yamaoka, S., Horiguchi, Y., Matsumoto, A., & Miyahara, Y. (2017). Specific recognition of human influenza virus with PEDOT bearing sialic acid-terminated trisaccharides. *ACS Applied Materials and Interfaces*, *9*(16), 14162–14170. https://doi.org/10.1021/acsami.7b02523.

He, H., & Gao, C. (2010). General approach to individually dispersed, highly soluble, and conductive graphene nanosheets functionalized by nitrene chemistry. *Chemistry of Materials*, *22*(17), 5054–5064. https://doi.org/10.1021/cm101634k.

He, Q., Wu, S., Yin, Z., & Zhang, H. (2012). Graphene-based electronic sensors. *Chemical Science*, *3*(6), 1764–1772. https://doi.org/10.1039/c2sc20205k.

He, R. X., Zhang, M., Tan, F., Leung, P. H. M., Zhao, X. Z., Chan, H. L. W., … Yan, F. (2012). Detection of bacteria with organic electrochemical transistors. *Journal of Materials Chemistry*, *22*(41), 22072–22076. https://doi.org/10.1039/c2jm33667g.

Hernández, R., Vallés, C., Benito, A. M., Maser, W. K., Xavier Rius, F., & Riu, J. (2014). Graphene-based potentiometric biosensor for the immediate detection of living bacteria. *Biosensors and Bioelectronics*, *54*, 553–557. https://doi.org/10.1016/j.bios.2013.11.053.

Holzinger, M., Goff, A. L., & Cosnier, S. (2014). Nanomaterials for biosensing applications: A review. *Frontiers in Chemistry*. *2*, https://doi.org/10.3389/fchem.2014.00063.

Hone, J. (2004). Carbon nanotubes: Thermal properties. In *Dekker encyclopedia of nanoscience and nanotechnology* (pp. 603–610). .

Huang, C. S., Huang, B. R., Jang, Y. H., Tsai, M. S., & Yeh, C. Y. (2005). Three-terminal CNTs gas sensor for N2 detection. *Diamond and Related Materials Taiwan*. https://doi.org/10.1016/j.diamond.2005.09.006.

Iqbal, A., Labib, M., Muharemagic, D., Sattar, S., Dixon, B. R., & Berezovski, M. V. (2015). Detection of Cryptosporidium parvum oocysts on fresh produce using DNA aptamers. *PLoS One*. *10*(9)https://doi.org/10.1371/journal.pone.0137455.

Kaushik, B. K., & Majumder, M. K. (2015). Carbon nanotube based VLSI interconnects: Analysis and design. In *Springer Briefs in Applied Sciences and Technology*. https://doi.org/10.1007/978-81-322-2047-3 (9788132220466), i–iv.

Kim, B., Lee, J., Namgung, S., Kim, J., Park, J. Y., Lee, M. S., & Hong, S. (2012). DNA sensors based on CNT-FET with floating electrodes. *Sensors and Actuators, B: Chemical*, *169*, 182–187. https://doi.org/10.1016/j.snb.2012.04.063.

Kim, S. N., Rusling, J. F., & Papadimitrakopoulos, F. (2007). Carbon nanotubes for electronic and electrochemical detection of biomolecules. *Advanced Materials*, *19*(20), 3214–3228. https://doi.org/10.1002/adma.200700665.

Kim, P., Shi, L., Majumdar, A., & McEuen, P. L. (2001). Thermal transport measurements of individual multiwalled nanotubes. *Physical Review Letters*, *87*(21), 2155021–2155024.

King, T., Osmond-McLeod, M. J., & Duffy, L. L. (2018). Nanotechnology in the food sector and potential applications for the poultry industry. *Trends in Food Science and Technology*, *72*, 62–73. https://doi.org/10.1016/j.tifs.2017.11.015.

Klumpp, C., Kostarelos, K., Prato, M., & Bianco, A. (2006). Functionalized carbon nanotubes as emerging nanovectors for the delivery of therapeutics. *Biochimica et Biophysica Acta - Biomembranes*, *1758*(3), 404–412. https://doi.org/10.1016/j.bbamem.2005.10.008.

Kong, J., Franklin, N. R., Zhou, C., Chapline, M. G., Peng, S., Cho, K., & Dai, H. (2000). Nanotube molecular wires as chemical sensors. *Science*, *287*(5453), 622–625. https://doi.org/10.1126/science.287.5453.622.

Koziol, K., Boskovic, B. O., & Yahya, N. (2010). Synthesis of carbon nanostructures by CVD method in carbon and oxide. *Nanostructures*, *5*, 23–49.

Lan, L., Yao, Y., Ping, J., & Ying, Y. (2017). Recent advances in nanomaterial-based biosensors for antibiotics detection. *Biosensors and Bioelectronics*, *91*, 504–514. https://doi.org/10.1016/j.bios.2017.01.007.

Lawal, A. T. (2016). Synthesis and utilization of carbon nanotubes for fabrication of electrochemical biosensors. *Materials Research Bulletin*, *73*, 308–350. https://doi.org/10.1016/j.materresbull.2015.08.037.

Lee, I., & Jun, S. (2016). Simultaneous detection of E. coli K12 and S. aureus using a continuous flow multijunction biosensor. *Journal of Food Science*, *81*(6), N1530–N1536. https://doi.org/10.1111/1750-3841.13307.

Lee, C., Wei, X., Kysar, J. W., & Hone, J. (2008). Measurement of the elastic properties and intrinsic strength of monolayer graphene. *Science*, *321*(5887), 385–388. https://doi.org/10.1126/science.1157996.

Li, X. X., Cao, C., Han, S. J., & Sim, S. J. (2009). Detection of pathogen based on the catalytic growth of gold nanocrystals. *Water Research*, *43*(5), 1425–1431. https://doi.org/10.1016/j.watres.2008.12.024.

Li, Z., Wang, L., Li, Y., Feng, Y., & Feng, W. (2019). Carbon-based functional nanomaterials: Preparation, properties and applications. *Composites Science and Technology*, *179*, 10–40. https://doi.org/10.1016/j.compscitech.2019.04.028.

Lian, Y., He, F., Wang, H., & Tong, F. (2015). A new aptamer/graphene interdigitated gold electrode piezoelectric sensor for rapid and specific detection of Staphylococcus aureus. *Biosensors and Bioelectronics*, *65*, 314–319. https://doi.org/10.1016/j.bios.2014.10.017.

Liu, Y., Dong, X., & Chen, P. (2012). Biological and chemical sensors based on graphene materials. *Chemical Society Reviews*, *41*(6), 2283–2307. https://doi.org/10.1039/c1cs15270j.

Liu, X., Su, L., Zhu, L., Gao, X., Wang, Y., Bai, F., … Li, J. (2016). Hybrid material for enrofloxacin sensing based on aptamer-functionalized magnetic nanoparticle conjugated with upconversion nanoprobes. *Sensors and Actuators, B: Chemical*, *233*, 394–401. https://doi.org/10.1016/j.snb.2016.04.096.

Lv, M., Liu, Y., Geng, J., Kou, X., Xin, Z., & Yang, D. (2018). Engineering nanomaterials-based biosensors for food safety detection. *Biosensors and Bioelectronics*, *106*, 122–128. https://doi.org/10.1016/j.bios.2018.01.049.

Madani, S. Y., Naderi, N., Dissanayake, O., Tan, A., & Seifalian, A. M. (2011). A new era of cancer treatment: Carbon nanotubes as drug delivery tools. *International Journal of Nanomedicine*, *6*.

Mahmoudpour, M., Ezzati Nazhad Dolatabadi, J., Torbati, M., Pirpour Tazehkand, A., Homayouni-Rad, A., & de la Guardia, M. (2019). Nanomaterials and new biorecognition molecules based surface plasmon resonance biosensors for mycotoxin detection. *Biosensors and Bioelectronics*. *143*, https://doi.org/10.1016/j.bios.2019.111603.

Majdinasab, M., Hayat, A., & Marty, J. L. (2018). Aptamer-based assays and aptasensors for detection of pathogenic bacteria in food samples. *TrAC, Trends in Analytical Chemistry*, *107*, 60–77. https://doi.org/10.1016/j.trac.2018.07.016.

Malekzad, H., Sahandi Zangabad, P., Mirshekari, H., Karimi, M., & Hamblin, M. R. (2017). Noble metal nanoparticles in biosensors: Recent studies and applications. *Nanotechnology Reviews*, *6*(3), 301–329. https://doi.org/10.1515/ntrev-2016-0014.

Mannoor, M. S., Tao, H., Clayton, J. D., Sengupta, A., Kaplan, D. L., Naik, R. R., … McAlpine, M. C. (2012). Graphene-based wireless bacteria detection on tooth enamel. *Nature Communications*. *3*, https://doi.org/10.1038/ncomms1767.

Mathur, R. B. (2016). Carbon nanomaterials: Synthesis, structure, properties and applications. In *Carbon Nanomaterials: Synthesis, Structure, Properties and Applications* (pp. 1–266). India: CRC Press. https://doi.org/10.1201/9781315371849.

Mohammadian, N., & Faridbod, F. (2018). ALS genosensing using DNA-hybridization electrochemical biosensor based on label-free immobilization of ssDNA on Sm2O3 NPs-rGO/PANI composite. *Sensors and Actuators, B: Chemical*, *275*, 432–438. https://doi.org/10.1016/j.snb.2018.07.103.

Muniandy, S., Teh, S. J., Thong, K. L., Thiha, A., Dinshaw, I. J., Lai, C. W., … Leo, B. F. (2019). Carbon nanomaterial-based electrochemical biosensors for foodborne bacterial detection. *Critical Reviews in Analytical Chemistry*, *49*(6), 510–533. https://doi.org/10.1080/10408347.2018.1561243.

Muñoz, R., & Gómez-Aleixandre, C. (2013). Review of CVD synthesis of graphene. *Chemical Vapor Deposition*, *19*(10–12), 297–322. https://doi.org/10.1002/cvde.201300051.

Mustafa, F., Hassan, R., & Andreescu, S. (2017). Multifunctional nanotechnology\tenabled sensors for rapid capture and detection of pathogens. *Sensors*, *17*(9).

Neto, A. C., Guinea, F., Peres, N. M., Novoselov, K. S., & Geim, A. K. (2009). The\telectronic properties of graphene. *Reviews of Modern Physics*, *81*(1).

Novoselov, K. S., Geim, A. K., Morozov, S. V., Jiang, D., Zhang, Y., Dubonos, S. V., … Firsov, A. A. (2004). Electric field effect in atomically thin carbon films. *Science*, 666–669. https://doi.org/10.1126/science.1102896.

Pandey, P., & Dahiya, M. (2016). Carbon nanotubes: Types, methods of preparation and applications. *Carbon*, *4*, .

Paredes, J. I., Villar-Rodil, S., Martínez-Alonso, A., & Tascón, J. M. D. (2008). Graphene oxide dispersions in organic solvents. *Langmuir*, 10560–10564. https://doi.org/10.1021/la801744a.

Potonik (2010). *Commission recommendation of 18 October 2011 on the definition of nanomaterial*: (pp. 38–40). .

Prasek, J., Drbohlavova, J., Chomoucka, J., Hubalek, J., Jasek, O., Adam, V., & Kizek, R. (2011). Methods for carbon nanotubes synthesis - review. *Journal of Materials Chemistry*, *21*(40), 15872–15884. https://doi.org/10.1039/c1jm12254a.

Pushpendra, K., Arun, K. S., Sajjad, H., Kwun, N. H., Kwan, S. H., Jonghwa, E., … Jai, S. (2013). Graphene: Synthesis, properties and application in transparent electronic devices. *Reviews in Advanced Sciences and Engineering*, 238–258. https://doi.org/10.1166/rase.2013.1043.

Ramnani, P., Saucedo, N. M., & Mulchandani, A. (2016). Carbon nanomaterial-based electrochemical biosensors for label-free sensing of environmental pollutants. *Chemosphere*, *143*, 85–98. https://doi.org/10.1016/j.chemosphere.2015.04.063.

Ray, S., Biswas, R., Banerjee, R., & Biswas, P. (2020). Gold nanoparticle intercalated mesoporous silica based nanozyme for selective colorimetric detection of dopamine. *Nanoscale Advances*, *2*, 734–745. https://doi.org/10.1039/C9NA00508K.

Riu, J., & Giussani, B. (2020). Electrochemical biosensors for the detection of pathogenic bacteria in food. *TrAC, Trends in Analytical Chemistry*. *126*, https://doi.org/10.1016/j.trac.2020.115863.

Safoura, H., Hamideh, R., Hossein, P., & Soheila, K. (2020). Modeling of ultrasensitive DNA hybridization detection based on gold nanoparticles/carbon-nanotubes/chitosan-modified electrodes. *Colloids and Surfaces A: Physicochemical and Engineering Aspects*, 124219. https://doi.org/10.1016/j.colsurfa.2019.124219.

Sapna, J. (2012). Development of an antibody functionalized carbon nanotube biosensor for foodborne bacterial pathogens. *Journal of Biosensors & Bioelectronics*. https://doi.org/10.4172/2155-6210.S11-002.

Sharma, R., Baik, J. H., Perera, C. J., & Strano, M. S. (2010). Anomalously large reactivity of single graphene layers and edges toward electron transfer chemistries. *Nano Letters*, *10*(2), 398–405. https://doi.org/10.1021/nl902741x.

Singh, R., Hong, S., & Jang, J. (2017). Label-free detection of influenza viruses using a reduced graphene oxide-based electrochemical immunosensor integrated with a microfluidic platform. *Scientific Reports*. *7*, https://doi.org/10.1038/srep42771.

Stanisavljevic, M., Krizkova, S., Vaculovicova, M., Kizek, R., & Adam, V. (2015). Quantum dots-fluorescence resonance energy transfer-based nanosensors and their application. *Biosensors and Bioelectronics*, *74*, 562–574. https://doi.org/10.1016/j.bios.2015.06.076.

Stankovich, S., Dikin, D. A., Piner, R. D., Kohlhaas, K. A., Kleinhammes, A., Jia, Y., ... Ruoff, R. S. (2007). Synthesis of graphene-based nanosheets via chemical reduction of exfoliated graphite oxide. *Carbon*, *45*(7), 1558–1565. https://doi.org/10.1016/j.carbon.2007.02.034.

Subramanian, S., Aschenbach, K. H., Evangelista, J. P., Najjar, M. B., Song, W., & Gomez, R. D. (2012). Rapid, sensitive and label-free detection of Shiga-toxin producing Escherichia coli O157 using carbon nanotube biosensors. *Biosensors and Bioelectronics*, *32*(1), 69–75. https://doi.org/10.1016/j.bios.2011.11.040.

Suehiro, J., Ikeda, N., Ohtsubo, A., & Imasaka, K. (2009). Bacterial detection using a carbon nanotube gas sensor coupled with a microheater for ammonia synthesis by aerobic oxidisation of organic components. *IET Nanobiotechnology*, *3*(2), 15–22. https://doi.org/10.1049/iet-nbt.2008.0011.

Sun, P., Wang, M., Liu, L., Jiao, L., Du, W., Xia, F., ... Yun, M. (2019). Sensitivity enhancement of surface plasmon resonance biosensor based on graphene and barium titanate layers. *Applied Surface Science*, *475*, 342–347. https://doi.org/10.1016/j.apsusc.2018.12.283.

Swaidan, A., Addad, A., Tahon, J. F., Barras, A., Toufaily, J., Hamieh, T., & Boukherroub (2020). Ultrasmall CuS-BSA-Cu3 (PO4) 2 nanozyme for highly efficient colorimetric sensing of H2O2 and glucose in contact lens care solutions and human serum. *Analytica Chimica Acta*, *1109*, 78–89. https://doi.org/10.1016/j.aca.2020.02.064.

Thévenot, D. R., Toth, K., Durst, R. A., & Wilson, G. S. (2001). Electrochemical biosensors: Recommended definitions and classification. *Analytical Letters*, *34*(5), 635–659. https://doi.org/10.1081/AL-100103209.

Vaibhav, R., Pragya, Y., Sankar, B. S., Kumar, M. A., Navneet, V., Anurag, V., & Kumar, P. J. (2014). Carbon nanotubes: An emerging drug carrier for targeting cancer cells. *Journal of Drug Delivery*, 1–23. https://doi.org/10.1155/2014/670815.

Vander Wal, R. L., Berger, G. M., & Ticich, T. M. (2003). Carbon nanotube synthesis in a flame using laser ablation for in situ catalyst generation. *Applied Physics A: Materials Science and Processing*, *77*(7), 885–889. https://doi.org/10.1007/s00339-003-2196-3.

Viculis, L. M., Mack, J. J., & Kaner, R. B. (2003). A chemical route to carbon nanoscrolls. *Science*, 1361. https://doi.org/10.1126/science.1078842.

Viculis, L. M., Mack, J. J., Mayer, O. M., Hahn, H. T., & Kaner, R. B. (2005). Intercalation and exfoliation routes to graphite nanoplatelets. *Journal of Materials Chemistry*, *15*(9), 974–978. https://doi.org/10.1039/b413029d.

Wang, M., Abbineni, G., Clevenger, A., Mao, C., & Xu, S. (2011). Upconversion nanoparticles: Synthesis, surface modification and biological applications. *Nanomedicine: Nanotechnology, Biology, and Medicine*, *7*(6), 710–729. https://doi.org/10.1016/j.nano.2011.02.013.

Warner, J. H., Schaffel, F., Rummeli, M., & Bachmatiuk, A. (2012). *Graphene: Fundamentals and emergent applications*. Newnes.

WHO (2015). *WHO estimates of the global burden of foodborne diseases: foodborne disease burden epidemiology reference group 2007-2015*. World Health Organization.

Wong, E. W., Sheehan, P. E., & Lieber, C. M. (1997). Nanobeam mechanics: Elasticity, strength, and toughness of nanorods and nanotubes. *Science*, *277*(5334), 1971–1975. https://doi.org/10.1126/science.277.5334.1971.

Wu, G., Meyyappan, M., & Lai, K. W. C. (2016). Graphene field-effect transistors-based biosensors for Escherichia coli detection. In: *16th International conference on nanotechnology - IEEE NANO 2016*, Hong Kong: Institute of Electrical and Electronics Engineers Inc. https://doi.org/10.1109/NANO.2016.7751414.

Wu, S., Zhang, H., Shi, Z., Duan, N., Fang, C. C., Dai, S., & Wang, Z. (2015). Aptamer-based fluorescence biosensor for chloramphenicol determination using upconversion nanoparticles. *Food Control*, *50*, 597–604. https://doi.org/10.1016/j.foodcont.2014.10.003.

Xia, Z. H., Guduru, P. R., & Curtin, W. A. (2007). Enhancing mechanical properties of multiwall carbon nanotubes via sp 3 interwall bridging. *Physical Review Letters*. *98*(24) https://doi.org/10.1103/PhysRevLett.98.245501.

Xu, C., Akakuru, O. U., Zheng, J., & Wu, A. (2019). Applications of iron oxide-based magnetic nanoparticles in the diagnosis and treatment of bacterial infections. *Frontiers in Bioengineering and Biotechnology*. *7*, https://doi.org/10.3389/fbioe.2019.00141.

Xue, L., Huang, F., Hao, L., Cai, G., Zheng, L., Li, Y., & Lin, J. (2020). A sensitive immunoassay for simultaneous detection of foodborne pathogens using MnO2 nanoflowers-assisted loading and release of quantum dots. *Food Chemistry*, *322*(30), 126719. https://doi.org/10.1016/j.foodchem.2020.126719.

Xue, J., Wang, X., Jeong, J. H., & Yan, X. (2019). Fabrication, photoluminescence and applications of quantum dots embedded glass ceramics. *Chemical Engineering Journal*, *383*, 123082.

Xue, Z., Zhang, Y., Yu, W., Zhang, J., Wang, J., Wan, F., ... Kou, X. (2019). Recent advances in aflatoxin B1 detection based on nanotechnology and nanomaterials-A review. *Analytica Chimica Acta*, *1069*, 1–27. https://doi.org/10.1016/j.aca.2019.04.032.

Yang, N., Chen, X., Ren, T., Zhang, P., & Yang, D. (2015). Carbon nanotube based biosensors. *Sensors and Actuators, B: Chemical*, *207*, 690–715. https://doi.org/10.1016/j.snb.2014.10.040.

Yao, B., Huang, H., & Liu, Kang Z. (2019). Carbon dots: A small conundrum, Trends in Chemistry. *1*(2), 235–246. https://doi.org/10.1016/j.trechm.2019.02.003.

Yoo, M. S., Shin, M., Kim, Y., Jang, M., Choi, Y. E., Park, S. J., ... Park, C. (2017). Development of electrochemical biosensor for detection of pathogenic microorganism in Asian dust events. *Chemosphere*, *175*, 269–274. https://doi.org/10.1016/j.chemosphere.2017.02.060.

Yu, M. F., Files, B. S., Arepalli, S., & Ruoff, R. S. (2000). Tensile loading of ropes of single wall carbon nanotubes and their mechanical properties. *Physical Review Letters*, *84*(24), 5552–5555. https://doi.org/10.1103/PhysRevLett.84.5552.

Yu, S., Wei, Q., Du, B., Wu, D., Li, H., Yan, L., ... Zhang, Y. (2013). Label-free immunosensor for the detection of kanamycin using Ag@Fe3O4 nanoparticles and thionine mixed graphene sheet. *Biosensors and Bioelectronics*, *48*, 224–229. https://doi.org/10.1016/j.bios.2013.04.025.

Zeng, Y., Zhu, Z., Du, D., & Lin, Y. (2016). Nanomaterial-based electrochemical biosensors for food safety. *Journal of Electroanalytical Chemistry*, *781*, 147–154. https://doi.org/10.1016/j.jelechem.2016.10.030.

Zhang, Z., Tian, Y., Huang, P., & Wu, F. Y. (2020). Using target-specific aptamers to enhance the peroxidase-like activity of gold nanoclusters for colorimetric detection of tetracycline antibiotics. *Talanta*. *208*, https://doi.org/10.1016/j.talanta.2019.120342.

Zhang, R., Zhang, Y., & Wei, F. (2017). Horizontally aligned carbon nanotube arrays: Growth mechanism, controlled synthesis, characterization, properties and applications. *Chemical Society Reviews*, *46*(12), 3661–3715. https://doi.org/10.1039/c7cs00104e.

Zhao, H., & Aluru, N. R. (2010). Temperature and strain-rate dependent fracture strength of graphene. *Journal of Applied Physics*. 064321https://doi.org/10.1063/1.3488620.

Zhou, M., Wang, Y., Zhai, Y., Zhai, J., Ren, W., Wang, F., & Dong, S. (2009). Controlled synthesis of large-area and patterned electrochemically reduced graphene oxide films. *Chemistry - A European Journal*, *15*(25), 6116–6120. https://doi.org/10.1002/chem.200900596.

Zhu, Y., Murali, S., Cai, W., Li, X., Suk, J. W., Potts, J. R., & Ruoff, R. S. (2010). Graphene and graphene oxide: Synthesis, properties, and applications. *Advanced Materials*, *22*(35), 3906–3924. https://doi.org/10.1002/adma.201001068.

Zou, D., Jin, L., Wu, B., Hu, L., Chen, X., Huang, G., & Zhang, J. (2019). Rapid detection of Salmonella in milk by biofunctionalised magnetic nanoparticle cluster sensor based on nuclear magnetic resonance. *International Dairy Journal*, *91*, 82–88. https://doi.org/10.1016/j.idairyj.2018.11.011.

Extraction and analytical methods for the identification of parasites in food

---

Introduction

Food is one of the essential components of daily life to provide human life with energy. Various benefits of food consumption, such as calorie-containing food, are used by the body for energy that enables people to move, breathe, and do their daily work. Consumption of food is a basic need for people to continue to live healthy lives. Nutrients such as carbohydrates, fats, and proteins are the most important intakes for humans as they help in the development of the body's healthy organ and nervous system. However, food safety disturbances can be fatal as they can cause food contamination from harmful bacteria or even parasites (Lothar, 2000). Infected or contaminated food products may potentially cause foodborne illness due to the miss-handling of raw products and contamination of food products before or after cooking (Kalyoussef & Feja, 2014). The foodborne disease becomes a serious issue, when production, food imports, and exports are growing considerably. Increased cases related to parasitic foodborne diseases were mainly due to parasitic worms found in various food products.

It is imperative to understand the contributing factors to the contamination of foods. Rockland and Nishi (1980) mentioned that improper handling of raw materials might contribute to the growth of harmful bacteria, which often occur at 0.9 water activity content and above. However, low water activity does not always promise food safety as there is still the presence of mold that can grow as low as 0.6 of water activity. Thus, the water activity content present in raw material plays a vital role in the determination of food safety. Additionally, the methods of food being processed can leads to major contributing factors as well. This is because each parasite has its unique characteristic, where few parasites might be resistant to heat. In this case, high heat treatment must be made to destroy the parasite and ensuring the safety of the food. Through understanding its features in terms of temperature and pH changes, the division of parasite can be inhibited. The common harmful bacteria raid processed food is *C. botulinum* that is mostly found in canned food. The presence of *C. botulinum* frequently found indented canned food as the temperature of the internal packaging was abused that contributes to induce a suitable environment for the growth of *C. botulinum* (Evancho, Tortorelli, & Scott, 2009).

101

Advanced Food Analysis Tools. https://doi.org/10.1016/B978-0-12-820591-4.00006-2

Moreover, improper food storage may lead to the initiation of a favorable environment for the growth of parasites. Most food products that are kept under room temperature have a higher tendency to be contaminated. The moisture content in the room temperature is often slightly higher than the food product. This phenomenon may cause the migration of moisture content to the food via osmotic pressure and leads to higher water activity in the food products. The incident causes harmful bacteria able to penetrate the food products (Rockland & Nishi, 1980). Therefore, by looking into these concerns and factors, evaluation of the best detection method of potential pathogens to ensure food safety is vital as they aid in the prevention of diseases. The presence of parasites, microbes, mites, and insects in food makes it undesirable for consumption, and due to that, there has been an increase in food product loss every year.

The occurrence of foodborne diseases has become a significant concern for human health. There have been continuously reported cases of foodborne diseases affecting the public due to poor sanitation practices during the processing of food products and cross-contamination that could take place during the transporting and storage process. One of the examples of food products that often are reported with such cases is the contamination of canned sardine with nematodes. Anisakis is a genus of nematodes that commonly associated with the consumption of fishery products as it has become a health risk on gastrointestinal infections and hypersensitive reactions. It belongs to the family of Anisakidae together with other genera, including *Pseudoterranova, Phocascaris*, and *Contracaecum*. These worms make fish as main transport hosts and aquatic crustaceans as intermediate hosts. It has been reported that species related to human infection are *A. simplex* and *Pseudoterranova decipiens*. Eating fish or cephalopods containing the larvae could infect the primary host (EFSA Panel on Biological Hazards [BIOHAZ], 2010).

Previous studies in the detection of anisakis parasite residue in food products have shown a positive result wherein *Anisakis* spp. were abundant and were found in food dairy products and minced fish products. This shows how vital strict inspection is towards food products as it might be contaminated unrealized. Typically *Anisakis* spp. will be found in fish muscle and fish-derived food products, even though proper handling methods were applied during the food processing or harvesting. This problem may occur because of the fish used for food production may lose its freshness and has low quality of fish stocks (Mossali et al., 2010). In 2018, there was a reported case of worm detection in the canned sardines from China that was brought in through Penang in mid of May. These worms have been detected through physical examination and sampling that was done on several sardine cans. It is proven that these worms are disease-carrying parasites in humans, and they are called the *Anisakis spp*, which is the reason why Anisakiasis disease can occur in humans when raw fish or fish that is partially cooked and infected with this parasite is consumed. The fish that becomes the host of these nematodes can cause parasitic and zoonotic diseases in humans when accidentally consumed by giving symptoms such as abdominal pain, diarrhea, nausea, and vomiting. This case was investigated for further action as it is an offense under the Malaysian Quarantine and Inspection

Services Act 2011. where it includes the importing of any of this agricultural or fisheries product with pests or contaminants (The Straits Time, September 29, 2018); besides that Dawson (2005) had listed several outbreaks of waterborne and foodborne diseases that took place in various locations mainly in the United States. In most western countries, the outbreaks of foodborne diseases caused by parasites have been detected in fresh foods, especially those that are harder to clean entirely and are directly consumed without undergoing processing that can keep the protozoan parasites active. Despite the number of reported cases of the presence of parasitic worms in food products, there is a lack of specific method invented specifically for detecting parasites as a preventative measure.

Parasites

Parasites are organisms that live in a host organism and obtain their food from its host. Typically, parasites are much smaller in size compared to their food source, which is the host organism, and this differentiates them from predators. Some parasites live in only one species of animal. However, many parasites, particularly the worms, spend part of their lives reproducing sexually in a final or definitive host and developing asexually as larvae during another part of their life in an intermediate host of a different species. Parasites that can cause disease in humans can be categorized into three main classes of protozoa, helminths, and ectoparasites. Parasites had infected millions of people all across the globe. These parasitic diseases are often associated with poverty and underdeveloped countries, as most of them can be combated by the improvement of surroundings and facilities such as clean water, sanitation, and hygiene. For instance, sickness such as dysentery and giardiasis are both closely related to the availability of clean water and poverty (Carrion, Hamer, & Evans, 2016). In underdeveloped countries, parasites are to be blamed for being the primary cause of diarrhea in children and stunted growth, which significantly impacts the economic losses, especially in terms of health and agriculture.

Foods associated with parasitic contamination

Parasites that are causing the most concern in terms of food safety include worms such as cestodes, nematodes and trematodes, and protozoans as well as single-celled organisms. These parasites can cause asymptomatic infections, causing an acute effect and other chronic diseases, which can lead to a fatality. Poultries and fishes are the common food product that involves in cases of foodborne illness. It is because certain parasites have used this particular product as their host, or those parasites were unwittingly transmitted. According to Adams, Murrell, and Cross (1997), nematodes, cestodes, trematodes, and acanthocephalans are the parasites that were found in seafood. While for poultry, protozoa, nematodes, cestodes, acanthocephalans, trematodes, and ectoparasites are the parasites found in poultry (Ruff, 1999).

Recently, a case regarding the nematodes worms, *Anisakis spp.* in canned sardines, had gone viral. The Malaysian Quarantine and Inspection Services (Maqis) had revealed the case when they did a sampling on one of the sardines brand from China. The problem may occur when the method of handling is insufficient and is not adequately managed. Besides that, eating raw fish or consuming uncooked food also can cause foodborne illness arising from these parasites. High temperature is needed when cooking them to make sure that all the pathogens or parasites are thoroughly killed. Certain parasites are immune to a specific high temperature. It is essential to know what temperature is suitable to apply in cooking fish or poultry. Thus, appropriate ways of handling fish and poultry during harvesting, storage, or processing are essential. Large food industries that use poultry and fish in their product can apply for various programs that are involved with food health such as Good Manufacturing Practices (GMP) or Hazard Analysis and Critical Control Point (HACCP) to avoid or prevent the risks.

Parasitic diseases also can be caused by the parasites coming from fruits and vegetables. Several types of parasites are capable of living and hosting the plants. One of the examples is tapeworms that may be found in fruits and vegetables due to farmers who have used human and animal wastes as fertilizer. Furthermore, nematodes also can exist in food plants such as *angiostrongylus* that is hosting in snail and leafy vegetables. Based on (Simpson, 1995), snails also infect the fruits or vegetables leave with the existence of the larvae in their mucus. Flatworm is one of the examples of a trematode that could host watery vegetables like water spinach. Some parasites do not host in fruits and vegetables but were transmitted to the plant food, which will infect humans and animals who ingested them. For example, *Ascaris* can live in contaminated water that is used to clean the fruits and vegetables (Doyle, 2003). Eating uncooked vegetables or unwashed fruits can be unhealthy and not encouraged as oocysts from cat feces might be spread by wind or water, which is harder to be controlled and prevented. The infection of *Toxoplasma gondii* oocysts on berries can lead to illnesses (Kniel et al., 2002). Therefore, it is crucial to clean the fruits and vegetables before consumption, as some consumers have the assumption that food plants are safe to be eaten raw. Leafy vegetables such as cabbage, which is more difficult to be washed can be soaked in vinegar as a disinfectant.

The probability risk related to raw milk consumption has been featured by quite a lot of authors (Fratini et al., 2016), which is caused by the presence of several zoonotic pathogens of which characterize as tick-borne encephalitis virus (TBEV) and *Coxiella burnetii*. The rickettsia is affecting fever in humans that most usually reported as contributory factors of milk-borne illness that linked to the consumption of milk in goat (Van den Brom et al., 2009). The protagonist of milk-borne toxicities in humans by further zoonotic pathogens besides TBEV and *C. burnetii*, including *Anaplasma phagocytophilum*, *Rickettsia spp.*, and *Toxoplasma gondii* have a lesser amount of investigating (Utech, Wharton, & Kerr, 1978). Economic destruction could be happened due to decreasing weight, meat and milk manufacture, fertility, and leather excellence while also accumulate the incidences of heard illness, pathogens spread, skin injury, animal pressure, and death (De Campos-Pereira, Bahia-Labruna, Szabó, & Marcondes-Klafe, 2008). According to a study by Cisak et al.

(2017), they suggested the possible threat of milk-borne *Toxoplasma* infection was by intake of raw cow milk. The milk-borne blowout might not imply in the case of *C. burnetii*, *A. phagocytophilum*, and *Rickettsia spp.* However, currently, the intake of raw bovine milk in the distribution of toxoplasmosis is still a case of argument (Cisak et al., 2017).

Classification of parasitic foodborne diseases
Amebiasis

Amebiasis, which is also known as amoebic dysentery, is instigated by the infection of the parasite *Entamoeba histolytica*, which is a protozoan with the pseudopod-forming and they are nonflagellated. *E. histolytica* was discovered to be present in fruits, vegetables, and drinking water that is contaminated. This organism can either exist as an infectious cyst or invasive trophozoite (Shirley, Farr, Watanabe, & Moonah, 2018). The main route of transmission of *E. histolytica* is through the ingestion of the infectious cysts, which commonly arise out of fecally contaminated hands, food, drinking water, and most interestingly during sexual contacts, especially among bisexuals group (Hung, Chang, & Ji, 2012). Recent analysis utilizing polymerase chain reaction (PCR) diagnostics had discovered that *E. histolytica* was among the top seven pathogens initiating dysentery (Liu et al., 2016).

Anisakiasis

Anisakis spp. larvae live in primary and intermediate hosts who are crustaceans and fish, respectively. However, it stops developing and maturing in an accidental host, which is human yet, and they are capable of stimulating fish-borne illnesses. The specific disease is called anisakiasis. Mattiucci, Cipriani, Levsen, Paoletti, and Nascetti (2018) determined that when this parasite has arrived on the gastrointestinal part, it may invite some diseases that can be categorized into several types of anisakiasis. The symptoms are that the patient will experience severe abdominal pain, nausea, vomiting, or diarrhea within 48 h after consumption (Nieuwenhuizen & Lopata, 2013). A more severe case is where the *Anisakis spp.* have infected the hosts by attaching themselves to the intestinal mucosa and penetrate the gastrointestinal tract. This severe infection of the mucosa can lead to tissue damage and gastric ulcers. Bouree, Paugam, and Petithory (1995) suggested that these symptoms of anisakiasis are similar and resemble in having a gastrointestinal disorder such as tumors, acute appendicitis, and gastric ulcer. Furthermore, some results from studies demonstrate that a person who has ingested Anisakis larvae through infected seafood may have experienced some allergic reactions, whether the nematode is alive or dead (Audicana, Ansotegui, De Corres, & Kennedy, 2002). According to Nieuwenhuizen et al. (2006), indirect contact with the parasite during fish processing or preparations can generate allergy, including asthma, conjunctivitis, and contact dermatitis. There are currently 12 discovered allergens in *Anisakis spp.*

Ascariasis

Ascariasis is an infection caused by *Ascaris lumbricoides* belonging to a class of parasites, often referred to as soil-transmitted helminths (Jourdan, Lamberton, Fenwick, & Addiss, 2018). These parasites may occur in foods in the form of eggs, larvae, or other immature forms (Gebrie, & Engdaw, 2015). Infection by this parasite is typically due to the transmission usually occurs subsequently after ingestion of food or water that is contaminated with *A. lumbricoides* eggs. The occurrence of symptoms may be varied subject to the phase of the parasite's life cycle and level of intensity of infection. Those with eosinophilic pneumonia are most probably to experience the symptoms 10–14 days after infection due to the self-limiting inflammatory reaction to larvae migrating through pulmonary tissue (Akuthota & Weller, 2012; Sultan, 1996). As for infections instigated from adult *Ascaris spp.*, it can cause acute abdomen, including upper gastrointestinal bleeding, small bowel obstruction, volvulus, peritonitis, and gastric ascariasis (Wang, Li, Huang, & Tang, 2013; Sultan, 1996; Das, 2014; Khuroo & Khuroo, 2010). As a public health control, WHO had made a commandment of administration of benzimidazole to control morbidity and eliminate ascariasis as a public health problem (Helminthiases, 2012).

Clonorchiasis

Clonorchis sinensis is a fish borne trematode that triggered foodborne disease, namely, clonorchiasis, to occur. The transmission of this parasite to humans is mostly through the consumption of raw freshwater fish. In a study by Bouvard et al. (2009), they mentioned that *C. sinensis* is categorized as a group I bio-carcinogen by the International Agency for Research on Cancer (IARC) of the WHO. Clonorchiasis is mostly ubiquitous in countries and regions of Asia, including South Korea, China, northern Vietnam, and far-eastern Russia (Lun et al., 2005; Rim, 2005; Qian, Chen, & Yan, 2013). Fully-grown worms of *C. sinensis* can occupy bile ducts for 20–25 years, and at the early stage of the infection, there are no noticeable clinical symptoms that often lead to overlooked diagnosis (Lun et al., 2005). Additionally, clonorchiasis is typically falsely diagnosed due to its generic symptoms, which include fatigue, inappetence, nausea, bellyache, jaundice, and hepatosplenomegaly (Qian et al., 2013). Clonorchiasis can be remedied meritoriously with praziquantel (PZQ) on immediate, accurate diagnosis, and exact species identification (Choi et al., 2003).

Cryptosporidiosis

A minimum of 23 species of *Cryptosporidium* have been recognized; however, the *Cryptosporidium parvum* is the only one to be considered as an etiologic agent of human infection. Transmission of *C. parvum* (Type II), which is commonly zoonotic, had been discovered to be abundant in many mammals, predominantly livestock. The majority of the first outbreaks of cryptosporidiosis have been closely associated with contaminated drinking water (MacKenzie et al., 1994). However, oocysts have also been retrieved from food, such as fresh vegetables and seafood as well as the possibility of transmission of *C. parvum* through human contacts. Subsequently, after infection, immunocompetent individuals might suffer from diarrhea, which typically lasts less than a fortnight. In immunodeficient or immunosuppressed individuals, diarrhea may be profuse and can result in significant morbidity and mortality due to disturbance of water and electrolytes (Centers for Disease Control and Prevention, 2015), specifically in AIDS patients. Immunodeficient patients are also more likely to have lymphomatic bile and pancreatic duct as well as lung infections (Lopez & Pardo, 2010).

Cyclosporiasis

Cyclospora cayetanensis is a coccidian protozoan parasite that recognized as pathogens that cause intestinal illness and other gastrointestinal symptoms (Bern et al., 2002). The cases reported due to foodborne illness concerning *Cyclospora cayetanensis* has totaled to 14,638 cases and is 0.1% of foodborne deaths cases caused by imported fresh products (Hikal & Said-Al Ahl, 2017). According to Ortega, Sterling, Gilman, Cama, and Diaz (1993), *Cyclospora cayetanensis* requires a period to sporulate into the infectious form, thus decreases the possibility of the direct spread between person-to-person. There are also cases of higher severity and duration of Cyclosporiasis on people with high-risk illnesses such as HIV, AIDS, and cancer. Major causes and risk factors for cyclosporiasis are such as the consumption of contaminated water or products (Hoge et al., 1993). Food products contaminated by *Cyclospora cayetanensis* will bring side effects such as diarrhea to the person consuming it. Higher susceptibility to *Cyclospora cayetanensis* may be due to individuals that are raising domestic animals, especially poultry by rural migrants with less exposure towards the danger of cyclosporiasis to their health (Bern et al., 2002). Prolonged exposure to this parasite may cause clinical manifestations such as prolonged diarrhea, nausea, abdominal cramps, anorexia, and weight loss (Ortega et al., 1997).

Diphyllobothriasis

Diphyllobothriasis is come mainly from the infection of the adult tapeworm of the genus Diphyllobothrium, specifically, *D. latum*. This species is the longest tapeworm to be found in humans that causes the disease (Rohela, Jamaiah, Chan, & Wan Yusoff, 2002). The human can suffer from diphyllobothriasis by consuming the infected fish product as most of the tapeworms were found in the flesh of the fish. The presence of diphyllobothriasis is mainly due to the development of plerocercoid larvae into an adult worm in the small intestine of the host, which consequently causes the immature operculated eggs to be discharged into the feces (Rohela et al., 2002). Subsequently, the transmission is more reliable when consuming raw materials or uncooked products. This disease can be detected by examining the presence of heavy proglottids in humans' feces where infected patients will display typical operculated eggs after the rupturing the heavy proglottids. Proglottid is the organ that presents in the tapeworm, which functions to attach to the host. Symptoms that were discovered in this disease were anemia, slightly abdominal pain, diarrhea, and vomiting as diphyllobothriasis causes the prevention of the absorption of vitamin B12 by the host that is responsible in regulating body's metabolism; the effective treatment is done by giving drugs which are known as PZQ or antihelminthic. PZQ drug prevents newly hatched insect larvae from multiply in the body (Rohela et al., 2002).

Fascioliasis

Fascioliasis is a parasitic disease affected by genus Fasciola, with *F. hepatica*, which uses freshwater snails of the family lymnaeidae as transitional hosts (Jennifer, Dirk, Gottfried, & Jürg, 2005). However, most patients were being infected by the consumption of water. Fascioliasis can be noticed based on the presence of Fasciola eggs in a stool or gallbladder sample from the patients as well as a positive serological test outcome. The two stages of this disease include acute fascioliasis and chronic fascioliasis. The acute fascioliasis punctured the liver capsule and initiated to migrate towards the biliary system. The relocation of larva effects damage in the inflammatory response, fever, and increases quadrant pain. As for the chronic fascioliasis, it will cultivate biliary obstruction, frank cholangitis, and pancreatitis symptoms. Saba et al. (2004) reported that the most symptoms experienced by patients that are infected with fascioliasis are commonly fatigue, fever, nausea, abdominal and body pains myalgia, arthralgia, weight loss, sweating pruritus, and cough. One of the treatments prepared to treated fascioliasis is by giving triclabendazole drugs. This drug enables in the prevention of protein synthesis, especially cathepsin L cysteine proteases that were released from the *F. hepatica* to attack its host (Jennifer et al., 2005).

Giardiasis

Giardiasis is one of the most common causes of diarrheal illness wide-reaching. It is an intestinal disease that affected by a flagellated protozoan parasite called *Giardia lamblia*, which can also be termed as *G. intestinalis* and *G. duodenalis*. Protozoan infections outbreak in humans has been reported to have a relation with raw fruits and vegetables. This is because food handler as the potential source of *Giardia lamblia* and raw sliced vegetables in epidemiological evidence has implicated an asymptomatic of transmission in an outbreak of Giardiasis (Mintz, Hudson-Wragg, Mshar, Cartter, & Hadler, 1993). Giardia transmission happened through the ingestion of the infective cyst stage shed in human or animal feces.

Consequently, water, food, or fomites might be fecally contaminated by the cyst present. The symptoms of the giardiasis are usually as well as diarrhea, flatulence, abdominal pain, and bloating (Ali & Hill, 2003). While according to research, the possibility of weight loss can be occurred because of malabsorption of nutrients on the bloodstream (Nygård et al., 2006). Commonly, the antibiotics used in the treatment of giardiasis are 5-Nitroimidazoles (5-NIs), which include metronidazole, tinidazole, secnidazole, and ornidazole. Specific alternative agents such as quinacrine, furazolidone, benzimidazole, paromycin, bacitracin zinc, chloroquine, and nitazoxanide are rarely used in the treatment of giardiasis (Gardner & Hill, 2001).

Nanophyetiasis

Nanophyetiasis is a disease caused by parasitic trematode name *Nanophyetus salmincola,* which infects salmonid fishes in freshwaters initially reported in the Pacific Northwest (Millemann & Knapp, 1970). The fully-grown worm lives mostly in the intestine of mammals, which are due to eating fish. Eggs shelter into the water by the host hatch into miracidia, which breaches the first intermediate host in one of two species of a snail named *Juga plicifera* or *J. silicula*. The snail has reproduced asexually then consequential in the progress of miracidia into redia then cercaria. Grown-up cercaria develops from the snail and pierce the piscine secondary intermediate host. The cercaria then encysts as metacercariae in several organs of the fish, such as in the gills, body's muscle, heart, and mainly in the posterior kidney (Millemann & Knapp, 1970). After being encysted, this metacercariae commonly will be survived the ocean phase in the salmonid life succession. *Nanophyetus salmincola* is the most probable cause of death to immature Coho Salmon *O. kisutch* during the early ocean-rearing phase (Jacobson, Teel, Van Doornik, & Casillas, 2008), and it is one of the most prevalent pathogens of out-migrating Chinook Salmon in estuaries throughout the Pacific Northwest (Arkoosh et al., 2004).

Opisthorchiasis

It has been noted that opisthorchiasis is a disease caused by *Opisthorchis viverrini* or known as liver fluke. In many cases that involved with tumor, it was found that liver fluke is the primary factor (Kurathong et al., 1985). This liver fluke infection has been widely spread in Thailand and Laos, it is also has been the leading public health problem there, and the concern has risen among the people (Sripa et al., 2011). Usually, those people who have been infected with *O. viverrini* will have abdominal pain, nausea, and diarrhea. Since *Opisthorchis viverrini* is the parasite worm; thus, it needs a host to stay alive. In this case, *O. viverrini* used fishes as their host. In an investigation of Opisthorchiasis and Opisthorchis-associated cholangiocarcinoma in Thailand and Laos, Sripa et al. (2011) reported the main factor of infection to occur, is because of those infected villagers had consumed raw fish or undercooked fish. Fish need to be fully cooked to kill all the parasites and bacteria. Lacking high temperatures in cooking will let them alive inside their host (fish).

Paragonimiasis

Paragonimiasis is an infectious disease caused by worm parasites such as *Paragonimus westermani* or known as lung fluke. *Paragonimus* has over more than 40 species, and *Paragonimus westermani* is the most common species in Asia. In another study of Paragonimiasis in the United States (A Report of Nine Cases in Hmong Immigrants) by (Johnson, Falk, Iber, & Davies, 1982), people who are having paragonimiasis will have few symptoms such as cough, hemoptysis, fever, dyspnea, pleurisy, and weight loss. The infections arise when a person consumed raw crustaceans that containing metacercariae and also eating the meat of paratenic hosts such as a pig. This is how the parasites were transmitted to the human body by staying in the host. Eating raw or uncooked meat is not a good habit, and it is crucial to cook them before consumption. In a study, stated that triclabendazole is the most effective drug for the treatment of Paragonimiasis (Keiser, Engels, Büscher, & Utzinger, 2005).

Taeniasis and cysticercosis

Taeniasis and cysticercosis are interrelated diseases that are infected by parasites of the tapeworm group. *Taenia saginata* sp. and *Taenia asiatica* sp. host only on animals, whereas *Taenia solium* sp. hosts mainly in humans, but in some cases, they have reported to harbor mammals like dogs and bear as their intermediate hosts. The *T. solium* usually causes taeniasis in humans after the ingestion of undercooked pork that has been infected by cysticerci (García, Gonzalez, Evans, Gilman, & Cysticercosis Working Group in Peru, 2003). The life cycle of a Taenia involves two mammal hosts at a time. It is also how Taeniasis occurs. The adult of *T. solium* may live in human intestines for more than 20 years, and their eggs multiply daily and are passed out through feces. When an intermediate host accidentally consumes these, the eggs grow into larvae, which is also known as (cysticerci) which will be deposited in the muscles. When human consumes these raw or undercooked beef or pork, the larvae are transmitted into their intestines where they eventually grow into adult worms. Some of the symptoms that may be faced by the patient with taeniasis is having an abnormal appetite, abdominal pain, diarrhea, or constipation.

One of a widespread case is when adult worms can also carry cysticercosis, whether directly or through contaminated food or water, which indicates the fecal-oral transmission. Furthermore, untreated urban sewage sludge can cause cysticercosis in cattle or hogs, whereas untreated human waste that has *T. solium* eggs could cause cysticercosis in humans (Doyle, 2003). However, the most severe stage of this disease is when the larvae reach the brain, where the term is known as neurocysticercosis. The symptoms of this disease are frequent headaches, seizures, and other neurological symptoms. This is the primary parasitic disease that occurs in the central nervous system. There is also cysticercosis that can occur outside the nervous system; however, they do not cause any significant symptoms. There will be small, movable, and painless nodules present in arms or chest and irritate but will gradually disappear. Lastly, ophthalmic cysticercosis is not very common, where it may cause visual disturbance and damage to the retinal tissue (García et al., 2003).

Toxoplasmosis and congenital toxoplasmosis

Toxoplasma gondii, which is a parasite that leads to this illness called toxoplasmosis, is a protozoan parasite that can be found in cat feces where the cats also eliminate oocysts in them. This disease can infect humans through the ingestion of the oocytes through contaminated food such as vegetables and even contaminated water. It also can be transmitted from raw meat and unpasteurized milk. The oocysts can sustain for a long time and can be spread by the wind and even insects and earthworms, which contaminate the soil (Doyle, 2003). Children who got this disease will show some symptoms of sore throat, mild flu, and myalgia (Kalyoussef & Feja, 2014). Congenital toxoplasmosis often transmits to the fetus in pregnant women, especially during the first pregnancy through the penetration of the placenta. Maternal diagnosis can be detected by serological screening, or the unusual condition of the fetus can be shown through ultrasound scanning (Bollani, Strocchio, & Stronati, 2013). This disease can cause abortion, causing blindness to the infant after birth and even resembles congenital infections such as rubella and herpes (Bollani et al., 2013). For infected pregnant women, the treatment can be done by giving them spiramycin, while for the fetus, pyrimethamine, sulfadoxine, and folinic acid can be given to the baby after birth. Infants who had vision loss because of hemorrhage need to undergo photodynamic therapy (Khan & Khan, 2018). Prevention is also essential where the separation of cats from the storage of food like vegetables and animals is made to avoid unwanted contamination. Cat litter should be managed well and thrown in enclosed garbage so that it will not be exposed to any areas near the water supply or reservoir.

Trichinellosis

Trichinellosis is caused by the ingestion of Trichinella larvae that are encysted in muscle tissue of meat from domestic or wild animals (Gottstein, Pozio, & Nöckler, 2009). Pathological mechanisms of lesions in trichinellosis are complex and relate to both developments of two generations of *Trichinella* sp. in the host and immunopathological events initiated by antigens released by the parasite (Koci, 2000). Some of the primary sources for *Trichinella* sp. include pigs, foxes, bears, and wild boars. The epidemiology of this disease is strongly associated with the consumption of raw or undercooked meat; thus, traditional dishes made with raw and undercooked meats are some of the factors by which this disease is widely transmitted (Gottstein et al., 2009). According to Gottstein et al. (2009), trichinellosis symptoms would be nonspecific such as uneasiness, headache, headache, fever that would last for 1–3 weeks depends on the severity and occasionally gastrointestinal illnesses. There are some methods to reduce the possibility of this disease to spread, such as cooking, freezing, irradiation, and curing, to inactivate the *Trichinella* sp. (Gamble et al., 2004).

Extraction methods

The extraction process is vital before the detection methods to proceed. The extraction method of nematodes is compulsory to detect the presence of anisakis species further. Nematode extraction varies in methods and has its limitations and advantages. Nematodes not only can be found in fish but also soil and plants. Nematology is the science of identifying and determining the kinds of nematodes available in the environment. Generally, anisakis species can be found in crustaceans and vertebrates, for example, fish as well as soils of plants. Extraction procedure or process can be done by either using naked eyes or involving DNA extraction of the target. Consideration must be taken in terms of size, density, and motility of the nematodes to separate them from plant tissue and soil particles (Luc, Sikora, & Bridge, 2005). The most common body parts available and used to extract nematodes are the larvae. The larvae are commonly found in the fish body cavity (Dzido, Kijewska, & Rokicki, 2012).

DNA extraction

DNA extraction is the process where DNA is separated from proteins, membranes, and other cellular material (Butler, 2012). According to Rice (2018), the method involves three necessary steps, namely, lysed, precipitation, and purification. The first step is lysed to break down the cells so the DNA in the nucleus will be released after the cell membrane is disrupted. The second step is precipitation. To get pure DNA, the DNA will be separated from proteins and other cells component by degrading the DNA and protein with ethanol or isopropanol. The next step is purification. At this stage, DNA is no longer precipitate with the aqueous phase, and DNA can be redissolved with water to ease the handling process and storage. Genomic DNA from individual nematode larvae of various types of fishes infected with anisakis species was extracted by the method of SDS/proteinase K treatment. Next, the DNA extracted was purified using DNA clean-up columns. Lastly, the purified DNA was eluted into $50\,\mu L$ ddH$_2$O and kept at $-20°C$ (Fang et al., 2010). According to Seesao et al. (2017), DNA extraction methods using Nucleobond Column (NC) and Wizard Genomic (WG) have great results in extracting nematodes DNA technique. Both methods correspondingly produce better results extracting smaller size and complex cuticle structure fish species that are infected with anisakis. However, comparing these two methods, WG has a higher yield of extracted DNA, and NC was better in removing solvent traces due to the anion-exchange resin. The extraction of nematodes DNA may as well use the QIAamp DNA Mini Kit according to the manufacturer's instructions. Extracted DNA is eluted in elution buffer and kept at $-20°C$ (Umehara, Kawakami, Araki, & Uchida, 2008).

Dissection method

The extraction of nematode can apply dissection method that is usually that extracted by dissecting and observing under a microscope. This method involves visible nematodes and is commonly used in plant material. The sample needs to be washed and placed in a water-filled petri dish, followed by dissecting using dissecting needles and forceps under the microscope with 15–50 × magnification. Handling a needle or paintbrush can be used to pick the larvae or eggs of the new nematode.

Furthermore, detecting nematodes can be done by staining the sample, but the mobility of nematodes can vanish (Van Bezooijen, 2006). This method was applied in a study by Cabrera et al. (2018) dissection method or sectioning to visualize host–parasite structure before microscopic observation from the plant. However, nematodes viscous eggs were extracted without involving the dissection method. Nematode's length observed using eyepiece micrometer after dissection method was applied to some of Galleria larvae (Akhurst, 1980). The larvae were dissected in water to estimate the number of nematodes available from agitated suspension. Bait insect dissection method was included to compare with the other two methods in terms of extraction and infectivity measures in a study by Hass, Griffin, and Downes (1999). The recovery of nematodes from soil using dissection method of bait insect in this study is 19.8% and stated as the least efficient method to extract infective juveniles (IJ) from the soil compared to the other two methods due to depending on the capability of IJ to infect bait insects.

Funnel spray method

Funnel spray methods principal is the importance of nematode mobility and sedimentation rate, which commonly applied in plant material. The apparatus used to extract nematodes in this method is identified as a mist chamber or mystifier. Different plant sample sizes and nematodes size uses a different diameter of the funnel. Extraction of nematode happens in this method when infected plant material is moistened in water, nematodes in the plant material will crawl out and sink. The apparatus includes 16 Baermann funnels (10 cm diameter) that are placed in a supporting frame under a spray nozzle. The constant supply of mist of fine water droplets is provided to avoid oxygen depletion (Van Bezooijen, 2006). According to Van Bezooijen (2006), some advantages of funnel spray methods are high efficiency, solid proofs that nematodes keep crawling out from the infected plant materials, and yield of nematodes in better condition due to the accumulation of microorganisms and oxygen depletion are prevented. However, disadvantages of this method are such as continuous water supply, hard to keep away from algae and fungi, and can affect the air humidity in the room. Examples of nematodes that can be extracted from this method are endoparasites such as *Hirschmanniella, Radopholus*, and *Bursaphelenchus* that will emerge and can be found at the bottom of the dish (Luc et al., 2005). A past study was done by researchers Brinkman, Duyts, Karssen, van der Stoel, and van der Putten (2015) on plant-feeding nematodes. By using the funnel spray method, nematodes extraction was extracted from roots that have been separated from the soil. It was processed for 48 h. Following (Bongers, 1988), nematodes characterized as plant feeding were the only ones to identify and calculate according to their genus and group of species.

Blender nematode filter method

The extraction of nematode using this method is by making use of nematode mobility. The homogenized sample using a domestic blender is placed on a nematode filter that is placed in a shallow water-filled tray. Nematodes are expected to move out of materials and into the water. The maximum size sample depends on the type of material used, and frequently only a few tens of grams can be extracted at once. This method uses less time compare to other methods and more effective due to the large surface of the tray used to extract nematodes. Disadvantages are that this method is more labor exhaustive and causes rapid decomposition of plants used to extract nematode that releases toxic wastes to the nematode that could cause nematode to die (Van Bezooijen, 2006). Some nematodes that are suitable to be extracted using this method are *Hirschmanniella* spp., *Radopholus similis*, *Nacobbus aberrans*, and other endoparasites (Hallmann & Viaene, 2013). This method was used in a study by Kanagy and Kaya (1996) to find out the possible role of marigold roots and $\propto$ − terthienyl in mediating host-finding by nematode *Steinernema carpocapsae*. The aqueous root extracts of tomato and marigold were prepared using this method before the nematodes were applied. Entomopathogenic nematodes functions may be inhibited by the presence of $\propto$ − terthienyl in the soil can be concluded resulted from this study.

Blender centrifugal flotation method

This extraction method can extract active and inactive nematodes from plant materials. Similar to the blender nematode filter method, the extraction sample yield only a few tens of grams at once. This method uses the specific gravity application between nematodes and other elements in the sample. Nematodes will float in extraction fluid that has a higher specific gravity, and the other element or particles will sink. The centrifugation process is to increase the rate of the separation process. This method enables the extraction of inactive and active nematodes. Besides, a short time needed to do extraction compared to other methods. However, the equipment used for this method is expensive, and the extraction fluid may affect the nematode shape (Van Bezooijen, 2006). According to Favoreto et al. (2018), on the research of plant pathogenic nematodes named *Aphelenchoides* besseyi, the blender centrifugal flotation method is used to process leaves and stems samples in approximately 10 g. Aphelenchoides is a derived genus from nematodes that were extracted at new tissue densities of 41 specimens in the experiment. In their research, each specimen was gathered, then they were narcotized inside distilled water along with slight heat.

Cobb's decanting and sieving method

Cobb's decanting and sieving method is an extraction method used when the sample was mixed with soil or sediment (Van Bezooijen, 2006). The purpose of this method is to discard rock or any unwanted particles before proceeding to further analysis. To separate the nematodes from soil or sediment, the sample obtained will be stirred, decanted, and sieved. Those nematodes will remain on sieves; however, those tiny particles will pass through. In this method, the sieves process is carried out several times with different sizes of mesh. The reason is to gather all the nematodes at different sizes separately. Once the process is done, nematodes will be transferred through the filter to water and decanted as an apparent suspension once extraction time is over. There is research that used Cobb's decanting and sieving in their research. It is about the efficiency of the extraction of meiofauna from sandy and muddy sediments. In the research, they were mixing samples manually with tap water and decanted immediately. The process was repeated for 10 times. While for muddy sediments, two sets were prepared and were labeled as method 1 and method 2. Method 1 is involving with decanting samples, while for method 2 it demands more time compared to the first method (Armenteros, García, Angulo, & Williams, 2011). At this rate, the researcher was preferred more on method 1. This method was also applied in a study of a method for estimating numbers of eggs of *Meloidogyne* spp. by Byrd, Ferris, and Nusbaum (1972). The study found that eight egg masses that were extracted and aliquots processed has obtained $12,259 \pm 864$ mean egg counts.

Baermann funnel method

Baermann funnel is a device designated to extract nematode from soil and plant. For the sample size, it varies since it depends on the diameter of funnel and type of material used. The principle used by the Baermann Funnel method is when an infected plan is placed into the water, the nematodes will crawl out (Van Bezooijen, 2006). Thus, the methods are likely more for the mobility of nematodes. In previous research of modification of the centrifugal-flotation technique for the isolation and concentration of nematodes and their eggs from the soil and plant tissue, one of the extraction methods used is the Baermann Funnel method. According to Caveness and Jensen (1955), the Baermann Funnel method has yielded the highest numbers for both eggs compare to other methods, but not for nematodes from plant tissue as the yield number is higher and more precise by using another method. The method is straightforward and cheapest method compare to others. However, many nematodes are dead during the process because of insufficient oxygen at the bottom caused the accumulation of metabolic corrects and microorganisms.

Oostenbrink elutriator

Nematodes are not only can be found in seafood, plant, and soil. It also can make liver silt, manure, litter, and other substrates as their host. Oostenbrink Elutriator method is a method that can be used to the harbor and wash the nematodes into suspension. However, the method is depending on the sample type and size (Van Bezooijen, 2006). In the Oostenbrink Elutriator, it will make nematodes and fine particles floating at the extraction column because of the upwards water stream. The more massive particles will be sat at the bottom of the apparatus. In the extraction column, the suspension is decanted through the side-outlet, and the fine particles were sieved out. That debris can be placed on the nematodes filter once done wash. Once the extraction time is over, nematodes can be decanted as an apparent suspension. Previous studies have reported that the Oostenbrink method has the least loss of nematodes amount compare to other methods, as the nematodes can be isolated from the soil without losing the number of nematodes. It may lose but in a small amount, like 5% though the sample is large (Verschoor & De Goede, 2000).

Detection methods

The conventional detection method is known for an innovative approach for parasite detection, especially in contaminated food products rather than the usual uses of agar plate for analyzing viable parasite or bacteria. Most conventional detection methods have few limitations that drawback to its reliability, novelty, and cost; the novelty indicates the detection of the parasite of interest that are continually being reported; conventionally, there is few rapid and sensitive conventional detection method which include mass spectrometry, ultrasonic testing, PCR, and UV transillumination that are quite often used to detect parasite as it has its specificity towards certain parasites (Gracias & McKillip, 2004).

Mass spectrometry

Mass spectrometry can be used to detect parasites through the accessibility of parallel reaction monitoring (PRM) of the peptide from the parasites. Parallel reaction monitoring is responsible for analyzing the existence of ion traps mass. For instance, each precursor ion noticed will react to the major charge state of the ion; thus, by tracing the ions transition for every peptide biomarkers in SEQUEST-HT searching, it is manageable to discover the existence of parasite (Mónica, José, Santiago, Ángel, & Isabel, 2016). Consequently, peptide biomakers are referred to as the selection of proteins from the parasite species based on its resistance towards heat. The selection of proteins undergoes an extraction method where the strains of protein were heated up for an equivalent range of time at different temperatures. For example, the proteins that are corresponded to SXP/RAL-2 protein family were selected to evaluate the presence of anisakis parasite; this is because SXP/RAL-2 protein specifically belongs to Anisakis spp. (Mónica et al., 2016). It appears that most parasite has a heat resistant characteristic which may be the cause of its presence in food products.

Equivalence to this detection method, Mónica et al. (2016) reported that monitoring for at least four peptide biomakers from the parasites through parallel reaction monitoring in a linear ion trap mass spectrometry allows in accelerating the detection. *P. falciparum* detection using mass spectrometry, the mass spectrometry chooses 1 to 3 stages of proteome analysis, which identifies 714 proteins in asexual blood stages, 931 and 645 in gametocytes and gametes stages, respectively. Both in gametocytes and gametes stage provide insights into the biological sexual stage of *P. falciparum* that include secreted and membrane-associated with proteins. The subset of protein may consist of domains that aid in the role in cell interaction indication. During the analysis, the result attained a typical gametocyte extraction revealed that most of the *P. falciparum* and red blood cell (RBC) proteins were existing in the soluble fraction. In contrast, membrane proteins such as the gametocyte of specific cell surface protein happen to be Pfs48/45 that indicates the presence of *P. falciparum*. The well-characterized, sexual stage-specific surface antigen, Pfs48/45 highlighted in the analysis. The assimilation of the peptide ion currents and a quantity coarsely proportional to the molar amount of peptide species generated a protein abundance ratio of more than eight between the two stages. Thus, the mass spectrometry used to indicate the presence of *P. falciparum* is dependent on its ionic condition (Mann et al., 2002).

Ultrasonic testing

Ultrasonic testing is a method where it will look into the thickness of the internal structure, usually intestine with the aid of high-frequency sound waves. The ultrasonic method may be useful as parasites often select its breeding place in the host's intestine; the presence of parasites, for instance, the presence of Anisakis spp. in the intestinal wall cause tissue impairment due to the invasion of the gut wall which leads to the acute abdomen (Caramello et al., 2003). Additionally, the acute abdomen takes place due to the involvement of terminal ileum that intersects small intestine with large intestine together. Often ultrasonic method reveals bloody abdominal fluid closed to the abdominal region; bloody fluid abdomen are the cause of thickening in the ileum (Caramello et al., 2003). Based on the previous study on patients that were diagnosed with parasite *C. sinensis* infection by Mei et al. (2016), ultrasonic testing was used to examine the thickness of the internal cell wall. The larger the thickness concludes that there were cells that were infected by the parasite. This is because, during the infection development of *C. sinensis*, the immunological balance exists between the host and the parasite; the parasitic infection will activate Th2 which produces cytokines IL-6 that inhibit the immunocompetence of macrophage activation and leads to internal body damage; since the IL-6 mediate autoimmune response against the liver cell, it causes thickening in the cell wall (Mei et al., 2016). *C. sinensis* infection may lead to changes of protein cell and caspase-3 in the apoptotic pathway as well or also known as the irregular condition of cells' death;

the programmed cell death will destroy the liver functional mechanism as the parasite may produce a morbid substance that may be the apoptosis signal to stimulate the liver cells apoptosis and lead to liver damage such as the change of the serum enzyme as well as cell wall thickening (Mei et al., 2016).

Polymerase chain reaction (PCR)

PCR is a type of molecular method of detection where it undergoes molecular hybridization. It uses a specific primer-probe as it was able to recognize the specific complementary DNA sequence or known as target DNA. The probe often uses oligonucleotide primers, which generally contain 20 base pairs. In the reaction, PCR experience repeated cycle that is initiated from exposing heat to double strain of DNA that cause denaturing, followed by annealing of primer through cooling the mixture and lastly elongation of DNA by Taq polymerase; the results obtained will be detected by gel electrophoresis for visual identification (Bhunia, 2018; McMeekin, 2003; Simjee, 2007). The detection conducted through the presence of fragments restriction. Research by Lopez and Pardo (2010), to detect *Anisakis simplex* was done based on the evaluation of a real-time PCR. This method was successfully conducted, and the detection of the nematode was able to be done. However, there is a limitation to the utilization of this method in detecting allergen produced by nematodes as the amount of allergen must be in the range of the threshold levels. Thus, the detection limits for various food products have to be in between the range of 1 to 100 ppm depending upon the type of food (Poms, Klein, & Anklam, 2004). Chen et al. (2018) also utilized PCR further molecular identification in the detection of ascaridoid parasites in *Conger myriaster*, whereby through PCR analysis, the six ascaridoid larval types classified herein were identified genetically as nine species. This marine species is commonly available in fish markets in Asian countries, especially Korea and Japan, where the consumption of sashimi or raw fish is very much favored (Choi et al., 2003).

UV transillumination

UV transillumination is a fast detection method that can be used to observe the presence of parasites in fishery products. The original method which was used by Karl and Leinemann (1993), was altered for this method of detection to be conducted is as follows: (1) At 30°C, saline solution with the ratio of 1:5 *w/v* was added to the samples. It was homogenized for 1–2 min by using a stomacher, (2) The homogenate was pressed to a thickness of 5 mm and examined in a dark room under UV light at 366 nm. Upon treatments applied to the samples, the larvae were still intact, and it can be observed that the parasites will appear to bluish-white fluorescence (Levsen & Lunestad, 2010). In 2006, Dixon proposed the procedures of isolating and identifying of roundworms in fish by using transillumination with UV. However, this method is found to have drawbacks as it is more laborious and expensive, and it is not applicable to be used in the analysis of processed products. However, research by Celano, Paparella, Fransvea, Balzaretti, and Celano (2013), suggested that UV transillumination a rapid and reliable method to detect Anisakis in fish when compared to other methods.

Conclusion

This chapter brings significant value to the study of instruments application along with the knowledge of the previous study gathered by a lot of researchers and scientists. Even though conventional techniques are deliberated as reliable standard methods, they took a long time and complicated process. A proper inspection must be made either before or after food production has done. The inspection must be made not only over-processed food products but also towards raw material products to ensure its quality. The food industry could also strengthen its regulations in processing foods to provide safe, nutritious, and high in quality foods. This step can be considered by the food industry actors when they are well aware and exposed to the whole truth related to the significance of detection methods of parasites and its harmful effects on food products. Therefore, new techniques are necessary to be introduced to overcome these weaknesses in conventional techniques and improved properties in experimental research.

References

Adams, A. M., Murrell, K. D., & Cross, J. H. (1997). Parasites of fish and risks to public health. *Revue Scientifique et Technique (International Office of Epizootics)*, *16*(2), 652–660. https://doi.org/10.20506/rst.16.2.1059.

Akhurst, J. R. (1980). Morphological and functional dimorphism in Xenorhabdus spp., bacteria symbiotically associated with the insect pathogenic nematodes neoaplectana and heterorhabditis. *Microbiology*, 303–309. https://doi.org/10.1099/00221287-121-2-303.

Akuthota, P., & Weller, P. F. (2012). Eosinophils and disease pathogenesis. *Seminars in Hematology*, *49*(2), 113–119. https://doi.org/10.1053/j.seminhematol.2012.01.005.

Ali, S. A., & Hill, D. R. (2003). Giardia intestinalis. *Current Opinion in Infectious Diseases*, *16* (5), 453–460. https://doi.org/10.1097/00001432-200310000-00012.

Armenteros, M., García, J. P., Angulo, A. P., & Williams, J. P. (2011). Efficiency of extraction of meiofauna from sandy and muddy marine sediments. *Revista de Investigaciones Marinas*, *29*(2), 113–118.

Arkoosh, M. R., Clemons, E., Kagley, A. N., Stafford, C., Glass, A. C., Jacobson, K., Reno, P., Myers, M. S., Casillas, E., Loge, F., & Johnson, L. L. (2004). Survey of pathogens in juvenile salmon *Oncorhynchus* spp. migrating through Pacific Northwest estuaries. *Journal of Aquatic Animal Health*, *16*(4), 186–196. https://doi.org/10.1577/H03-071.1.

Audicana, M. T., Ansotegui, I. J., De Corres, L. F., & Kennedy, M. W. (2002). Anisakis simplex: Dangerous—Dead and alive? *Trends in Parasitology*, *18*(1), 20–25. https://doi.org/10.1016/S1471-4922(01)02152-3.

Bern, C., Ortega, Y., Checkley, W., Roberts, J. M., Lescano, A. G., Cabrera, L., … Gilman, R. H. (2002). Epidemiologic differences between cyclosporiasis and cryptosporidiosis in peruvian children. *Emerging Infectious Diseases*, *8*(6), 581–585. https://doi.org/10.3201/eid0806.01-0331.

Bhunia, A. K. (2018). *Foodborne microbial pathogens: Mechanisms and pathogenesis.* Springer.

Bollani, L., Strocchio, L., & Stronati, M. (2013). Congenital toxoplasmosis. *Early Human Development*, *89*, S70–S72.

Bongers, A. M. T. (1988). De Nematoden van Nederland (Pirola, Schoorl, The Netherlands). *Natuurhistorische Bibliotheek van de KNNV*,(46).

Bouree, P., Paugam, A., & Petithory, J. C. (1995). Anisakidosis: Report of 25 cases and review of the literature. *Comparative Immunology, Microbiology and Infectious Diseases*, *18*(2), 75–84. https://doi.org/10.1016/0147-9571(95)98848-C.

Bouvard, V., Baan, R., Straif, K., Grosse, Y., Secretan, B., El Ghissassi, F., Benbrahim-Tallaa, L., Guha, N., Freeman, C., Galichet, L., & Cogliano, V. (2009). A review of human carcinogens—Part B: Biological agents. *The Lancet Oncology*, *10*(4), 321. https://doi.org/10.1016/s1470-2045(09)70096-8.

Brinkman, E. P., Duyts, H., Karssen, G., van der Stoel, C. D., & van der Putten, W. H. (2015). Plant-feeding nematodes in coastal sand dunes: Occurrence, host specificity and effects on plant growth. *Plant and Soil*, *397*(1–2), 17–30. https://doi.org/10.1007/s11104-015-2447-z.

Butler, J. M. (2012). Chapter 2—DNA extraction methods. In *Advanced topics in forensic DNA typing*. Maryland: Elsevier.

Byrd, D. W., Jr, Ferris, H. O. W. A. R. D., & Nusbaum, C. J. (1972). A method for estimating numbers of eggs of *Meloidogyne* spp. in soil. *Journal of Nematology*, *4*(4), 266.

Cabrera, J., Olmo, R., Ruiz-Ferrer, V., Abreu, I., Hermans, C., Martinez-Argudo, I., … Escobar, C. (2018). A phenotyping method of giant cells from root-knot nematode feeding sites by confocal microscopy highlights a role for CHITINASE-LIKE 1 in Arabidopsis. *International Journal of Molecular Sciences*, *19*(2), 429. https://doi.org/10.3390/ijms19020429.

Caramello, P., Vitali, A., Canta, F., Caldana, A., Santi, F., Caputo, A., … Balbiano, R. (2003). Intestinal localization of anisakiasis manifested as acute abdomen. *Clinical Microbiology and Infection*, *9*(7), 734–737. https://doi.org/10.1046/j.1469-0691.2003.00660.x.

Carrion, M. N., Hamer, D. H., & Evans, D. (2016). Parasitic diseases, an overview. In *International encyclopedia of public health* (pp. 399–408). United States: Elsevier Inc. https://doi.org/10.1016/B978-0-12-803678-5.00241-1.

Caveness, F. E., & Jensen, H. J. (1955). Modification of the centrifugal flotation technique for the isolation and concentration of nematodes and their eggs from soil and plant tissue. *Proceedings of the helminthological society of Washington: Vol. 22*, (pp. 87–89).

Celano, G. V., Paparella, A., Fransvea, A., Balzaretti, C., & Celano, G. (2013). Rapid method for detection of anisakidae larvae in marine fishes, based on UV transillumination. *Biochemistry and Bioinformatics*, *3*(4), 392–394.

Centers for Disease Control and Prevention (2015). *Parasites-cyclosporiasis (cyclospora infection)*.

Chen, M. F., O'Neill, S. M., Carey, A. J., Conrad, R. H., Stewart, B. A., Snekvik, K. R., Ylitalo, G. M., & Hershberger, P. K. (2018). Infection by *Nanophyetus salmincola* and toxic contaminant exposure in out-migrating steelhead from Puget Sound, Washington: Implications for early marine survival. *Journal of Aquatic Animal Health*, *30*(2), 103–118. https://doi.org/10.1002/aah.10017.

Choi, P., Hur, J. W., Lim, J. H., Lee, J. Y., Kim, D. W., Park, M. I., Park, S. J., Chang, H. K., Oh, K. S., & Koo, J. Y. (2003). A case of gastric submucosal tumor suspected to be caused by Anisakis. *Clinical Endoscopy, 27*(1), 26–30.

Cisak, E., Zając, V., Sroka, J., Sawczyn, A., Kloc, A., Dutkiewicz, J., & Wójcik-Fatla, A. (2017). Presence of pathogenic rickettsiae and protozoan in samples of raw milk from cows, goats, and sheep. *Foodborne Pathogens and Disease, 14*(4), 189–194. https://doi.org/10.1089/fpd.2016.2203.

Das, A. K. (2014). Hepatic and biliary ascariasis. *Journal of Global Infectious Diseases, 6*(2), 65–72. https://doi.org/10.4103/0974-777X.132042.

Dawson, D. (2005). Foodborne protozoan parasites. *International Journal of Food Microbiology, 103*(2), 207–227. https://doi.org/10.1016/j.ijfoodmicro.2004.12.032.

De Campos-Pereira, M., Bahia-Labruna, M., Szabó, M. P. J., & Marcondes-Klafe, G. (2008). Rhipicephalus (Boophilus) microplus biologia, controle e resistência. In *Primeira edição. São Paulo. Editorial MedVet.*

Doyle, M. E. (2003). *Foodborne parasites: A review of the scientific literature.* UW-Madison: Food Research Institute.

Dzido, J., Kijewska, A., & Rokicki, J. (2012). Selected mitochondrial genes as species markers of the Arctic Contracaecum osculatum complex. *Journal of Helminthology.* https://doi.org/10.1017/S0022149X11000332 Poland.

EFSA Panel on Biological Hazards (BIOHAZ) (2010). Scientific opinion on risk assessment of parasites in fishery products. *EFSA Journal, 8*(4), 1543.

Evancho, G. M., Tortorelli, S., & Scott, V. N. (2009). Microbiological spoilage of canned foods. *Compendium of the microbiological spoilage of foods and beverages* New York, NY: Springer, pp. 185–221. https://doi.org/10.1007/978-1-4419-0826-1_7.

Fang, W., Xu, S., Zhang, S., Wang, Y., Chen, X., & Luo, D. (2010). Multiple primer PCR for the identification of anisakid nematodes from Taiwan Strait. *Experimental Parasitology, 124*(2), 197–201. https://doi.org/10.1016/j.exppara.2009.09.011.

Favoreto, L., Faleiro, V. D. O., Freitas, M. A., Brauwers, L. R., Galbieri, R., Homiak, J. A., Lopes-Caitar, V. S., Marcelino-Guimarães, F. C., & Meyer, M. C. (2018). First report of *Aphelenchoides besseyi* infecting the aerial part of cotton plants in Brazil. *Embrapa Soja-Nota Técnica/Nota Científica (ALICE), 102*(12), 2662.

Fratini, F., Turchi, B., Pedonese, F., Pizzurro, F., Ragaglini, P., Torracca, B., … Nuvoloni, R. (2016). Does the addition of donkey milk inhibit the replication of pathogen microorganisms in goat milk at refrigerated condition? *Dairy Science and Technology, 96*(2), 243–250. https://doi.org/10.1007/s13594-015-0249-y.

Gamble, H. R., Pozio, E., Bruschi, F., Nöckler, K., Kapel, C. M. O., & Gajadhar, A. A. (2004). International commission on trichinellosis: Recommendations on the use of serological tests for the detection of Trichinella infection in animals and man. *Parasite, 11*(1), 3–13. https://doi.org/10.1051/parasite/20041113.

García, H. H., Gonzalez, A. E., Evans, C. A., Gilman, R. H., & Cysticercosis Working Group in Peru (2003). Taenia solium cysticercosis. *The Lancet, 362*(9383), 547–556. https://doi.org/10.1016/S0140-6736(03)14117-7.

Gardner, T. B., & Hill, D. R. (2001). Treatment of giardiasis. *Clinical Microbiology Reviews, 14*(1), 114–128. https://doi.org/10.1128/CMR.14.1.114-128.2001.

Gebrie, M., & Engdaw, T. A. (2015). Review on Taeniasis and its zoonotic importance. *European Journal of Applied Sciences, 7*(14), 182–191. https://doi.org/10.5829/idosi.ejas.2015.7.4.96169.

Gottstein, B., Pozio, E., & Nöckler, K. (2009). Epidemiology, diagnosis, treatment, and control of trichinellosis. *Clinical Microbiology Reviews*, *22*(1), 127–145. https://doi.org/10.1128/CMR.00026-08.

Gracias, K. S., & McKillip, J. L. (2004). A review of conventional detection and enumeration methods for pathogenic bacteria in food. *Canadian Journal of Microbiology*, *50*(1), 883–886.

Hallmann, J., & Viaene, N. (2013). Nematode extraction: PM 7/119 (1). *OEPP/EPPO Bulletin*, *43*, 471–495.

Hass, B., Griffin, C. T., & Downes, M. J. (1999). Persistence of heterorhabditis infective juveniles in soil: Comparison of extraction and infectivity measurements. *Journal of Nematology*, *31*(4), 508–516.

Helminthiases, W. S. T. (2012). *Eliminating soil-transmitted helminthiases as a public health problem in children: progress report 2001–2010 and strategic plan 2011–2020*: (pp. 19–29). France: World Health Organization.

Hikal, W. M., & Said-Al Ahl, H. A. (2017). Food related parasitic infection: A review. *American Journal of Food Science and Health*, *3*(2), 30–34.

Hoge, C. W., Echeverria, P., Shlim, D. R., Rajah, R., Shear, M., Rabold, J. G., & Triplett, J. (1993). Epidemiology of diarrhoeal illness associated with coccidian-like organism among travellers and foreign residents in Nepal. *The Lancet*, *341*(8854), 1175–1179. https://doi.org/10.1016/0140-6736(93)91002-4.

Hung, C. C., Chang, S. Y., & Ji, D. D. (2012). Entamoeba histolytica infection in men who have sex with men. *The Lancet Infectious Diseases*, *12*(9), 729–736. https://doi.org/10.1016/S1473-3099(12)70147-0.

Jacobson, K. C., Teel, D., Van Doornik, D. M., & Casillas, E. (2008). Parasite-associated mortality of juvenile Pacific salmon caused by the trematode Nanophyetus salmincola during early marine residence. *Marine Ecology Progress Series*, *354*, 235–244. https://doi.org/10.3354/meps07232.

Jennifer, K., Dirk, E., Gottfried, B., & Jürg, U. (2005). Triclabendazole for the treatment of fascioliasis and paragonimiasis. *Expert Opinion on Investigational Drugs*, 1513–1526. https://doi.org/10.1517/13543784.14.12.1513.

Johnson, J. R., Falk, A., Iber, C., & Davies, S. (1982). Paragonimiasis in the United States. A report of nine cases in Hmong immigrants. *Chest*, *82*(2), 168–171. https://doi.org/10.1378/chest.82.2.168.

Jourdan, P. M., Lamberton, P. H. L., Fenwick, A., & Addiss, D. G. (2018). Soil-transmitted helminth infections. *The Lancet*, *391*(10117), 252–265. https://doi.org/10.1016/S0140-6736(17)31930-X.

Kalyoussef, S., & Feja, K. N. (2014). Foodborne Illnesses. *Advances in Pediatrics*, *61*(1), 287–312. https://doi.org/10.1016/j.yapd.2014.04.003.

Kanagy, J. M. N., & Kaya, H. K. (1996). The possible role of marigold roots and α-terthienyl in mediating host-finding by steinernematid nematodes. *Nematologica*, *42*(2), 220–231. https://doi.org/10.1163/004325996X00066.

Karl, H., & Leinemann, M. (1993). A fast and quantitative detection method for nematodes in fish fillets and fishery products. *Arch Lebensmittelhyg*, *44*(5), 124–125.

Keiser, J., Engels, D., Büscher, G., & Utzinger, J. (2005). Triclabendazole for the treatment of fascioliasis and paragonimiasis. *Expert Opinion on Investigational Drugs*, *14*(12), 1513–1526. https://doi.org/10.1517/13543784.14.12.1513.

Khan, K., & Khan, W. (2018). Congenital toxoplasmosis: An overview of the neurological and ocular manifestations. *Parasitology International*, *67*(6), 715–721. https://doi.org/10.1016/j.parint.2018.07.004.

Khuroo, N. S., & Khuroo, M. S. (2010). Gastric ascariasis presenting as unique dyspeptic symptoms in an endemic area. *American Journal of Gastroenterology*, *105*(7), 1675–1677. https://doi.org/10.1038/ajg.2010.112.

Kniel, K. E., Lindsay, D. S., Sumner, S. S., Hackney, C. R., Pierson, M. D., & Dubey, J. P. (2002). Examination of attachment and survival of toxoplasma gondii oocysts on raspberries and blueberries. *Journal of Parasitology*, *88*(4), 790–793. https://doi.org/10.1645/0022-3395(2002)088[0790:EOAASO]2.0.CO;2.

Koci, W. (2000). Trichinellosis: Human disease, diagnosis and treatment. *Veterinary Parasitology*, *93*(3–4), 365–383. https://doi.org/10.1016/S0304-4017(00)00352-6.

Kurathong, S., Lerdverasirikul, P., Wongpaitoon, V., Pramoolsinsap, C., Kanjanapitak, A., Varavithya, W., … Brockelman, W. Y. (1985). Opisthorchis viverrini infection and cholangiocarcinoma. A prospective, case-controlled study. *Gastroenterology*, *89*(1), 151–156. https://doi.org/10.1016/0016-5085(85)90755-3.

Levsen, A., & Lunestad, B. T. (2010). Anisakis simplex third stage larvae in Norwegian spring spawning herring (Clupea harengus L.), with emphasis on larval distribution in the flesh. *Veterinary Parasitology*, *171*(3–4), 247–253. https://doi.org/10.1016/j.vetpar.2010.03.039.

Liu, T., Wang, Y., Luo, X., Li, J., Reed, S. A., Xiao, H., … Schultz, P. G. (2016). Enhancing protein stability with extended disulfide bonds. *Proceedings of the National Academy of Sciences of the United States of America*, *113*(21), 5910–5915. https://doi.org/10.1073/pnas.1605363113.

Lopez, I., & Pardo, M. A. (2010). Evaluation of a real-time polymerase chain reaction (PCR) assay for detection of anisakis simplex parasite as a food-borne allergen source in seafood products. *Journal of Agricultural and Food Chemistry*, *58*(3), 1469–1477. https://doi.org/10.1021/jf903492f.

Lothar, L. (2000). Basic aspects of food preservation by hurdle technology. *International Journal of Food Microbiology*, 181–186. https://doi.org/10.1016/s0168-1605(00)00161-6.

Luc, M., Sikora, R. A., & Bridge, J. (2005). *Plant parasitic nematodes in subtropical and tropical agriculture*: (pp. 1–871) (2nd ed.). France: CABI Publishing.. Retrieved from *http://bookshop.cabi.org/*.

Lun, Z. R., Gasser, R. B., Lai, D. H., Li, A. X., Zhu, X. Q., Yu, X. B., & Fang, Y. Y. (2005). Clonorchiasis: A key foodborne zoonosis in China. *Lancet Infectious Diseases*, *5*(1), 31–41. https://doi.org/10.1016/S1473-3099(04)01252-6.

MacKenzie, W. R., Hoxie, N. J., Proctor, M. E., Gradus, M. S., Blair, K. A., Peterson, D. E., … Davis, J. P. (1994). A massive outbreak in Milwaukee of Cryptosporidium infection transmitted through the public water supply. *New England Journal of Medicine*, *331*(3), 161–167. https://doi.org/10.1056/NEJM199407213310304.

Mann, M., Ishihama, Y., Andersen, J. S., Vermunt, A. M. W., Pain, A., Sauerwein, R. W., … Stunnenbergt, H. G. (2002). Analysis of the plasmodium falciparum proteome by high-accuracy mass spedrometry. *Nature*, *419*(6906), 537–542. https://doi.org/10.1038/nature01111.

Mattiucci, S., Cipriani, P., Levsen, A., Paoletti, M., & Nascetti, G. (2018). Molecular epidemiology of Anisakis and Anisakiasis: An ecological and evolutionary road map. *Advances in parasitology* (pp. 93–263). Vol. 99(pp. 93–263). Italy: Academic Press. https://doi.org/10.1016/bs.apar.2017.12.001.

Detecting pathogens in food. McMeekin, T. A. (Ed.), (2003). Elsevier.

Mei, F., Lin, L., Chun, S., Mei, X., Ji-Mei, D., Pei, L., … Yan-Bing, F. (2016). Ultrasonic diagnosis of patients with clonorchiasis and preliminary study of pathogenic mechanism. *Asian*

Pacific Journal of Tropical Medicine, 694–697. https://doi.org/10.1016/j.apjtm.2016.05.009.

Millemann, R. E., & Knapp, S. E. (1970). Biology of nanophyetus salmincola and "Salmon poisoning" disease. *Advances in Parasitology*, *8*(C), 1–41. https://doi.org/10.1016/S0065-308X(08)60250-X.

Mintz, E. D., Wragg, M. H., Mshar, P., Cartter, M. L., & Hadler, J. L. (1993). Foodborne giardiasis in a corporate office setting. *Journal of Infectious Diseases*, *167*(1), 250–253. https://doi.org/10.1093/infdis/167.1.250.

Mónica, C., José, M. G., Santiago, P., Ángel, F. G., & Isabel, M. (2016). Protein biomarker discovery and fast monitoring for the identification and detection of Anisakids by parallel reaction monitoring (PRM) mass spectrometry. *Journal of Proteomics*, 130–137. https://doi.org/10.1016/j.jprot.2016.05.012.

Mossali, C., Palermo, S., Capra, E., Piccolo, G., Botti, S., Bandi, C., … Giuffra, E. (2010). Sensitive detection and quantification of anisakid parasite residues in food products. *Foodborne Pathogens and Disease*, *7*(4), 391–397. https://doi.org/10.1089/fpd.2009.0428.

Nieuwenhuizen, N. E., & Lopata, A. L. (2013). Anisakis—A food-borne parasite that triggers allergic host defences. *International Journal for Parasitology*, *43*(12 − 13), 1047–1057. https://doi.org/10.1016/j.ijpara.2013.08.001.

Nieuwenhuizen, N., Lopata, A. L., Jeebhay, M. F., Herbert, D. R., Robins, T. G., & Brombacher, F. (2006). Exposure to the fish parasite Anisakis causes allergic airway hyperreactivity and dermatitis. *Journal of Allergy and Clinical Immunology*, *117*(5), 1098–1105. https://doi.org/10.1016/j.jaci.2005.12.1357.

Nygård, K., Schimmer, B., Søbstad, Ø., Walde, A., Tveit, I., Langeland, N., Hausken, T., & Aavitsland, P. (2006). A large community outbreak of waterborne giardiasis-delayed detection in a non-endemic urban area. *BMC Public Health*, *6*(1), 141. https://doi.org/10.1186/1471-2458-6-141.

Ortega, Y. R., Nagle, R., Gilman, R. H., Watanabe, J., Miyagui, J., Quispe, H., … Sterling, C. R. (1997). Pathologic and clinical findings in patients with cyclosporiasis and a description of intracellular parasite life-cycle stages. *Journal of Infectious Diseases*, *176*(6), 1584–1589. https://doi.org/10.1086/514158.

Ortega, Y. R., Sterling, C. R., Gilman, R. H., Cama, V. A., & Diaz, F. (1993). Cyclospora species—A new protozoan pathogen of humans. *New England Journal of Medicine*, *328*(18), 1308–1312. https://doi.org/10.1056/NEJM199305063281804.

Poms, R. E., Klein, C. L., & Anklam, E. (2004). Methods for allergen analysis in food: A review. *Food Additives and Contaminants*, *21*(1), 1–31 https://doi.org/10.1080/02652030310001620423.

Qian, M. B., Chen, Y. D., & Yan, F. (2013). Time to tackle clonorchiasis in China. *Infectious Diseases of Poverty*, *2*(1).

Rice, G. (2018). DNA extraction. Retrieved from: https://serc.carleton.edu/microbelife/research_methods/genomics/dnaext.html (Retrieved 27 October 2018).

Rim, H. J. (2005). Clonorchiasis: An update. *Journal of Helminthology*. https://doi.org/10.1079/JOH2005300 South Korea.

Rockland, I. B., & Nishi, S. (1980). Fundamental of water activity. *Food Technology*, *34*, 42–59.

Rohela, M., Jamaiah, I., Chan, K. W., & Wan Yusoff, W. S. (2002). Diphyllobothriasis: The first case report from Malaysia. *Southeast Asian Journal of Tropical Medicine and Public Health*, *33*(2), 229–230.

Ruff, M. D. (1999). Important parasites in poultry production systems. *Veterinary Parasitology*. https://doi.org/10.1016/S0304-4017(99)00076-X United States.

Saba, R., Korkmaz, M. E. T. I. N., Inan, D., Mamikoğlu, L., Turhan, Ö., Günseren, F., Cevikol, C., & Kabaalioğlu, A. (2004). *Human fascioliasis*, *10*(5), 385–387. https://doi.org/10.1111/j.1469-0691.2004.00820.x.

Seesao, Y., Gay, M., Merlin, S., Viscogliosi, E., Aliouat-Denis, C. M., & Audebert, C. (2017). A review of methods for nematode identification. *Journal of Microbiological Methods*, *138*, 37–49. https://doi.org/10.1016/j.mimet.2016.05.030.

Shirley, D. A. T., Farr, L., Watanabe, K., & Moonah, S. (2018). *A review of the global burden, new diagnostics, and current therapeutics for amebiasis. Open forum infectious diseases: (Vol. 5)*. USA: Oxford University Presshttps://doi.org/10.1093/ofid/ofy161 No. 7, p. ofy161.

Simjee, S. (2007). *Foodborne diseases*. Humana Press.

Simpson, T. W. (1995). More on Angiostrongylus cantonensis infection. *The New England Journal of Medicine*, *333*(13), 882.

Sripa, B., Bethony, J. M., Sithithaworn, P., Kaewkes, S., Mairiang, E., Loukas, A., … Brindley, P. J. (2011). Opisthorchiasis and opisthorchis-associated cholangiocarcinoma in Thailand and Laos. *Acta Tropica*, *120*(1), S158–S168. https://doi.org/10.1016/j.actatropica.2010.07.006.

Sultan, K. M. (1996). ASCARIASIS. *Gastroenterology Clinics of North America*, 553–577. https://doi.org/10.1016/s0889-8553(05)70263-6.

Umehara, A., Kawakami, Y., Araki, J., & Uchida, A. (2008). Multiplex PCR for the identification of Anisakis simplex sensu stricto, Anisakis pegreffii and the other anisakid nematodes. *Parasitology International*, *57*(1), 49–53. https://doi.org/10.1016/j.parint.2007.08.003.

Utech, K. B. W., Wharton, R. H., & Kerr, J. D. (1978). Resistance to Boophilus microplus (Canestrini) in different breeds of cattle. *Australian Journal of Agricultural Research*, *29*(4), 885–895. https://doi.org/10.1071/AR9780885.

Van Bezooijen, J. (2006). *Methods and techniques for nematology (p. 20)*. Wageningen: The Netherlands: Wageningen University.

Van den Brom, R., Santman-Berends, I., Luttikholt, S., Moll, L., Van Engelen, E., & Vellema, P. (2009). Bulk tank milk surveillance as a measure to detect Coxiella burnetii shedding goat herds in the Netherlands between 2009 and 2014. *Journal of Dairy Science*, *98*(6), 3814–3825.

Verschoor, B. C., & De Goede, R. G. M. (2000). The nematode extraction efficiency of the Oostenbrink elutriator-cottonwool filter method with special reference to nematode body size and life strategy. *Nematology*, *2*(3), 325–342. https://doi.org/10.1163/156854100509204.

Wang, P., Li, R. Z., Huang, Z. Y., & Tang, C. W. (2013). Report on 16 cases of small intestine ascariasis diagnosed by capsule endoscopy. *Chinese Journal of Parasitology & Parasitic Diseases*, *31*(3), 242–243.

Biosensor technology to detect chemical contamination in food

Introduction

Food contamination can occur deliberately or inadvertently in foods and originate from several different sources such as naturally occurring toxicants (phytotoxins), bacterial contamination, the inappropriate usage of pesticides and veterinary drugs, and the addition of chemicals during processing techniques, as well as evolving chemical hazards. The pollution can influences food in three ways by physical, chemical, and microbiological as well as occurring at different stages, whether during collection, cleaning, processing, transporting, or even during storage. Hence, these food contaminations can lead to many severe illnesses and diseases, especially food-borne illnesses.

Microbiological contamination refers to non-intended or accidental infectious material, including bacteria, fungi, mold, and more. However, Salmonella and *Escherichia coli* are the most common examples of microbiological contamination, which regularly happen due *to the negligence of food handlers during* food preparation and processing, as well as from the consumer itself. For instance, when food is not adequately handled (stored and set at dangerous temperature), it may result in food spoilage due to the production of toxins.

Meanwhile, the physical contamination of food occurs at any stage of manufacture until the involvement of foreign materials (glass, metal components, hair, insects, and plastics) in food which generally can cause health hazards to the customer, where the contaminants may be introduced to foods due to negligence of food manufacturers or equipment.

Chemical contaminants are generally linked to agrochemical since the usage of fertilizers and pesticides is very widespread in this industry, and poses a significant public health issue when ingested by people. Recently, several cases have been recorded in the food industry, where fruits and vegetables have been polluted with pesticide residues. According to Nerín, Aznar, and Carrizo (2016), pesticide-infected food is possibly dangerous to human consumption because it can emit toxic substances or heavy metals such as arsenic, mercury, and lead, which are abundantly found in soil and water.

Therefore, a lot of research and methods have been performed to identify and prevent chemical contamination in foods, including high-performance liquid chromatography (HPLC), inductively coupled plasma mass spectrometry (ICP-MS),

127

Advanced Food Analysis Tools. https://doi.org/10.1016/B978-0-12-820591-4.00007-4

inductively coupled plasma atomic emission spectrometry (ICP-AES), atomic absorption spectrometry (AAS), and many more.

Biosensor technology has recently attracted the interest of many scientists in the food industry, where innovation and improvement in nanotechnology and biometrics schemes as well as materials boosting the biosensor market. Besides, this modern analytical method has provided many benefits for food analysis and also portable and straightforward to use to conduct the on-site detection for specified compounds.

Biosensor technology

IUPAC describes biosensors technology as an integrated receptor–transducer device capable of providing specific quantitative or semi-quantitative analytical data utilizing a biological recognition element. Biosensors are analytical devices used to detect specific analytes and have become the most widely researched discipline due to access, fast, low-cost, highly sensitive, and selective biosensors that lead to advancements in next-generation medicines such as individualized medicine and ultrasensitive point-of-care detection of markers for diseases.

Parkhey and Mohan (2019) defined biosensor was functionally composed of three components, namely, a biological element, a transducer, and electronic devices. The first component of the biosensor is called a biological element or also known as bioreceptor is responsible for sensing the analyte and producing a response signal. Then, the signal converted into the detectable response by the transducer, and eventually, the signal must be interpreted and amplifies by the detector before it is shown through the electronic device system. The steps for a biosensor process are pictorially represented in Fig. 7.1.

Throughout the decades, many biosensing technologies and similar devices have been established using the latest updated technology, and as well as promising monitoring and analytical methods with broad applications in clinical diagnosis, environmental research, food industry, and other fields where precise and rigorous analyses are primarily required. However, the most popular biosensors used today are home pregnancy tests and glucose detectors. Therefore, biosensors technology has been studied and developed to be used for the detection of different food components (food coloring, food additives, preservatives, and others), and toxicity biosensors may also be used to determine the risks of food pollution (Evtugyn, 2016).

Current status

In 1962, the first biosensor was invented, which consisted of an oxygen electrode modified with glucose oxidase and overlaying the Teflon membrane (Warriner, Reddy, Namvar, & Neethirajan, 2014). Since then, this technology has been further developed to enhance its capability and improve performance; thus, more target analyte can be discovered. The biosensor application is significant and has been

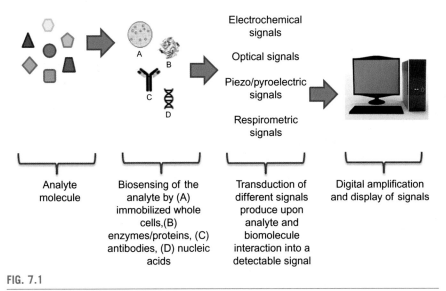

FIG. 7.1

The pictorial description for biosensor method.

implemented or applied in various fields especially in the food industry, as it is used to sustain food safety and quality, helping to distinguish between natural and artificial, shelf-life estimation, determining its safety, adulteration, and monitoring practice as well as in the fermentation industry.

Throughout the year, the biosensor technology has drawn interest and recognition from many food industries or companies as well as being accepted by academics to carry out their studies and also widely focused on healthcare and medical sector (monitoring glucose and lactose level, analytical measurement of folic acid, detection of molecular markers in real samples). Table 7.1 in the following section shows the example of analyte in determining food safety and quality.

Fundamentals and mechanism

Transducing elements, materials, and immobilization procedures are the manufacture of biosensors with a very high degree of scientific comprehension, notably in the fields of chemistry, biology, and engineering. According to Mehrotra (2016), there are three distinct groups of materials with different mechanisms are used in the biosensors process, including biocatalytic group (enzymes), bio affinity group (antibodies, and nucleic acids), and microbe-based containing microorganisms.

The biological recognition element is one of the components of the biosensor technology that is connected to electronic transducer devices (piezoelectric, optical, or physicochemical). The biochemical receptor immobilizes biological elements (nucleic acids, antibodies, proteins, enzymes, DNA, or whole cells) to the target

Table 7.1 Example of analyte in determining food and safety.

Purpose	Class	Example	Example food matrix/regulatory limit	References
Food safety	Bacteria	*Clostridium botulinum*	Low acid vacuum-packed foods/ Negative for growth within shelf-life of the product	Augustin (2011)
		Escherichia coli O157: H7	Beef trim/negative in 375 g sample	Bosilevac, Guerini, Brichta-Harhay, Arthur, and Koohmaraie (2007)
		Listeria monocytogenes	Deli meat/negative in 25 g sample	Crowley et al. (2014)
		Salmonella	Peanut butter/ Negative in 25 g sample	Lindhardt et al. (2010)
		Staphylococcus aureus	Yogurt/two out of five samples to have no more than 100 CFU/g	Anonymous (2005)
	Fecal indicators	Fecal coliforms	Water/negative in 100 mL sample	Anonymous (2012a)
		Escherichia coli	Lettuce/negative in 25 g sample	Anonymous (2012b)
		Enterobacteriaceae	Dried milk/one out of 5 samples permitted to have no more than 100 CFU/g	Anonymous (2007)
	Mycotoxins	Toxoplasma	No regulatory limit at this time	Berthiller et al. (2014), Tothill (2011)
		Aflatoxin	15 mg/kg	
		Deoxynivalenol	2 mg/kg	
		Fumonisin	2 mg/kg	
		Orchratoxin	0.2 mg/kg	
		Patulin	0.5 mg/kg	
		HT-2 toxin	0.025 mg/kg	
	Allergens	Peanut	15 mg/kg	Faeste, Roenning, Christians, and Granum (2011)
		Egg	15 mg/kg	
		Soy	15 mg/kg	
		Gluten	20 mg/kg	
		Sulfites	10 mg/kg	

Table 7.1 Example of analyte in determining food and safety—cont'd

Purpose	Class	Example	Example food matrix/regulatory limit	References
	Pesticides	Methyl bromide	Spices 400 mg/kg	Desmarchelier and Ren (1999)
		Picoxystrobin	Barley 0.2 mg/kg	Mikulikova, Svoboda, and Belakova (2008)
		Pinoxaden	Grain 0.01 mg/kg	Anonymous (2013)
	Virus	Norovirus	No regulatory limit at this time	N/A
		Rotavirus	No regulatory limit at this time	N/A
		Advenovirus	No regulatory limit at this time	N/A
	Protozoan	Cyclospora	No regulatory limit at this time	N/A
		Cryptosporidium	No regulatory limit at this time	N/A
Shelf-life	N/A	TMAO Oxygen	Not applicable	N/A
		Xanthine	Not applicable	N/A
Fermentation	N/A	Glucose	Not applicable	N/A
		Ethanol	Not applicable	N/A

Note: Regulatory limits may differ between geographical jurisdictions.

analyte, including antigens, substrates, enzyme-substrate complexes, and others. The transducer-connected receptor that converts the biochemical signals to the electrical and optical signal and then records the electronic device. The electrical signal generation may indicate the concentration of the analyte (Patra, Mahato, & Kumar, 2019).

Toxicological elements and risks analysis of biosensors
Different types of biosensor

There are numerous type of biosensor that can be used for the detection process, as shown in Table 7.2.

Mechanism of toxicity effects

Nowadays, many chemicals can be classified as dangerous substances as it is lead to a broad variety of toxicity cases (soil, water, and air) and also can create other environmental issues that may occur in the structure of the material. This toxic chemical

Table 7.2 Types of biosensors.

Biosensors	Description
Enzyme-based biosensor	Based on immobilization techniques that involve enzymes (oxidases, amino oxidases, polyphenol oxidases, oxidoreductases, and peroxidases) that are adsorbed using ionic bonding, van der Waals forces or covalent bonding
Microbe-based or cell-based biosensor	The sources of these sensors are from plant and animal, and the targeted analyte can serve as a substrate or inhibitor of these methods
Organelle-based biosensor	Sensors are made from intercellular components (mitochondria, chloroplasts, membranes, and microsomes) with high stability, longer detection time, and low specificity
Immunosensors biosensor	The mechanism of these sensors is based on the affinity of antibodies towards its particular antigens. For instance, the interaction of antibodies with the components in the host's immune system occurs when it is bound explicitly to particular contaminants or pathogens
DNA biosensor	Based on the recognition of single-strand nucleic acid and binding characteristics to its corresponding strand in a given sample. The interaction occurs when the stable hydrogen bond is formed between the two strands of nucleic acids
Magnetic biosensor	It is based on the principles of magnetoresistance effect with specific sensitivity and size for the nanoparticle detection in the microfluidic medium
Thermal or calorimetric biosensor	Assimilation of biosensor components into a physical transducer
Optical biosensor	Involved light sources and an abundance of optical materials to generate a light beam with specific features. The light is then transmitted to a modulating agent (the type of modified sensing head), which is connected to the photodetector

can, in particular, change the structure of biological processes as well as impair development and reproduction processes (Hassan, Van Ginkel, Hussein, Abskharon, & Oh, 2016). Table 7.3 shows the summarization of the mechanism for toxicity effects in fish, plants, and bacteria.

Factors that influence toxicity

A biosensor is one of the best tools for measuring the toxicity of materials as it provides a simple and accurate indicator of toxicity relative to traditional approaches. According to Hassan et al. (2016), toxic chemicals can exert a cumulative and synergistic impact on the development of microorganisms. Table 7.4 shows the details and summarization of five selected toxicity factors.

Table 7.3 List of the mechanism of toxicity effects.

Organisms	Types of species	Mechanism of toxicity effects
Fish	Zebrafish embryos	Larval growth and survival
	Fathead minnow	Mortality and motility
	Bluegill	Cell division and differentiation
	Salmonids	ATP levels
Plants	Chinese cabbage	Micronucleus production, genotoxicity
	Oats	Germination rate, biomass weight, enzymatic activity
	Vicia faba	
Bacteria	Nitrifying bacteria	The capacity of microorganisms to transform carbon, nitrogen, and sulfur enzymatic and microbial growth mortality, glucose uptake activity, respiration
	Nitrobacter	
	Nitrosomonas	

Table 7.4 The factors of toxicity.

Toxicity factors	Description
Form of materials	The form of materials may have a profound effect on its toxicity, particularly in the case of metallic materials, which are known as heavy metals. For example, the toxicity of mercury vapor differs significantly from methyl mercury and Chromium Cr3+ is nontoxic, whereas Cr6+ induces skin or nasal corrosion and lung cancer
Inhale chemical activity	The activity of natural chemicals often differs significantly which some can easily damage cells and cause instantaneous cell death, whereas others slowly interact with a cell's activity. For instance, the hydrogen cyanide binds to the enzyme cytochrome oxidase, causes cellular hypoxia and rapid death. Besides, the Nicotine binds to cholinergic receptors in the central nervous system (CNS), affects nerve conduction, and creates a slow onset of paralysis
Dosage	It is necessary to describe if the substance is acute or chronic toxicant. Logically, a large number of doses can cause acute toxicants. As an example, the toxicant effects for ethanol and arsenic are liver cirrhosis and skin/liver cancer, respectively. Also, excessive use of ethanol cause CNS depression while a high amount of arsenic consumption cause gastrointestinal damage
Exposure route	There are two significant routes exposure including ingestion and inhalation which differences in absorption and distribution within the body. The ingestion route, it is ingested specified chemicals, when absorbed from intestines, migrate first to the liver and can be detoxified instantly. Secondly, inhalation route, inhaled toxicants directly enter the general blood circulation and may disperse throughout the body until being detoxified by the liver

Continued

Table 7.4 The factors of toxicity—cont'd

Toxicity factors	Description
Absorption	Some chemical is easily absorbed, and some are partially absorbed. For instance, nearly all alcohols are readily consumed when ingested while the rates and extent of absorption can vary based on the type of the chemical and the route of exposure. For example, ethanol is easily consumed from the gastrointestinal tract but poorly absorbed through the skin but organic mercury is quickly absorbed from the gastrointestinal tract, but inorganic lead sulfate is not
Life span	An individual's age or life stage can be essential when determining his or her reaction towards toxicants as certain chemicals are more toxic to infants and the elderly compared to young adults

Application of biosensor technology in detection of chemical residues in food

Food safety and quality are crucial to the food industry because they are directly tied to human well-being. For instance, the pollutions from several sources, including pesticide residues, toxins, veterinary drug residues, hazardous food additives, or even migrating substances from packaging materials, can be found in food when handled carelessly or without adequate protection. Therefore, compared to the other recent analytical tool, biosensor technology is the most effective approach for detecting the presence of pollutants in food matrices with less time consuming, low cost, and portable detectors as well as real-time and in situ analysis.

Pesticides residues

Pesticides are widely used in the agricultural industry to destroy pests and weeds, however, the excessive use of these substances may contaminate crops by releasing their residues into the environment, which is then consumed by soil and water. This phenomenon has had a significant impact on food safety, quality, and cause foods not safe to consume. Thus, there are a variety of methods that have been introduced to tackle these problems but due to its minimum cost, accessible and high sensitivity, and less time-consuming process, biosensors have been the preferable approach compare to the conventional method like HPLC, ICP-MS, and GC–MS.

An enzyme-based biosensor is one of the biosensor techniques widely utilized by food scientists. Zhang, Arugula, Wales, Wild, and Simonian (2015) developed a rapid and straightforward approach with high specificity for pesticide residues analysis using inhibition of acetylcholine esterase (AChE). AChE hydrolyzed acetylthiocholine to thiocholine when immobilized on the electrode surface, and the oxidation peak was observed on the detection system.

Meanwhile, Oliveira et al. (2013) used enzyme biosensor analysis for carbamate-pesticides. The immobilization of the enzyme *Trametes versicolor* laccase was conducted on the graphene-doped carbon-paste electrode modified with Prussian blue films. The principle of this approach was based on the inhibition of laccase and 4-aminophenol activity.

Besides, Wei and Wang (2015) as well as Liu and Wei (2014) developed a detection system for organophosphorus pesticides using a boron-doped diamond electrode, and the electrode was designed using platinum-carbon aerogels (Pt-CAs) composites. The electron transfer rate increased, and the interfacial resistance decreased due to the usage of reinforced Pt-CAs, which raised the reactive surface area of the electrode. The inhibition of organophosphorus pesticides shows its concentration in the analyzed sample. However, the biosensor methods for pesticides identification in food matrices are summarized in Table 7.5.

Heavy metals

Heavy metals are well-known for their toxicity and ability to accumulate in the aquatic organism and even induce cancer owing to their carcinogenic properties (Rajeshkumar et al., 2018). According to Liang et al. (2016), overexposure to heavy metals such as consuming tainted food (seafood, fish) with heavy metals is vulnerable to adverse effects, including cause major cardiac problems, which at worst can cause death. Therefore, the biosensor is the most suitable device to apply for the identification of heavy metals in food matrices.

Besides, Chouteau et al. (2005) experimented to detect the existence of heavy metals by using a conductometric biosensor that uses the alkaline-phosphatase enzyme as a biorecognition element whereas heavy metals act as enzyme inhibitors. Then, the change in pH and conductivity was perceived by condumetric transducer in the presence of heavy metals and alkaline-phosphatase enzymes.

Bienzymatic biosensor method was created by Nadèje et al. (2014) by immobilizing the *Arthrospira platensis* species cell on the gold transducer. The principle of this approach was the phosphatase, and esterase activities were impaired in the presence of heavy metals and pesticides in the sample. However, the inhibition activities at various concentrations of heavy metals were then measured to determine the amount produced in the sample.

Besides, Tortolini et al. (2014) and Liu et al. (2015) created a method for the identification of mercury ion utilizing a DNA biosensor. The principle method used was the formation of complex thymine-Hg-thymine (T-Hg-T), which is produced when the mercury ions attach to the two thymines, causing the elevated peak of faradic current to be detected by the square-wave voltammetry. Meanwhile, in another study by Liu et al. (2015), cuprous oxide (Cu_2O), nanochitosan composites, and thymine-rich ssDNA are used to create a DNA biosensor while the detection process was performed by electrochemical impedance spectroscopy.

Other than that, the optic biosensors were successfully carried out by Li et al. (2015) for mercury ions detection. During this process, Graphene quantum dots with high conductivity and $CdTe@SiO_2$ quantum dots were used for the biosensor

Table 7.5 Types of biosensors for the detection of various residues

Residues	Target molecule	Immobilization steps	Biorecognition elements	Type of transducers	References
Pesticides	Paraxon	GCE/MWCNT-polyethyleneimine (PEI)/MWCNT-DNA/OPH + AChE	Enzyme	Electrochemical	Zhang et al. (2015)
	Carbofuran	Graphene doped carbon-paste electrode (GPE)/PB/laccase	Enzyme	Electrochemical	Oliveira et al. (2013)
	Methamidophos Monocrotophos	Boron doped diamond (BDD)/Pt-carbon aerogels (Pt-CAs)/AChE	Enzyme	Electrochemical	Liu and Wei (2014)
	Methyl parathion	FCE/NiNPs-CGR-NF/AChE-Chi/NF	Enzyme	Electrochemical	Yang, Wang, Liu, and Wang (2013)
Heavy metals	Cadmium ion	Sensor chips/Si$_3$N$_4$ layer/BSA	Enzyme	Electrochemical	Chouteau, Dzyadevych, Durrieu, and Chovelon (2005)
	Mercury ion	Graphene quantum dots	Chemical	Optic	Li, Wang, Ni, and Kokot (2015)
	Cadmium ion	Au/poly(allylamine hydrochloride)-coated	Cell	Electrochemical	Tekaya et al. (2014)
	Mercury ion	Au/2-mercaptoethanol/thiolated oligonucleotide/thymine/Hg^{2+}/thymine	DNA	Electrochemical	Tortolini et al. (2014)
	Mercury ion	Au/Cu$_2$O + nanochitosan (Cu$_2$O@NCs)-ssDNA	DNA	Electrochemical	Liu et al. (2015)
Food additives	Monosodium glutamate	Oxygen electrode/polypropylene film/L-glutamate oxidase (L-GLOD) + L-glutamate dehydrogenase (L-GLDH)	Enzyme	Electrochemical	Basu, Chattopadhyay, Roychudhuri, and Chakraborty (2006)
	Propyl gallate (PG)	Graphite-Teflon-tyrosinase-composite electrodes	Enzyme	Electrochemical	Morales et al. (2005)
	Benzoic acid	GCE/CaCO$_3$ nanomaterials/tyrosinase	Enzyme	Electrochemical	Shan et al. (2008)
	Nitrite	GCE/HRP/(ZnCrABTS)-catalase/(ZnAlCl)	Enzyme	Electrochemical	Chen (2008)
	Amaranth Ponceau 4R	GCE/CNT-ppy	Chemical	Electrochemical	Wang et al. (2015)

construction and resulted in a low detection limit was recorded. Therefore, the types of biosensor for heavy metals detection are summarized in Table 7.5.

Migrating substances from packaging materials

Proper packaging is capable of fulfilling all the essential functions of food packaging, including containment, protection, communication, and marketing into the product (Fuertes et al., 2016). Besides, the quality of the products or materials inside the packaging is entirely secure, not easily migrated to food (when it is subjected to any changes in condition), and can prevent any unintended harm from happening via the preservation process.

Bisphenol A or generally known as BPA is one of the materials that make up the packaging system (plastics and resins) and is mostly used in containers or water bottles to keep food and beverages in good condition. However, Liu, Liu, and Liu (2016) established an aptamer-based electrochemical biosensor for identification of BPA in the food packaging system by immobilizing gold nanoparticles (AuNPs) onto a glassy carbon electrode (GCE) surface. Besides, the thiolate-modified BPA aptamer was self-assembled to GCE, and the Au—S bond was formed. The components of the probe used in this process were streptavidin-modified horseradish peroxidase-functionalized gold nanoparticle (avidin-HRP-AuNP). In the presence of hydrogen peroxide, H_2O_2, the reaction will involve the oxidation of hydroquinone (HQ) and a rise in the concentration of BPA as the amounts of avidin-HRP-AuNP decreased. Also, Alam and Deen (2020) developed an electrochemical sensor for BPA detection in water using graphene oxide and β-cyclodextrin-functional multiwalled carbon nanotubes. The suggested electrochemical sensor may be convincing to design a simple cost-effective water quality monitoring system.

Endocrine-disrupting compounds (EDC) is a hazardous migrating substance comprising of NonylPhenols (NP), BisPhenol A (BPA), and phthalates (Vandermarken et al., 2019) which may impact human safety even at a shallow dose but has not been included in regulation as it is not widely discovered. Typically, these chemicals can be found in paperboard packaging, where it is potential to transfer or pass the chemicals into food and often used for the packaging of dried food products.

Besides, Vandermarken et al. (2019) developed a method using ERE-CALUX (Estrogen Responsive Elements Chemically Activated Luciferase Gene Expression) biosensor to investigate the migration of EDC from paperboard packaging into the foods. Throughout this research, the biosensor was focused on a human breast carcinoma cell line that carrying the ER-responsive luciferase reporter gene and is conducted by measuring the overall estrogenic activity, including both known and unknown estrogenic chemicals. Also, this method can identify the safeness of the paperboard as a recycled commodity.

Toxins

Toxins are secondary metabolites that primarily originated from fungi species (*Penicillium* and *Aspergillus)* that can contaminate foods such as fruits, nuts, cereal, beans, and many more. The presence of toxins in foodstuff is undoubtedly a severe health threat for humans and animals due to the carcinogenic and mutagenic properties. To detect the toxins in various food samples and matrices, a different type of biosensors is used, as shown in Table 7.6.

Daly et al. (2000) successfully detect the aflatoxin B1 by using the commercial surface plasmon resonance (SPR) sensor, which carried out based on a competitive inhibition immunoassay. Meanwhile, the development of the SPR sensor was done by Choi, Chang, Lee, Kim, and Chun (2009) for zearalenone detection, and the sensor system was used by using the molecular imprinting polymer method.

Table 7.6 Detection of toxins in various food matrices with different types of biosensors.

Types of biosensor	Toxins	Matrix	References
Electrochemical	Citrinin, Microcystin-LR, Aflatoxins (AFB1, T2, HT-2, AFMI)	Rice, lake water, corn, barley, grapes, milk	Arévalo, Granero, Fernández, Raba, and Zón (2011), Wang et al. (2009), Piermarini, Volpe, Micheli, Moscone, and Palleschi (2009), Vidal et al. (2013), Owino et al. (2008) and Bacher, Pal, Kanungo, and Bhand (2012)
	Staphylococcal enterotoxin B	Watermelon juice, apple juice, soy milk, pork	Tang, Tang, Su, and Chen (2010)
	Ricin	Milk, vegetable soup, tomato juice	Chai, Lee, and Takhistov (2010)
	Botulinum neurotoxin type A	Full and skim milk	Liu et al. (2014)
	Staphylococcal enterotoxin B	Milk	Chen (2008)
Electrochemical immunosensor	Fumonisin Deoxynivalenol, nivalenol Zearalenone Alternariul, alternariol monomethyl ether	Corn, cereals, maize, corn, baby food cereal, water	Abdul Kadir and Tothill (2010), Ricci et al. (2009), Hervas, López, and Escarpa (2009)
Electrochemical (square wave voltammetry)	Okadaic acid	Mussels	Eissa and Zourob (2012)
	Brevetoxin B	Mussels, razor clams, cockles	Tang et al. (2012)

Unapproved and hazardous food additives

Food additives are commonly used in the food industry to maintain and improve physicochemical, biological, sensory, and rheological properties of food as well as help to regulate color, flavor, sweetness, pH, stability, and overall product quality. Other than that, food additives tend to prolong the expiry date and allow the food products to last longer without any contamination (Martins, Sentanin, & De Souza, 2019).

There are several food additives that widely used, including glutamate, propyl gallate, benzoic acids, some food colorants, and others. Glutamate or commercially known as monosodium glutamate (MSG) is a well-known additive among the users as it is responsible for improving the taste and making food taste delicious. However, an excessive amount of MSG can be considered as one of the chemical pollutions in food due to the selfishness of food manufacturers to gain profit rather than reconsider the side effect of MSG on human health.

Both Pasco et al. (1999) and Batra, Kumari, and Pundir (2014) have discovered amperometric biosensor and enzyme biosensor (glutamate dehydrogenase and glutamate oxidase) were used to detect the presence of an excessive amount of MSG in food which can produce a significant risk to human health. There are two transducer components, such as oxygen and gold electrode, but the gold electrode is most preferable as it has high conductivity and enhanced the electron transfer between the bioreceptor and the transducer.

Propyl gallate (PG) is a synthetic phenolic antioxidant typically used in edible falts, oils, and dehydrated foodstuffs. In 2015, the amperometric PG biosensors method was established by Morales, González, Reviejo, and Pingarrón (2005) to accurately detect PG in food and tyrosinase were chosen as biological recognition substances. However, the detection process for this approach was based on the electrochemical oxidation of PG at the Graphite-Teflon-composite electrode (Martins et al., 2019).

Benzoic acid is one of the preservatives that widely used in the food industry to protect food from any harmful chemical changes and helps to regulate the growth of microbes better. However, excessive consumption of benzoic acid in food can pose a severe health effect on a human being. Therefore, Shan, Li, Xue, and Cosnier (2008) developed a detection method (amperometric biosensors) based on the use of mushroom tissue, tyrosinase, and polyphenol oxidase as biological recognition compounds. The working principle for this method is the inhibition of such substances by benzoic acids and inhibitory activity results in a drop in oxygen concentration.

Food colorants are classified as substances added to food to improve the poor color of food, preserve the color lost during food storage and processing, and to increase consumer's eating desires as most of the children are interested in foods and drinks with vibrant colors. The color additives have been lawfully applied to processed foods (soft drinks, bakery products, canned and vegetable products, dairy products, meat and fish products, wine and pastry) since 1880 under the guidance of different legislations such as EEC (European Economic Committee) and FDA (Food and Drug Administration).

Amaranth (E123) and Ponceau 4R (E124) are water-fat soluble synthetic colorants, which are among the hazardous food colorants that are broadly employed in the food industry as a food additive, despite, being prohibited by most developed countries. However, higher intakes of Amaranth and Ponceau may cause hyperactivity, asthma, skin rashes, and other disturbing behavior, particularly against children. Therefore, Wang, Gao, Sun, and Zhao (2015) established a biosensor for the simultaneous determination of both colorants based on the use of carbon nanotube (CNT) and polypyrrole (ppy-) composite modified electrode. Table 7.5 in the following section shows the summarization of the biosensor technology used for the detection of hazardous and unapproved food additives:

Regulations and legislations

Since chemical contaminations cause multiple health risks towards humans, the limited use of these chemicals and also the medium from which the chemicals originated must be enforced by statute and regulations. Other than that, the laws and regulations must be revised periodically to monitor the problems effectively.

National

Various government and nongovernment agencies, including the Ministry of Agriculture and Ministry of Health and Customs, are responsible for taking a significant part in the cycle of sustaining and controlling the safety and quality of the food sector in Malaysia. The primary food health legislation was implemented in the Food Act 1983 and came into force in October 1985 under the following Food Regulations or is also recognized as the Food Regulation 1985. To be honest, the stated law is not only intended to protect the public against the dangers of food security and food frauds but it also highly encourages the food manufacturer and handlers to prepare, manage and distribute the food in a high-quality manner (Philip, 2015).

Other than Food Act 1983 and Food Regulations 1985, Pesticide Act 1974, Fisheries Act 1983, Animal Ordinance 1953, and Veterinary Surgeon Act 1974 under Ministry of Agricultural and Agro-based Industry and Trade Description Act under Ministry of Domestic Trade and Consumer Affairs are also another legislation that can be applied in monitory food safety in Malaysia (WHO, n.d.).

Global

The World Health Organization (WHO) was established an internationally applicable food regulation, the Codex Alimentarius Commission, which comprises the community from 175 countries involved in the Codex Alimentarius Program. However, the establishment of the food standard was undoubtedly based on the international negotiations procedure between FAO and WHO, 2006.

The Codex Alimentarius Commission contains more than 200 guidelines, 50 of them are focused on food hygiene, technological codes of practice, and permissible concentration limits for additives, pesticides, and veterinary drugs. Besides, it also highlights the requirements for labeling, analysis, and sampling method (Development of Food Legislation around the World, 2010).

Recent updates

Generally, all laws need to be reviewed and keep on updating by considering the 14 steps of procedures in Codex standards. The Technical Advisory Committee, which is under the oversight of the Director of Food Quality Control Division of Ministry of Health is regularly revised and updated all the regulations, and also responsible for the enforcement and review legislation of Food Regulation 1985.

Public awareness and acceptance

Nowadays, most of the world population is well conscious of and accountable for ensuring the safety and quality of food by developed and discovered many methods to overcome, monitor, and solve the problems. Biosensors are one of the methods that offer versatile technology that is capable of estimating the permissible residue amount of permitted food additives and even detecting the possible food hazard that contaminates in food matrices. However, future research can be developed and improved, thus achieving the standard specifications accepted by the researchers and the public.

Hence, the biosensor technology has high selectivity, sensitivity, able to detect multiple contaminants, reduced false error, fast and also rapid without having complicated sample preparations. Besides, the sensor size also should be considered in nanosize as it is more portable, transportable, and also easy to use. This low-cost technology is genuinely helping the researchers to conduct their analysis when other analytical methods use costly equipment and involve extensive preparation. Thus, all of these features are to meet the new need for globalization and urbanization.

Conclusion and future perspectives

Biosensors technology should be employed by a wide variety of industries worldwide, primarily the food industry, to control and maintain quality and food safety, for food security purposes, and food composition analysis. On top of that, this approach has been the most favored technique in food quality analysis due to the high specificity and sensitivity, rapid and required less cost for analysis of various specified substances and compounds.

Since the present pollutants in food matrices have a very complicated and complex structure, the advancement, development as well as innovation in the field of the biosensor as well as the opportunities and threats of this field need to be created by food manufacturers to comply with the regulations and legislation. Therefore, food safety and quality can be ensured based on the health condition and well-being of customers.

References

Abdul Kadir, M. K., & Tothill, I. E. (2010). Development of an electrochemical immunosensor for fumonisins detection in foods. *Toxins*, *2*(4), 382–398. https://doi.org/10.3390/toxins2040382.

Alam, A. U., & Deen, M. J. (2020). Bisphenol A electrochemical sensor using graphene oxide and β-cyclodextrin-functionalized multi-walled carbon nanotubes. *Analytical Chemistry*, *92*(7), 5532–5539.

Anonymous (2005). *Enumeration of* Staphylococcus aureus *in foods in compendium of analytical methods. MFHPB-21.* http://www.hc-sc.gc.ca/fnan/resrech/analymeth/microbio/volume2-eng.php. Accessed 25 January 2019.

Anonymous (2007). *Enumeration of Enterobacteriaceae species in food and environmental samples using 3M_ Petrifilm_Enterobacteriaceae count plates in compendium of analytical methods.* http://www.hc-sc.gc.ca/fn-an/res-rech/analy-meth/microbio/volume3-eng.php. Accessed 25 January 2019.

Anonymous (2012a). *Screening bottled water (water in sealed containers) for the presence of indicator and pathogenic bacteria in Compendium of analytical methods. MFLP-60.* http://www.hc-sc.gc.ca/fn-an/res-rech/analy-meth/microbio/volume3-eng.php. Accessed 25 January 2019.

Anonymous (2012b). *Enumeration of Escherichia coli in foods by a direct plating (DP) method in compendium of analytical methods. MFHPB-27.* http://www.hc-sc.gc.ca/fn-an/resrech/analy-meth/microbio/volume2-eng.php. Accessed 25 January 2019.

Anonymous (2013). *40 CFR 150.17 protection of the environment. Code of Federal Regulations.* Pub Office of the Federal National Archives and Records of Administration.

Arévalo, F. J., Granero, A. M., Fernández, H., Raba, J., & Zón, M. A. (2011). Citrinin (CIT) determination in rice samples using a micro fluidic electrochemical immunosensor. *Talanta*, *83*(3), 966–973. https://doi.org/10.1016/j.talanta.2010.11.007.

Augustin, J. C. (2011). Challenges in risk assessment and predictive microbiology of food-borne spore-forming bacteria. *Food Microbiology*, *28*(2), 209–213. https://doi.org/10.1016/j.fm.2010.05.003.

Bacher, G., Pal, S., Kanungo, L., & Bhand, S. (2012). A label-free silver wire based impedimetric immunosensor for detection of aflatoxin M1 in milk. *Sensors and Actuators B: Chemical*, *168*, 223–230. https://doi.org/10.1016/j.snb.2012.04.012.

Basu, A. K., Chattopadhyay, P., Roychudhuri, U., & Chakraborty, R. (2006). A biosensor based on coimmobilized L-glutamate oxidase and L-glutamate dehydrogenase for analysis of monosodium glutamate in food. *Biosensors and Bioelectronics*, *21*(10), 1968–1972. https://doi.org/10.1016/j.bios.2005.09.011.

Batra, B., Kumari, S., & Pundir, C. S. (2014). Construction of glutamate biosensor based on covalent immobilization of glutmate oxidase on polypyrrole nanoparticles/polyaniline modified gold electrode. *Enzyme and Microbial Technology*, *57*, 69–77. https://doi.org/10.1016/j.enzmictec.2014.02.001.

Berthiller, F., Burdaspal, P. A., Crews, C., Iha, M. H., Krska, R., Lattanzio, V. M. T., MacDonald, S., Malone, R. J., Maragos, C., Solfrizzo, M., & Stroka, J. (2014). Developments in mycotoxin analysis: An update for 2012–2013. *World Mycotoxin Journal*, *7*(1), 3–33. https://doi.org/10.3920/WMJ2013.1637.

Bosilevac, J. M., Guerini, M. N., Brichta-Harhay, D. M., Arthur, T. M., & Koohmaraie, M. (2007). Microbiological characterization of imported and domestic boneless beef trim used for ground beef. *Journal of food protection*, *70*(2), 440–449. https://doi.org/10.4315/0362-028X-70.2.440.

Chai, C., Lee, J., & Takhistov, P. (2010). Direct detection of the biological toxin in acidic environment by electrochemical impedimetric immunosensor. *Sensors*, *10*(12), 11414–11427. https://doi.org/10.3390/s101211414.

Chen, Z. G. (2008). Conductometric immunosensors for the detection of staphylococcal enterotoxin B based bio-electrocalytic reaction on micro-comb electrodes. *Bioprocess and Biosystems Engineering*, *31*(4), 345–350. https://doi.org/10.1007/s00449-007-0168-2.

Choi, S. W., Chang, H. J., Lee, N., Kim, J. H., & Chun, H. S. (2009). Detection of mycoestrogen zearalenone by a molecularly imprinted polypyrrole-based surface plasmon resonance (SPR)sensor. *Journal of Agricultural and Food Chemistry*, *57*(4), 1113–1118. https://doi.org/10.1021/jf804022p.

Chouteau, C., Dzyadevych, S., Durrieu, C., & Chovelon, J. M. (2005). A bi-enzymatic whole cell conductometric biosensor for heavy metal ions and pesticides detection in water samples. *Biosensors and Bioelectronics*, *21*(2), 273–281. https://doi.org/10.1016/j.bios.2004.09.032.

Crowley, E., Bird, P., Flannery, J., Benzinger, M. J., Jr, Fisher, K., Boyle, M., Huffman, T., Bastin, B., Bedinghaus, P., Judd, W., & Hoang, T. (2014). Evaluation of VIDAS® UP listeria assay (LPT) for the detection of listeria in a variety of foods and environmental surfaces: First action 2013.10. *Journal of AOAC International*, *97*(2), 431–441.

Daly, S. J., Keating, G. J., Dillon, P. P., Manning, B. M., O'Kennedy, R., Lee, H. A., & Morgan, M. R. A. (2000). Development of surface plasmon resonance-based immunoassay for aflatoxin B1. *Journal of Agricultural and Food Chemistry*, *48*(11), 5097–5104. https://doi.org/10.1021/jf9911693.

Desmarchelier, J. M., & Ren, Y. L. (1999). Analysis of fumigant residues—A critical review. *Journal of AOAC International*, *82*(6), 1261–1280. https://doi.org/10.1093/jaoac/82.6.1261.

Eissa, S., & Zourob, M. (2012). A graphene-based electrochemical competitive immunosensor for the sensitive detection of okadaic acid in shellfish. *Nanoscale*, *4*(23), 7593–7599. https://doi.org/10.1039/C2NR32146G.

Evtugyn, G. A. (2016). Biosensor to ensure food security and environmental control. *Comprehensive Analytical Chemistry*, *74*, 121–152. https://doi.org/10.1016/bs.coac.2016.03.017.

Faeste, C. K., Roenning, H. T., Christians, U., & Granum, P. E. (2011). Liquid chromatography and mass spectrometry in food allergen detection. *Journal of Food Protection*, *74*(2), 316–345. https://doi.org/10.4315/0362-028X.JFP-10-33.

Fuertes, G., Soto, I., Carrasco, R., Vargas, M., Sabattin, J., & Lagos, C. (2016). Intelligent packaging systems: Sensors and nanosensors to monitor food quality and safety. *Journal of Sensors*. https://doi.org/10.1155/2016/4046061.

Hassan, S. H. A., Van Ginkel, S. W., Hussein, M. A. M., Abskharon, R., & Oh, S. E. (2016). Toxicity assessment using different bioassays and microbial biosensors. *Environment International*, *92–93*, 106–118. https://doi.org/10.1016/j.envint.2016.03.003.

Hervás, M., López, M. Á., & Escarpa, A. (2009). Electrochemical immunoassay using magnetic beads for the determination of zearalenone in baby food: An anticipated analytical tool for food safety. *Analytica Chimica Acta*, *653*(2), 167–172. https://doi.org/10.1016/j.aca.2009.09.02.

Liang, P., Wu, S. C., Zhang, J., Cao, Y., Yu, S., & Wong, M. H. (2016). The effects of mariculture on heavy metal distribution in sediments and cultured fish around the Pearl River Delta region, South China. *Chemosphere*, *148*, 171–177. https://doi.org/10.1016/j.chemosphere.2015.10.110.

Lindhardt, C., Schönenbrücher, H., Slaghuis, J., Bubert, A., Ossmer, R., Junge, B., Harzman, C., & Berghof-Jäger, K. (2010). " Salmonella" detection in peanut butter: Validación of a real-time PCR method. *Alimentaria: Revista de Tecnología e Higiene de Los Alimentos*, 85–88 (413).

Liu, J., Guan, Z., Lv, Z., Jiang, X., Yang, S., & Chen, A. (2014). Improving sensitivity of gold nanoparticle based fluorescence quenching and colorimetric aptasensor by using water resuspended gold nanoparticle. *Biosensors and Bioelectronics*, *52*, 265–270. https://doi.org/10.1016/j.bios.2013.08.059.

Liu, S., Kang, M., Yan, F., Peng, D., Yang, Y., He, L., … Zhang, Z. (2015). Electrochemical DNA biosensor based on microspheres of cuprous oxide and nano-chitosan for Hg(II) detection. *Electrochimica Acta*, *160*, 64–73. https://doi.org/10.1016/j.electacta.2015.02.030.

Liu, Y., Liu, Y., & Liu, B. (2016). A dual-signaling strategy for ultrasensitive detection of bisphenol A by aptamer-based electrochemical biosensor. *Journal of Electroanalytical Chemistry*, *781*, 265–271. https://doi.org/10.1016/j.jelechem.2016.06.048.

Liu, Y., & Wei, M. (2014). Development of acetylcholinesterase biosensor based on platinum-carbon aerogels composite for determination of organophosphorus pesticides. *Food Control*, *36*(1), 49–54. https://doi.org/10.1016/j.foodcont.2013.08.005.

Li, Z., Wang, Y., Ni, Y., & Kokot, S. (2015). A rapid and label-free dual detection of Hg (II) and cysteine with the use of fluorescence switching of graphene quantum dots. *Sensors and Actuators B: Chemical*, *207*, 490–497. https://doi.org/10.1016/j.snb.2014.10.071.

Martins, F. C. O. L., Sentanin, M. A., & De Souza, D. (2019). Analytical methods in food additives determination: Compounds with functional applications. *Food Chemistry*, *272*, 732–750. https://doi.org/10.1016/j.foodchem.2018.08.060.

Mehrotra, P. (2016). Biosensors and their applications—A review. *Journal of Oral Biology and Craniofacial Research*, *6*(2), 153–159. https://doi.org/10.1016/j.jobcr.2015.12.002.

Mikulikova, R., Svoboda, Z., & Belakova, S. (2008). Monitoring of residues of fungicides used in malting barley protection. *Kvasny Prumysl (Czech Republic)*, *54*(11-12), 332–337.

Morales, M. D., González, M. C., Reviejo, A. J., & Pingarrón, J. M. (2005). A composite amperometric tyrosinase biosensor for the determination of the additive propyl gallate in foodstuffs. *Microchemical journal*, *80*(1), 71–78. https://doi.org/10.1016/j.microc.2004.10.023.

Nadèje, T., Olga, S., Ben, O. H., Florence, L., Philippe, N., Ben, O. H., & Nicole, J. -R. (2014). Bi-enzymatic conductometric biosensor for detection of heavy metal ions and pesticides in water samples based on enzymatic inhibition in *Arthrospira platensis*. *Journal of Environmental Protection*, 441–453. https://doi.org/10.4236/jep.2014.55047.

Nerín, C., Aznar, M., & Carrizo, D. (2016). Food contamination during food process. *Trends in Food Science and Technology*, *48*, 63–68. https://doi.org/10.1016/j.tifs.2015.12.004.

Oliveira, T. M., Barroso, M. F., Morais, S., Araújo, M., Freire, C., de Lima-Neto, P., Correia, A. N., Oliveira, M. B., & Delerue-Matos, C. (2013). Laccase-Prussian blue film-graphene doped carbon paste modified electrode for carbamate pesticides quantification. *Biosensors & Bioelectronics 47*, 292–299. https://doi.org/10.1016/j.bios.2013.03.026.

Owino, J. H., Arotiba, O. A., Hendricks, N., Songa, E. A., Jahed, N., Waryo, T. T., Ngece, R. F., Baker, P. G., & Iwuoha, E. I. (2008). Electrochemical immunosensor based on polythionine/gold nanoparticles for the determination of aflatoxin B1. *Sensors, 8*(12), 8262–8274. https://doi.org/10.3390/s8128262.

Parkhey P. and Mohan S.V., Biosensing applications of microbial fuel cell: Approach toward miniaturization. In *Microbial electrochemical technology* (pp. 977-997). Elsevier. https://doi.org/10.1016/B978-0-444-64052-9.00040-6

Pasco, N., Jeffries, C., Davies, Q., Downard, A. J., Roddick-Lanzilotta, A. D., Gorton, L., et al. (1999). Characterisation of a thermophilic L-glutamate dehydrogenase biosensor for amperometric determination of L-glutamate by flow injection analysis. *Biosensors and Bioelectronics, 14*(2), 171–178. https://doi.org/10.1016/s0956-5663(98)00120-1.

Patra, J. K., Mahato, D. K., & Kumar, P. (2019). Biosensor technology—Advanced scientific tools, with special reference to nanobiosensors and plant- and food-based biosensors. In *Nanomaterials in plants, algae and microorganisms* (pp. 287–303). Academic Press. https://doi.org/10.1016/B978-0-12-811488-9.00014-7.

Philip, A. (2015). [Malaysia] Food safety in Malaysia. *Japan Medical Association Journal, 58*(4), 180–184.

Piermarini, S., Volpe, G., Micheli, L., Moscone, D., & Palleschi, G. (2009). An ELIME-array for detection of aflatoxin B1 in corn samples. *Food Control, 20*(4), 371–375. https://doi.org/10.1016/j.foodcont.2008.06.003.

Rajeshkumar, S., Liu, Y., Zhang, X., Ravikumar, B., Bai, G., & Li, X. (2018). Studies on seasonal pollution of heavy metals in water, sediment, fish and oyster from the Meiliang Bay of Taihu Lake in China. *Chemosphere, 191*, 626–638. https://doi.org/10.1016/j.chemosphere.2017.10.078.

Ricci, F., Pino, F., Abagnale, M., Messia, M., Marconi, E., Volpe, G., Moscone, D., & Palleschi, G. (2009). Direct electrochemical detection of trichothecenes in wheat samples using a 96-well electrochemical plate coupled with microwave hydrolysis. *World Mycotoxin Journal, 2*(2), 239–245. https://doi.org/10.3920/WMJ2008.1133.

Shan, D., Li, Q., Xue, H., & Cosnier, S. (2008). A highly reversible and sensitive tyrosinase inhibition-based amperometric biosensor for benzoic acid monitoring. *Sensors and Actuators, B: Chemical, 134*(2), 1016–1021. https://doi.org/10.1016/j.snb.2008.07.006.

Tang, D., Tang, J., Su, B., & Chen, G. (2010). Ultrasensitive electrochemical immunoassay of staphylococcal enterotoxin B in food using enzyme-nanosilica-doped carbon nanotubes for signal amplification. *Journal of Agricultural and Food Chemistry, 58*(20), 10824–10830. https://doi.org/10.1021/jf102326m.

Tang, J., Hou, L., Tang, D., Zhou, J., Wang, Z., Li, J., & Chen, G. (2012). Magneto-controlled electrochemical immunoassay of brevetoxin B in seafood based on guanine-functionalized graphene nanoribbons. *Biosensors and Bioelectronics, 38*(1), 86–93. https://doi.org/10.1016/j.bios.2012.05.006.

Tekaya, N., Saiapina, O., Ouada, H. B., Lagarde, F., Namour, P., Ouada, H. B., & Jaffrezic-Renault, N. (2014). *Bi-enzymatic conductometric biosensor for detection of heavy metal ions and pesticides in water samples based on enzymatic inhibition in arthrospira platensis*. https://doi.org/10.4236/jep.2014.55047.

Tortolini, C., Bollella, P., Antonelli, M. L., Antiochia, R., Mazzei, F., & Favero, G. (2014). DNA-based biosensors for Hg2+ determination by polythymine-methylene blue modified electrodes. *Biosensors & Bioelectronics*, *67*, 524–531.

Tothill, I. (2011). Biosensors and nanomaterials and their application for mycotoxin determination. *World Mycotoxin Journal*, *4*(4), 361–374. https://doi.org/10.3920/WMJ2011.1318.

Vandermarken, T., Boonen, I., Gryspeirt, C., Croes, K., Van Den Houwe, K., Denison, M. S. , … Elskens, M. (2019). Assessment of estrogenic compounds in paperboard for dry food packaging with the ERE-CALUX bioassay. *Chemosphere*, *221*, 99–106. https://doi.org/10.1016/j.chemosphere.2018.12.192.

Vidal, J. C., Bonel, L., Ezquerra, A., Hernández, S., Bertolín, J. R., Cubel, C., & Castillo, J. R. (2013). Electrochemical affinity biosensors for detection of mycotoxins: A review. *Biosensors and Bioelectronics*, *49*, 146–158. https://doi.org/10.1016/j.bios.2013.05.008.

Wang, L., Chen, W., Xu, D., Shim, B. S., Zhu, Y., Sun, F., Liu, L., Peng, C., Jin, Z., Xu, C., & Kotov, N. A. (2009). Simple, rapid, sensitive, and versatile SWNT—paper sensor for environmental toxin detection competitive with ELISA. *Nano Letters*, *9*(12), 4147–4152. https://doi.org/10.1021/nl902368r.

Wang, M., Gao, Y., Sun, Q., & Zhao, J. (2015). Ultrasensitive and simultaneous determination of the isomers of Amaranth and Ponceau 4R in foods based on new carbon nanotube/polypyrrole composites. *Food Chemistry*, *172*, 873–879. https://doi.org/10.1016/j.foodchem.2014.09.157.

Warriner, K., Reddy, S. M., Namvar, A., & Neethirajan, S. (2014). Developments in nanoparticles for use in biosensors to assess food safety and quality. *Trends in Food Science and Technology*, *40*(2), 183–199. https://doi.org/10.1016/j.tifs.2014.07.008.

Wei, M., & Wang, J. (2015). A novel acetylcholinesterase biosensor based on ionic liquids-AuNPs-porous carbon composite matrix for detection of organophosphate pesticides. *Sensors and Actuators, B: Chemical*, *211*, 290–296. https://doi.org/10.1016/j.snb.2015.01.112.

WHO, WHO regional conference on food safety for Asia and the Pacific. (n.d.).

Yang, L., Wang, G., Liu, Y., & Wang, M. (2013). Development of a biosensor based on immobilization of acetylcholinesterase on NiO nanoparticles–carboxylic graphene–nafion modified electrode for detection of pesticides. *Talanta*, *113*, 135–141. https://doi.org/10.1016/j.talanta.2013.03.025.

Zhang, Y., Arugula, M. A., Wales, M., Wild, J., & Simonian, A. L. (2015). A novel layer-by-layer assembled multi-enzyme/CNT biosensor for discriminative detection between organophosphorus and non-organophosphrus pesticides. *Biosensors and Bioelectronics*, *67*, 287–295. https://doi.org/10.1016/j.bios.2014.08.036.

Nanotechnology-based optical biosensors for food applications

Introduction

There is a high demand for alternative methods in the food sector to ensure the authenticity of food products cost-effectively. It was a significant issue that challenged scientists to develop more reliable and feasible technologies. The advancement of biosensors in response is promising that rapid progress has been made, and the optical biosensor subfield is showing impressive results during this time. Biosensors consist of several components that integrate a biorecognition component such as biological material, a biomic or a biologically derived material bind to the sample, electrical interference where the signal is generated, a transducer that converts the biochemical reaction to a measurable signal, a signal processor that converts the signal to a physical parameter, and an interface that displays the results (Inan et al., 2017; Jayanthi, Das, & Saxena, 2017; Patel, Nanda, Sahoo, & Mohapatra, 2016). The biosensors have different operation modes of signal transduction, which had been designated into an optical, electrochemical, thermometric, piezoelectric, and magnetic biosensor. Current progress in the strategy of a biosensor is linked with nanomaterials to improved sensitivity and efficiency, as well as the development of various new signal transduction technologies because of their unique optical, mechanical, electrical, and chemical features (Pandit, Dasgupta, Dewan, & Prince, 2016).

Optical biosensors have gained much attention as effective research instruments with a wide range of applications and deliver significant advantages due to excellent stability and accurate measurement accuracy (Sadani, Nag, & Mukherji, 2019). It is one of the devices that had been widely utilized in many industries, including the health care industry, the food industry as well as environmental sciences. It required the transduction of optical for the desired components or any substances in a biological system, which extensively used such as chromatography and spectrophotoscopy techniques due to its simplicity, sensitivity, accuracy, and for the acquisition of data. However, the conventional method involves expensive equipment, well-trained personnel, and a prolonged period for sample pretreatment. There are comprehensive efforts have obtained for the development of fast, low-cost, sensitive, selective, and portable biosensors and bioassays to overcome the limitations mentioned above. The transduction via optical will provide a quantitative determination of the characteristics in the radiation of lights, including amplitude, polarization, phase, and frequency. Brecht and Gauglitz (1995) mentioned the detection of transduction

Advanced Food Analysis Tools. https://doi.org/10.1016/B978-0-12-820591-4.00008-6

characteristics is often based on the principles of surface plasmon resonance (SPR), grating couplers (GCP), total internal reflection fluorescence (TIRF), waveguide-based SPR (WSPR), Ellipsometry (ELL), and integrated optical interferometers (IO) and all of these methods will respond to any changes in optical density.

Optical sensors

The research and technological development of optical biosensors have experienced exponential growth over the last decade. An analytical optical biosensor is a versatile tool that includes a combination of biorecognition sensing features and transducer systems. An optical biosensor is known to produce a signal that is proportionate to the level of the measured analyte. The optical biosensor can use various biological materials, including enzymes, antibodies, antigens, receptors, nucleic acids, whole cells, and tissues, as elements of biorecognition (Baoyi & Zhongdang, 2020; Damborský, Švitel, & Katrlík, 2016; Majdinasab, Mishra, Tang, & Marty, 2020). An optical biosensor is to identify the magnitude and frequency of the electrical signal which is generated by the reaction of analytes that bind on the biosensing membrane (Turner, Chang, Fang, Brandow, & Murphy, 1995) and the manipulation of the optical biosensor are essential for commercial and economical means also known to be as a multidiscipline detection which includes the nanobiotechnology. Generally, there are two classes of detection protocols for optical biosensing, namely label-free and label-based detection modes. Concisely, the signal detected from label-free mode is produced directly from the interaction between analyzed material and transducer. In contrast, label-based sensing requires the use of a label to generate an optical signal by the colorimetric, fluorescent, or luminescent procedure (Damborský et al., 2016; Khansili, Rattu, & Krishna, 2018). Optical biosensors offer great benefits such as direct, real-time, and label-free detection of many biological and chemical substances that show high specificity and sensitivity, fast response, remote control, cost-effectiveness as well as strong adaptability.

Fig. 8.1 offers a graphical description of these approaches, where a change in optical intensity controls most. Although fiber optics has been the most promising and adapted biosensing research method in the last decade, it has had an enormous possibility to improve real-time, direct, and label-free detection methods (Luo, Xu, Zhao, & Chen, 2004). This provides significant benefits over electronic biosensing and other traditional means by creating more accurate, sensitive, small-scale, low-cost, and most reliable biosensing tools that are ideal for extreme environments and have higher tolerance and versatility as with electromagnetic interference or sensing formats. Besides, optical biosensors are considered to be versatile in the production of commercial and economical for multidisciplinary approaches, including microelectronics, microelectromechanical systems (MEMSs), and advanced food

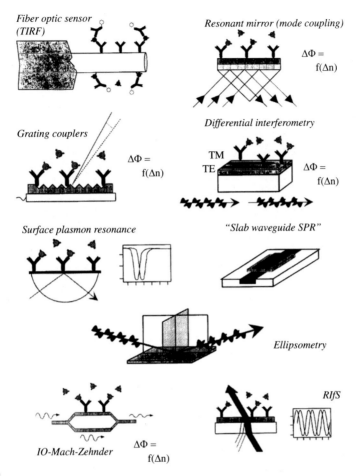

FIG. 8.1

Schematic of optical transducer theories.

nanobiotechnology (Damborský et al., 2016; Singh, 2017). Optical biosensors are capable of evaluating chemical and biological reactions through the evaluation of few parameters such as light absorption, fluorescence, reflectance, and luminescence. These biosensor approaches use the electromagnetic effects of light for the identification, quantification, and analysis of high-sensitivity biochemical interactions and the functionality of label-free and real-time assays (Soler, Huertas, & Lechuga, 2019; Zanchetta, Lanfranco, Giavazzi, Bellini, & Buscaglia, 2017). Fig. 8.2 shows a summary of the taxonomy multiplexed optical biosensors, which include modern and conventional optics-based sensors.

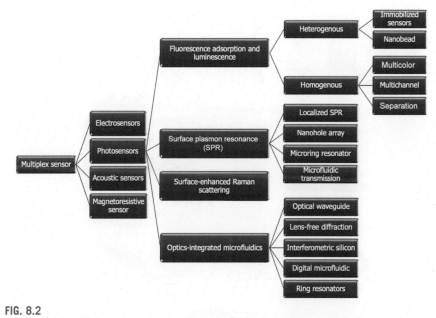

FIG. 8.2

Taxonomic of optical sensors and microfluidic for multiplex bioassays.

Principles and classification of optical biosensor
Surface plasmon resonance (SPR) biosensors

SPR-based biosensor is a recognized optical sensor for biological protein interaction for food safety and quality control in the food industry. SPR is a confined electromagnetic wave guided along a surface of noble metals known as chemically stable gold. There is a popular SPR sensor chip sold by GE healthcare company called Qflex Kits that have been produced for monitoring beneficial in food products such as folic acid, biotin, pantothenic acid, vitamin B2 and B12 (O'Kane & Wahlström, 2011). The Qflex Kits can be used to detect a variety of drug residues in food such as chloramphenicol (J. Ferguson et al., 2005), sulfonamides in Honey (Pastor-Navarro, Gallego-Iglesias, Maquieira, & Puchades, 2007), sulfadiazine and sulfamethazine (McGrath, Baxter, Ferguson, Haughey, & Bjurling, 2005), streptomycin (Ferguson et al., 2002), clenbuterol and ractopamine (Blanca et al., 2005) in various matrixes of food.

Surface plasmon resonance imaging (SPRi)

Surface plasmon resonance imaging (SPRi) is classified as an optical biosensor method that had been utilized to identify the interaction between biorecognition elements with the analyte in real-time. Spoto and Minunni (2012) stated that the technique had been fully developed due to its significant achievement in terms of instrumentation, processing of data, and analysis. The sensitivity of SPR imaging is higher compared to conventional SPR, which enables multiple different interactions simultaneously on an array of specifically patterned molecules (Erickson, Mandal, Yang, & Cordovez, 2008). SPR imaging technique is based on a label-free mode where it is applied to identify the reactions between the molecules in real-time. It also makes it possible to operate in a multiplex format by immobilizing various kinds of ligands used on a single SPRi-Biochip and allows the analysis of different parameters in only time. SPR imaging devices classified into four categories: (i) angle modulation, (ii) wavelength modulation, (iii) amplitude modulation, and (iv) phase modulation (Couture, Zhao, & Masson, 2013; Peng et al., 2014).

For angle modulation, the angle at which the SPR occurs is to identify and describe the prism configuration. Angle modulation is the most used type of modulation compared to other types of modulation. Monochromatic light radiates the metallic film, scans the full range of angles by using a scanning source and a rotating light source at a particular angle. Meanwhile, the angle of beam light will diverge for a fixed source (Homola, 2008; Wang, Zhan, Huang, & Hong, 2013). The modulation of wavelength is the modified angle of the incident light at a given value, where the reflected light wavelength is modulated as the sensing principle. Zhang et al. (2013) reported that the reflected intensity dip is being quantified against the difference between the refractive index (RI) and the incident wavelength range.

The SPRi method for amplitude modulation is to measure the reflectivity of the monochromatic incident p-polarized light at a fixed angle. However, this technique has its disadvantage where the presence of output noise will increase the resolution by the production of noise from the light source (Homola, 2008). Somehow, the light source noise may be reduced by referencing (Homola, 2008; Piliarik & Homola, 2009). The variations of intensity of reflected light in SPRi are being measured by using 2D detectors, and it is expressed as percent reflectivity, % R (Spoto & Minunni, 2012). SPRi is consistent with phase modulation because it can conduct multiplex detection with simultaneous identification of thousands of channels (Kashif, Bakar, Arsad, & Shaari, 2014).

Localized surface plasmon resonance (LSPR)

According to Willets and Van Duyne (2007), LSPR is a visual phenomenon created by a trapped light wave within conductive nanoparticles that is shorter than the light wavelength. It is light coupling to the resonance oscillation of the charge density on the nanostructured surface due to the interaction between the incident light and the conduction band. As a result, coherent localized plasmon oscillations are generated with a resonant frequency that depends on the physical characteristics of the nanoparticles (Petryayeva & Krull, 2011). LSPR turns out on nanoscopic structures such as spheres, disks, holes, rods, shells, and many more (Puiu & Bala, 2016). This technique usually intensifies the process-related to optical observation, including fluorescence, plasmon resonance energy transfer (PRET), and surfaced-enhanced Raman spectroscopy (SERS). The photons from the interaction between nanoparticles and light are absorbed, and some of them may be dispersed. The nanoparticles can achieve high molar extinction absorption coefficients and provide a wide range of Rayleigh dispersion in the LSPR (Jensen, Malinsky, Haynes, & Van Duyne, 2000). According to Petryayeva and Krull (2011), LSPR induces exceptionally intense and highly localized electromagnetic fields that have produced slight changes in the local RI to allow nanoparticles to become more sensitive transducers. Usually, the application of NPs will promote sharp peaks in the spectral absorbance for LSPR at visible also near-infrared frequencies. Somehow, gold nanoparticles often altered by using thiol or disulfide-terminated molecules during the synthesis of nanoparticles to displace stabilizing ligands. The spectral information is enhanced for SERS, PRET, and metal-enhanced fluorescence (MEF) (Choi, Kang, & Lee, 2009; Choi, Park, Kang, & Lee, 2009) and nanoplasmonic molecular rulers (Sönnichsen, Reinhard, Liphardt, & Alivisatos, 2005; Thaxton & Mirkin, 2005) as the electromagnetic field become stronger.

LSPR is based on the characteristics of nanoparticles, distance separation, and proximity to nanoparticles. The shapes and sizes of the metallic nanoparticles impart spectral properties as the surface polarization varies. Assorted shapes such as triangles, bipyramids, cubes, spheres, octahedrons, prisms, nanoshells, nanotubes, nanostars, and structured array films are being produced to modify the absorption of LPSR. Lu, Rycenga, Skrabalak, Wiley, and Xia (2009) stated that the separation of charges is directly proportional to the edges or sharpness of nanoparticles, resulting in the extinction spectra. Symmetrically, the intensity of LSPR also increases. Thus, the relative magnitude between the absorption cross-section and the scatter cross-section are influenced by nanoparticle size and are expressed as a ratio (scattering: absorption). Also, the polarization of nanoparticles will enable the determination of resonance absorption peaks number (Liz-Marzán, 2006; Lu et al., 2009). The instruments of LSPR are designed to run specific experiments and applications. In general, the device used in LSPR consists of a light source, which is either white light or laser, sample, and a detector. UV–vis spectroscopy is utilized among other technologies to measure the spectrum of nanoparticles with excitation relies on a white light source. At a high angle, the surface is hit by the incident white light, and the scattered light will be collected at the region of a low angle. Petryayeva and Krull (2011) showed that the spectrometer and detector received scattered light from a low angle and a camera that uses a CCD chip to measure light intensity.

Recently, Sadani et al. (2019) developed a U-bend optical fiber sensor based on LSPR for the ultrasensitive detection of mercury in various types of samples such as vegetables, fish tissue, water, and fossil fuel soil. The LSPR integrated gold nanoparticles with chitosan capped and immobilized on bovine serum albumin for mercury detection, which is abundantly present in animal origin proteins and polysaccharides. Furthermore, Zhu et al. (2020) designed various multi-tapered LSPR optical fiber sensors based on ascorbic acid to increase the sensitivity for tremendous potential in practical routine diagnostics. The proposed sensor, with an optimum number of tapered areas, is an excellent option for the efficient identification of ascorbic acid due to the broad range of comparative studies on structural progress and nanomaterials.

Evanescent wave fluorescence

The evanescent wave, known as the electromagnetic field, appears as a phenomenon of light trapped in the optical waveguide or fiber. The light is internally reflected and travels through the waveguide and the surrounding medium, which has a lower RI and creates an evanescent wave. The light that goes entering the waveguide has a higher incidence angle than the critical angle, which reflects all the light inside the waveguide (Taitt, Anderson, & Ligler, 2005, 2016). Evanescent waves have been applied to other types of biosensors due to their surface selectivity, including resonant mirrors, interferometers, SPR sensors, fiber optic, and flat array fluorescence sensors, all of which are capable of measuring the event of surface-specific binding in real-time. The waveguide must be made of suitable materials with ideal characteristics that match the optical properties and can be easily adjusted for the attachment of the recognition molecules.

The phenomenon of the evanescent field only at the surface and any interactions that occur other than in the evanescent field will not be detected significantly. Since this phenomenon occurs only at the surface, the signal will be generated by the excitation of the evanescent wave which only excites the fluorescent molecules on the surface (Damborský et al., 2016) and this will limit the signal from the unwanted background while only enhance the signal from the captured fluorophores on the surface. The excitation of fluorophore will be determined based on the light wavelength. A diode laser with a longer wavelength will be utilized as it is inexpensive and will give a longer distance between the fluorescence and dye-labeled species and fluorophore that occurs naturally. The recognition of the molecule and binding process will occur within the evanescent wave limits.

Surface-enhanced Raman scattering biosensor (SERS)

Raman spectroscopy is used to measure inelastically dispersed light by allowing the interrogation and identification of the vibrational states of molecules capable of giving fingerprinting of the molecular structure and also of the material composition (Raman & Krishnan, 1928). The utilization of surface-enhanced Raman scattering (SERS) effect is to improve the intensity of the Raman signal produced by the molecules. Raman scattering, which occurs in the SERS effect, is caused by two factors, namely the location of optical fields in metallic nanostructures, which create an electromagnetic field, and the enhancement of chemical or electronic areas, which are influenced by the combination of molecular and metal nanostructure, which will increase the Raman cross-section. Somehow, foreign molecules that are not in contact with the metal surface may also be enhanced. The intensity of the Raman signal would be improved and depends on the particles of metal nanoparticle's surface. It is crucial in controlling the properties of SERS structures such as size, shape, the distance between nanoparticles, the interaction of nanoparticles with the substrate, solvent, dielectric overlayers, and molecular absorbates throughout the process to optimize the desired characteristics of SERS (Tian, Ren, & Wu, 2002).

The properties of nanoparticles may affect the intensity of the SERS; thus, different features of nanoparticles will determine the final peak plasmon-resonance wavelength and its performance. The Coulomb attraction of electrons and nuclei can cause the electron cloud to oscillate in enhancing electromagnetics. The sum of the incident field with the particle dipoles would thus result in an improvement of the local electric field (Kelly, Coronado, Zhao, & Schatz, 2003). The surface-enhanced Raman effect can occur on the metallic surface when the Raman scattering field is intensified by the coupling action between the plasmonic-electromagnetic resonance and the electromagnetic light field (Metiu & Das, 1984). Besides, chemical enhancement can also improve the SERS effect where the adsorbed Raman polarizability molecule on the metal surface is increased (Wu, Li, Ren, & Tian, 2008). As the photon exerts on the metal, electron in the metal excites to a certain degree, which is absorbed by the molecule on the metal surface. Otto, Billmann, Eickmans, Ertürk, and Pettenkofer (1984) claimed that after moving back from the excited state, the electron would interact with a metal hole, while the excited molecule remained at the excited state. This process can induce charge transfer (CT) and establish chemical enhancement, contributing to SERS development. Recently, H. Li et al. (2020) proposed a dual-channel biosensor (SERS and fluorescence) strategy for fast and highly responsive detection of mercury in ion tap water and milk samples. A dual-channel biosensor using core magnetite collide nanocrystal clusters of polymethacrylic acid magnetic beads were conjugated with aptamer to capture mercury ions.

Thin-film deposition
Langmuir–Blodgett technology

Irving Langmuir and Katherine Blodgett developed Langmuir–Blodgett films in the early 20th century. Langmuir–Blodgett conducted an experiment where a constant surface pressure held the Langmuir monolayer during the migration onto a solid substrate. The properties of the monolayers are maintained during the conveying of Langmuir film, which creates chances to produce an array of multilayer structures with different types of compositions. Organic molecules are used to process and transmit information, as well as preparing the molecular electronic devices (Roberts, 1990). Langmuir–Blodgett film widely applied in various areas such as electronics, optics, microlithography, chemical sensors, and biosensors as well as biochemical probes (Deb, Biswas, Hussain, & Bhattacharjee, 2005; Petty, 1996). The Langmuir–Blodgett films used the transferring process, where the layers moved from the subphase of the water were moved by vertical deposition to the reliable support. Additionally, the horizontal method, also known as Langmuir–Schaeffer deposition, has been applied to make the layer (Ulman, 2013). The formation of Langmuir–Blodgett film is made up of two components which are "head" and "tail" part, where "head" part is hydrophilic which has the properties of warm water, meanwhile, "head" part has a substantial measure towards the molecule polarity and able to form a bond with hydrogen atom such as –OH, –COOH, and –NH$_2$. For the "tail" part, it is hydrophobic, which will repel from water and usually has a long aliphatic compound. For molecules that are possessed by hydrophilic and hydrophobic regions are known as amphiphiles.

A volatile organic solvent such as chloroform, hexane, and toluene, which could prevent reaction between the molecules of interest and subphase, is required to dissolve the particles of interest. The method of deposition for Langmuir–Blodgett required the immersion and pulling off a solid substrate by the vertical process through the coating monolayer, where the surface pressure is being sustained at a specific value. The best solid substrates can be made of glass, silicon, quartz or mica and can be used at any pressure. However, the immersion and pulling off the substrate through the monolayer must be assessed in controlled and constant value, which is in the range from 1 to 5 mm/min (Hussain, 2009). Langmuir–Blodgett films have properties in optical applications, which as a conductive part and photo-responsive part. Ferreira et al. (2007) stated that a film produces a polymer light-emitting diode (PLED) when a polyfluorene is made up of film monolayers. The upper photo-responsive structure is responsible for conductive component conduction. The photo-responding structure will change when exposed to UV light, and the conduction of the film will increase. In any case, when exposed to visible light, the structure will return to its original form and allow the film's conduction to return to its low value (Hussain, 2009). However, the development of Langmuir–Blodgett films can be affected by many factors, as well as the form and characteristics of the solid substrate, such as the nature of the spread film, the composition of the subphase and temperature, the surface pressure and the rate of deposition.

Layer by layer (LbL)

SPR is a valuable instrument for real-time immunoreactions investigation based on monitoring local RI changes resulting from the interaction between a target and the biorecognition factor that is immobilized on the surface of the sensor. Layer-by-layer (LbL) approaches used in SPR to enhance sensing performance, with low detection limits for the specific analyte (de Almeida, de Barros, Mazali, & Ferreira, 2020; Miyazaki, Camilo, Shimizu, & Ferreira, 2019). Shimazaki, Mitsuishi, Ito, and Yamamoto (1997) stated that the CT of electron-donating carbazolyl groups and electron-accepting 3,5-dinitrobenzene groups in methylene chloride would form the LbL film. The use of thin films is surpassing compared to a powder form or by using a solution. The use of thin films enables the formation of the organized structure at the molecular level and controls the thickness of the films at once based on the required films.

Substantially, the formation of multiple layers in the LbL technique is the charge–charge interaction of substrate and monolayers that are bonded by electrostatic forces. Also, the interaction of donor or acceptor, hydrogen bonding, adsorption/drying cycles, covalent bonds, stereocomplex formation, or specific recognition are also other driving forces that can create a multilayer besides electrostatic force (Decher & Schlenoff, 2003). However, there is at least one of the interactions present to form a multilayer film. Thus, the formation of the multilayer system is due to the interaction between the various film layers. The process of creating the films is only by dipping a substrate into a solution that consists of positive and negative charged particles to form a uniform and stable layer, which this process is simple and inexpensive. The process is repeated several times to create multiple layers of thin films. According to Kumara, Tripp, and Muralidharan (2007), the forces that held the thin films is not only specified to electrostatic forces but also can be bonded by noncovalent bonds, such as hydrogen bonds and hydrophobic interactions.

Solid support for use in optical biosensors and other immobilization strategies

The detection of the sample using a biosensor required the immobilization of the biological compound on the transducer surface. The interaction between the sample and the transducer will generate an electrical signal resulting in the contact information to be collected. The results may be shown to change the optical properties, such as absorption, reflectance, emission, or any pattern changes in interferometric when the transducer responds to the analyte. The photodetector will detect and record any changes that occur and convert to an electrical signal. In optical biosensors, three types of supports are usually used to trigger the covalent immobilization of biocomponent: (i) an inert example which is utilized as mechanical support so the handling of planar sensors will become more comfortable, (ii) optical waveguide which is the crucial part that involves a visual interrogation process of the sensor material, (iii) an active substance such as fluorescent nanoparticles, metal films, beads of noble metals, and nanoparticles as well as inorganic or organic micro-substances. The immobilization of biomolecule must be made on a reactive surface in which the layer must be layered by coating it with either polymer or with biorecognition elements such as antibodies. The attachment of biomolecule to the support is made by attaching them covalently, which is commonly used other than physical absorption (Choi, 2004; Tedeschi, Domenici, Ahluwalia, Baldini, & Mencaglia, 2003). For Enzymes, there are immobilized onto membrane support such as Immunodyne, Biodyne (Gautier, Blum, & Coulet, 1989; Xie, Suleiman, & Guilbault, 1992), and Immobilon (Mascini, 1995). Generally, the bio components are being immobilized by using hydrophilic polymer, also used as optical indicators. Solgels are usually used for enzyme immobilization as well as receptors (Aylott, Richardson, & Russell, 1997) and even whole cells (Kwok, Dong, Lo, & Wong, 2005; Lin et al., 2006) immobilization. Aside from that, Hydrogels are also widely used and becoming the most popular since there no restriction of the biological component needed.

Application of optical biosensor in food

Optical bioassays are commonly used to identify residues in food products due to their sensitivity and specificity. The optical sensor is based on a change in optical characteristics when the target analyte is explicitly bound to the bioreceptor, where the signal is measured by light. Optical technologies are divided into a few groups based on various optical concepts such as SPR, SERS, fluorescence, chemiluminescence (CL), electrochemiluminescence (ECL), colorimetric and immunochromatographic biosensors.

Colorimetric sensor

The colorimetric sensor is popular among the various forms of optical sensors due to their simplicity, easy to use, practicality, cost-effectiveness, and observation by the naked eye. The practical theory of colorimetric assays is to transform the detection phase into a change of color. Metal nanomaterials such as gold and silver nanoparticles have gained a great deal of interest in developing colorimetric assays. Gold nanoparticles, as an intensively investigated nanomaterial, have been widely applied in the fabrication of biosensors because of the unique physical and optical properties, which has high SPR absorption. The strong SPR is related to the effect of the quantum size caused by the interaction between electromagnetic radiation and conduction band electrons of gold nanoparticles (Jain, Huang, El-Sayed, & El-Sayed, 2008; Saha, Agasti, Kim, Li, & Rotello, 2012).

Recently, Veríssimo, Gamelas, Fernandes, Evtuguin, and Gomes (2020) presented a sensor composed of an optical fiber with the exposed tip coated with the polyoxometalate salt specifically designed to be insoluble in water that experiences a color change while in contact with formaldehyde. The sensor has been successfully tested for quantification formaldehyde in milk and compared to the conventional method. Bener, Şen, and Apak (2020) designed a simple, quick, and sensitive colorimetric approach based optical sensor using acidified pararosaniline hydrochloride for monitoring the level of sulfite (allergen) in food extracts without pretreatment. The optical sensor performed less sensitive to interferences from turbidity and colored components of the complex food matrix. Casanueva-Marenco, Díaz-de-Alba, Herrera-Armario, Galindo-Riaño, and Granado-Castro (2020) developed a single-use optical sensor using 2-acetylpyridine benzoylhydrazone in a polymer-inclusive membrane immobilized on an inert rectangular polyester strip to monitor heavy metals in food and beverage, dietary supplements and health products. The single-use configuration is useful for regular assessment, providing excellent optical and mechanical characteristics, user-friendly, low-cost, and simple tools.

Fluorescence biosensor

Fluorescence biosensors are attractive and highly influential optical diagnostic strategies due to their unique advantages like ease of operation, multiplexing capability, wide dynamic range, and nondestructive nature. Fluorescence is the emission of visible light in a substance such as fluorescent dye or nanomaterial by excited atoms until returned to the ground (Majdinasab, Hayat, & Marty, 2018). Förster Resonance Energy Transfer (FRET) is a widely used mechanism in fluorescence techniques. The fluorogenic probes, including the fluorophore as a donor and the quencher as an acceptor, form the FRET pair, where the fluorescence of the donor is extinguished by the acceptor when the FRET pair is located nearby (Hirata & Kiyokawa, 2016).

For instance, Ren et al. (2019) designed FRET biosensor based on a four-way branch migration hybridization chain reaction (HCR) for the detection of *Vibrio parahaemolyticus*. It has great potential for detecting pathogens in clinical infection and food safety. Furthermore, Zhong, Gao, Chen, and Jia (2020) manufactured optical biosensors using a dopamine self-polymerization and cross-linking of the fluorescent probe for the detection of *Pseudomonas aeruginosa* to ensure food safety. The proposed optical sensor offers an alternative platform for detecting bacteria in milk, juices, and ice cream samples. (Yue et al., 2018) constructed sensitive and selective fluorescent sensors based metal–organic framework using organic linker 4,4′-(1H-pyrazole-1,3-diyl) dibenzoic acid for detection of ascorbic acid. (Y. Wang et al., 2019) combine the advantages of ratiometric fluorometry and colorimetry to develop a dual-mode method for the determination of ascorbic acid and of ascorbic acid oxidase activity. Similarly, Lah, Jamaludin, Rokhani, Rashid, and Noo (2019) introduced graphene quantum dots coated with gold nanoparticles/cysteamine used to enhance the fluorescence sensing process to detect lard in pig meat. The current sensor has an enormous application to identify and quantify lard for the prospective innovation of food technology.

Chemiluminescence biosensor

CL-based sensors and biosensors are widely used in a variety of fields exclusively for sensitive optical sensor systems to enhance the effectiveness of analytical performance. The concept of luminescence depends on the production of light from an electronically agitated complex that returns to its ground state. The basis of the excitation force serves as the basis for sorting the range of luminescence. CL shows high sensitivity and is capable of detecting a low level of an analyte when the light is generated by a chemical reaction (Blum & Marquette, 2006). Literally, two chemical compounds react to form a high-energy medium which breaks and releases some of its energy as light photons to reach its ground state (Cho, Park, Chong, Kim, & Lee, 2014). CL procedure not using external light sources and longer duration compared to traditional fluorescence techniques (Li, Liu, & Cui, 2014). Currently, CL biosensor has emerged among the sensitive analytical methods which incorporated with nanotechnology.

Surface plasmon resonance (SPR)

SPR is extensively applied that focus on the oscillation takes place at the edge between two components that can be induced by electrons and photons (Situ, Mooney, Elliott, & Buijs, 2010). SPR is 2.5 times higher than that of other optical methods due to its robustness, responsiveness, its applicability to rapid analysis, consistency, and cost-effectiveness. SPR is very sensitive to the dielectric RI that can be attached to the metal surface. In the meantime, the RI is the inherent nature of the materials, and any dielectric integrated into the metal can be seen. As a result, based on this principle, SPR-based biosensors generally combine a wide range of biomolecules such as an enzyme, antibody, and nucleic acid on the metal surface (Rajan, Chand, & Gupta, 2007). Molecules can be recognized directly by relying on values received by the SPR binding reaction. In the last couple of years, SPR-based biosensors have acquired consideration in the detection of specific analyte due to their compact design, cost of testing and ability to analyze in real-time and label-free analysis (Homola, 2003).

Conclusion and future perspectives

Food residues become a significant concern for high quality and healthy food production. Currently, many analytical methods have been developed in various fields to find the ideal method for identifying and quantifying contamination of various analytes, such as pesticide, drug residues, pathogens, heavy metal, and toxic residues. Alternatively, Optical biosensor includes modern analytical tools for reduced size and large-scale, as well as high-throughput screening of a wide range of samples for many different parameters. Different sensitivity-enhancing techniques have been developed for optical biosensors that enhance the signal-to-noise ratio of a simple, compact, and low-cost analytical tool with comprehensive range detection. Nanotechnology has been linked in biosensors for the production of the commercial product at the point of care to overcome the current obstacles of biosensors. The incorporation of nanomaterials is capable of increasing optical and magnetic properties and paves the way for increased sensitivity and precision sensing.

Future efforts should also be focused on improving the aspects of biorecognition to boost their sensitivity towards specific environmental conditions. The binding behavior of almost all forms of biorecognition elements can be influenced by sample conditions, including pH, temperature, viscosity, and strength of ions. Moreover, the interaction of nonspecific bioreceptors with interfering compounds present in biological samples such as food remains a major problem making multiple sample preparation steps inevitable. In this context, high stability, long shelf life, simple to synthesize, low manufacturing costs, molecularly influenced polymers, and in vitro processing can be provided to establish advanced food science and technology biosensors. Finally, the application of enhanced nanomaterial and biorecognition elements can yield upgraded transducer with improved performance.

References

Aylott, J. W., Richardson, D. J., & Russell, D. A. (1997). Optical biosensing of gaseous nitric oxide using spin-coated sol - gel thin Films. *Chemistry of Materials*, *9*(11), 2261–2263. https://doi.org/10.1021/cm970324v.

Baoyi, S., & Zhongdang, X. (2020). Recent achievements in exosomal biomarkers detection by nanomaterials-based optical biosensors—A review. *Analytica Chimica Acta*. https://doi.org/10.1016/j.aca.2020.02.041.

Bener, M., Şen, F. B., & Apak, R. (2020). Novel pararosaniline based optical sensor for the determination of sulfite in food extracts. *Spectrochimica Acta Part A: Molecular and Biomolecular Spectroscopy*. *226*, https://doi.org/10.1016/j.saa.2019.117643.

Blanca, J., Muñoz, P., Morgado, M., Méndez, N., Aranda, A., Reuvers, T., & Hooghuis, H. (2005). Determination of clenbuterol, ractopamine and zilpaterol in liver and urine by liquid chromatography tandem mass spectrometry. *Analytica Chimica Acta* https://doi.org/10.1016/j.aca.2004.09.061 Spain.

Blum, L. J., & Marquette, C. A. (2006). *Chemiluminescence-based sensors*: (pp. 157–178). *Optical chemical sensors* Dordrecht: Springer. https://doi.org/10.1007/1-4020-4611-1_8.

Brecht, A., & Gauglitz, G. (1995). Optical probes and transducers. *Biosensors and Bioelectronics*, *10*(9–10), 923–936. https://doi.org/10.1016/0956-5663(95)99230-I.

Casanueva-Marenco, M. J., Díaz-de-Alba, M., Herrera-Armario, A., Galindo-Riaño, M. D., & Granado-Castro, M. D. (2020). Design and optimization of a single-use optical sensor based on a polymer inclusion membrane for zinc determination in drinks, food supplement and foot health care products. *Materials Science and Engineering: C*, *110*, 110680. https://doi.org/10.1016/j.msec.2020.110680.

Cho, S., Park, L., Chong, R., Kim, Y. T., & Lee, J. H. (2014). Rapid and simple G-quadruplex DNA aptasensor with guanine chemiluminescence detection. *Biosensors and Bioelectronics*, *52*, 310–316. https://doi.org/10.1016/j.bios.2013.09.017.

Choi, M. M. F. (2004). Progress in enzyme-based biosensors using optical transducers. *Microchimica Acta*, *148*(3–4), 107–132. https://doi.org/10.1007/s00604-004-0273-8.

Choi, Y., Kang, T., & Lee, L. P. (2009). Plasmon resonance energy transfer (PRET)-based molecular imaging of cytochrome C in living cells. *Nano Letters*, *9*(1), 85–90. https://doi.org/10.1021/nl802511z.

Choi, Y., Park, Y., Kang, T., & Lee, L. P. (2009). Selective and sensitive detection of metal ions by plasmonic resonance energy transfer-based nanospectroscopy. *Nature Nanotechnology*, *4*(11), 742–746. https://doi.org/10.1038/nnano.2009.258.

Couture, M., Zhao, S. S., & Masson, J. F. (2013). Modern surface plasmon resonance for bioanalytics and biophysics. *Physical Chemistry Chemical Physics*, *15*(27), 11190–11216. https://doi.org/10.1039/c3cp50281c.

Damborský, P., Švitel, J., & Katrlík, J. (2016). Optical biosensors. *Essays in Biochemistry*, *60*(1), 91–100. https://doi.org/10.1042/EBC20150010.

de Almeida, J. C., de Barros, A., Mazali, I. O., & Ferreira, M. (2020). Influence of gold nanostructures incorporated into sodium montmorillonite clay based on LbL films for detection of metal traces ions. *Applied Surface Science*, *507*, 144972. https://doi.org/10.1016/j.apsusc.2019.144972.

Deb, S., Biswas, S., Hussain, S. A., & Bhattacharjee, D. (2005). Spectroscopic characterizations of the mixed Langmuir-Blodgett (LB) films of 2,2′-biquinoline molecules: Evidence of dimer formation. *Chemical Physics Letters*, *405*(4–6), 323–329. https://doi.org/10.1016/j.cplett.2005.02.060.

Decher, G., & Schlenoff, J. B. (2003). *Multilayer thin films: Sequential assembly of nanocomposite materials.* Weinheim: Wiely-VCH.

Erickson, D., Mandal, S., Yang, A. H. J., & Cordovez, B. (2008). Nanobiosensors: Optofluidic, electrical and mechanical approaches to biomolecular detection at the nanoscale. *Microfluidics and Nanofluidics, 4*(1–2), 33–52. https://doi.org/10.1007/s10404-007-0198-8.

Ferguson, J. P., Baxter, G. A., McEvoy, J. D. G., Stead, S., Rawlings, E., & Sharman, M. (2002). Detection of streptomycin and dihydrostreptomycin residues in milk, honey and meat samples using an optical biosensor. *Analyst, 127*(7), 951–956. https://doi.org/10.1039/b200757f.

Ferguson, J., Baxter, A., Young, P., Kennedy, G., Elliott, C., Weigel, S., … Sharman, M. (2005). Detection of chloramphenicol and chloramphenicol glucuronide residues in poultry muscle, honey, prawn and milk using a surface plasmon resonance biosensor and Qflex® kit chloramphenicol. *Analytica Chimica Acta.* https://doi.org/10.1016/j.aca.2004.11.042 United Kingdom.

Ferreira, M., Olivati, C. A., MacHado, A. M., Assaka, A. M., Giacometti, J. A., Akcelrud, L., & Oliveira, O. N. (2007). Langmuir and Langmuir-Blodgett films of polyfluorenes and their use in polymer light-emitting diodes. *Journal of Polymer Research, 14*(1), 39–44. https://doi.org/10.1007/s10965-006-9078-2.

Gautier, S. M., Blum, L. J., & Coulet, P. R. (1989). Fibre-optic sensor with co-immobilised bacterial bioluminescence enzymes. *Biosensors, 4*(3), 181–194. https://doi.org/10.1016/0265-928X(89)80019-7.

Hirata, E., & Kiyokawa, E. (2016). Future perspective of single-molecule FRET biosensors and intravital FRET microscopy. *Biophysical Journal, 111*(6), 1103–1111. https://doi.org/10.1016/j.bpj.2016.01.037.

Homola, J. (2003). Present and future of surface plasmon resonance biosensors. *Analytical and Bioanalytical Chemistry, 377*(3), 528–539. https://doi.org/10.1007/s00216-003-2101-0.

Homola, J. (2008). Surface plasmon resonance sensors for detection of chemical and biological species. *Chemical Reviews, 108*(2), 462–493. https://doi.org/10.1021/cr068107d.

Hussain, S. A. (2009). *Langmuir-Blodgett films a unique tool for molecular electronics.* arXiv preprint arXiv:0908.1814.

Inan, H., Poyraz, M., Inci, F., Lifson, M. A., Baday, M., Cunningham, B. T., & Demirci, U. (2017). Photonic crystals: Emerging biosensors and their promise for point-of-care applications. *Chemical Society Reviews, 46*(2), 366–388. https://doi.org/10.1039/c6cs00206d.

Jain, P. K., Huang, X., El-Sayed, I. H., & El-Sayed, M. A. (2008). Noble metals on the nanoscale: Optical and photothermal properties and some applications in imaging, sensing, biology, and medicine. *Accounts of Chemical Research, 41*(12), 1578–1586. https://doi.org/10.1021/ar7002804.

Jayanthi, V. S. P. K. S. A., Das, A. B., & Saxena, U. (2017). Recent advances in biosensor development for the detection of cancer biomarkers. *Biosensors and Bioelectronics, 91*, 15–23. https://doi.org/10.1016/j.bios.2016.12.014.

Jensen, T. R., Malinsky, M. D., Haynes, C. L., & Van Duyne, R. P. (2000). Nanosphere lithography: Tunable localized surface plasmon resonance spectra of silver nanoparticles. *Journal of Physical Chemistry B, 104*(45), 10549–10556.

Kashif, M., Bakar, A. A. A., Arsad, N., & Shaari, S. (2014). Development of phase detection schemes based on surface plasmon resonance using interferometry. *Sensors (Switzerland), 14*(9), 15914–15938. https://doi.org/10.3390/s140915914.

Kelly, K. L., Coronado, E., Zhao, L. L., & Schatz, G. C. (2003). *The optical properties of metal nanoparticles: The influence of size, shape, and dielectric environment.* https://doi.org/10.1021/jp026731y.

Khansili, N., Rattu, G., & Krishna, P. M. (2018). Label-free optical biosensors for food and biological sensor applications. *Sensors and Actuators, B: Chemical, 265,* 35–49. https://doi.org/10.1016/j.snb.2018.03.004.

Kumara, M. T., Tripp, B. C., & Muralidharan, S. (2007). Layer-by-layer assembly of bioengineered flagella protein nanotubes. *Biomacromolecules, 8*(12), 3718–3722. https://doi.org/10.1021/bm7005449.

Kwok, N. Y., Dong, S., Lo, W., & Wong, K. Y. (2005). An optical biosensor for multi-sample determination of biochemical oxygen demand (BOD). *Sensors and Actuators, B: Chemical, 110*(2), 289–298. https://doi.org/10.1016/j.snb.2005.02.007.

Lah, C. N. H. C., Jamaludin, N., Rokhani, F. Z., Rashid, S. A., & Noor, A. S. M. (2019). Lard detection using a tapered optical fiber sensor integrated with gold-graphene quantum dots. *Sensing and Bio-Sensing Research, 26,* 100306. https://doi.org/10.1016/j.sbsr.2019.100306.

Li, H., Huang, X., Mehedi Hassan, M., Zuo, M., Wu, X., Chen, Y., & Chen, Q. (2020). Dual-channel biosensor for Hg2+ sensing in food using Au@Ag/graphene-upconversion nanohybrids as metal-enhanced fluorescence and SERS indicators. *Microchemical Journal. 154,* https://doi.org/10.1016/j.microc.2019.104563.

Li, N., Liu, D., & Cui, H. (2014). Metal-nanoparticle-involved chemiluminescence and its applications in bioassays. *Analytical and Bioanalytical Chemistry, 406*(23), 5561–5571. https://doi.org/10.1007/s00216-014-7901-x.

Lin, L., Xiao, L. L., Huang, S., Zhao, L., Cui, J. S., Wang, X. H., & Chen, X. (2006). Novel BOD optical fiber biosensor based on co-immobilized microorganisms in ormosils matrix. *Biosensors and Bioelectronics, 21*(9), 1703–1709. https://doi.org/10.1016/j.bios.2005.08.007.

Liz-Marzán, L. M. (2006). Tailoring surface plasmons through the morphology and assembly of metal nanoparticles. *Langmuir, 22*(1), 32–41. https://doi.org/10.1021/la0513353.

Lu, X., Rycenga, M., Skrabalak, S. E., Wiley, B., & Xia, Y. (2009). Chemical synthesis of novel plasmonic nanoparticles. *Annual Review of Physical Chemistry, 60,* 167–192. https://doi.org/10.1146/annurev.physchem.040808.090434.

Luo, X. L., Xu, J. J., Zhao, W., & Chen, H. Y. (2004). Glucose biosensor based on ENFET doped with SiO2 nanoparticles. *Sensors and Actuators, B: Chemical, 97*(2–3), 249–255. https://doi.org/10.1016/j.snb.2003.08.024.

Majdinasab, M., Hayat, A., & Marty, J. L. (2018). Aptamer-based assays and aptasensors for detection of pathogenic bacteria in food samples. *TrAC Trends in Analytical Chemistry, 107,* 60–77. https://doi.org/10.1016/j.trac.2018.07.016.

Majdinasab, M., Mishra, R. K., Tang, X., & Marty, J. L. (2020). Detection of antibiotics in food: New achievements in the development of biosensors. *TrAC Trends in Analytical Chemistry. 127,* https://doi.org/10.1016/j.trac.2020.115883.

Mascini, M. (1995). Enzyme-based optical-fibre biosensors. *Sensors and Actuators B: Chemical, 29*(1–3), 121–125. https://doi.org/10.1016/0925-4005(95)01672-4.

McGrath, T., Baxter, A., Ferguson, J., Haughey, S., & Bjurling, P. (2005). Multi sulfonamide screening in porcine muscle using a surface plasmon resonance biosensor. *Analytica Chimica Acta.* https://doi.org/10.1016/j.aca.2004.10.054 United Kingdom.

Metiu, H., & Das, P. C. (1984). The electromagnetic theory of surface enhanced spectroscopy. *Annual Review of Physical Chemistry, 35*(1), 507–536. https://doi.org/10.1146/annurev.pc.35.100184.002451.

Miyazaki, C. M., Camilo, D. E., Shimizu, F. M., & Ferreira, M. (2019). Improved antibody loading on self-assembled graphene oxide films for using in surface plasmon resonance immunosensors. *Applied Surface Science*, *490*, 502–509. https://doi.org/10.1016/j.apsusc.2019.06.095.

O'Kane, A., & Wahlström, L. (2011). Biosensors in vitamin analysis of foods. In *Fortified foods with vitamins: Analytical concepts to assure better and safer products* (pp. 65–75). Wiley-VCHUnited Kingdom. https://doi.org/10.1002/9783527634156.ch4.

Otto, A., Billmann, J., Eickmans, J., Ertürk, U., & Pettenkofer, C. (1984). The \adatom model\ of SERS (surface enhanced Raman scattering): The present status. *Surface Science*, *138* (2–3), 319–338. https://doi.org/10.1016/0039-6028(84)90251-6.

Pandit, S., Dasgupta, D., Dewan, N., & Prince, A. (2016). Nanotechnology based biosensors and its application. *The Pharma Innovation*, *5*(6, Part A), 18.

Pastor-Navarro, N., Gallego-Iglesias, E., Maquieira, A., & Puchades, R. (2007). Development of a group-specific immunoassay for sulfonamides. Application to bee honey analysis. *Talanta*, *71*(2), 923–933. https://doi.org/10.1016/j.talanta.2006.05.073.

Patel, S., Nanda, R., Sahoo, S., & Mohapatra, E. (2016). Biosensors in health care: The milestones achieved in their development towards lab-on-chip-analysis. *Biochemistry Research International*. *2016*, https://doi.org/10.1155/2016/3130469.

Peng, W., Liu, Y., Fang, P., Liu, X., Gong, Z., Wang, H., & Cheng, F. (2014). Compact surface plasmon resonance imaging sensing system based on general optoelectronic components. *Optics Express International*, *22*(5), 6174–6185. https://doi.org/10.1364/OE.22.006174.

Petryayeva, E., & Krull, U. J. (2011). Localized surface plasmon resonance: Nanostructures, bioassays and biosensing-A review. *Analytica Chimica Acta*, *706*(1), 8–24. https://doi.org/10.1016/j.aca.2011.08.020.

Petty, M. C. (1996). *Langmuir-Blodgett films: An introduction.* Cambridge University Press.

Piliarik, M., & Homola, J. (2009). Surface plasmon resonance (SPR) sensors: Approaching their limits? *Optics Express*, *17*(19), 16505–16517. https://doi.org/10.1364/OE.17.016505.

Puiu, M., & Bala, C. (2016). SPR and SPR imaging: Recent trends in developing nanodevices for detection and real-time monitoringof biomolecular events. *Sensors (Switzerland). 16* (6). https://doi.org/10.3390/s16060870.

Rajan, Chand, S., & Gupta, B. D. (2007). Surface plasmon resonance based fiber-optic sensor for the detection of pesticide. *Sensors and Actuators, B: Chemical*, *123*(2), 661–666. https://doi.org/10.1016/j.snb.2006.10.001.

Raman, C. V., & Krishnan, K. S. (1928). A new type of secondary radiation. *Nature*, *121* (3048), 501–502.

Ren, D., Sun, C., Huang, Z., Luo, Z., Zhou, C., & Li, Y. (2019). A novel FRET biosensor based on four-way branch migration HCR for *Vibrio parahaemolyticus* detection. *Sensors and Actuators B: Chemical*, *296*, 126577. https://doi.org/10.1016/j.snb.2019.05.054.

Roberts, C. G. (Ed.), (1990). *Potential applications of Langmuir-Blodgett films* (pp. 317–411). In *Langmuir-Blodgett films*Boston, MA: Plenum Press, Springer.

Sadani, K., Nag, P., & Mukherji, S. (2019). LSPR based optical fiber sensor with chitosan capped gold nanoparticles on BSA for trace detection of Hg (II) in water, soil and food samples. *Biosensors and Bioelectronics*, *134*, 90–96. https://doi.org/10.1016/j.bios.2019.03.046.

Saha, K., Agasti, S. S., Kim, C., Li, X., & Rotello, V. M. (2012). Gold nanoparticles in chemical and biological sensing. *Chemical Reviews*, *112*(5), 2739–2779. https://doi.org/10.1021/cr2001178.

Shimazaki, Y., Mitsuishi, M., Ito, S., & Yamamoto, M. (1997). Preparation of the layer-by-layer deposited ultrathin film based on the charge-transfer interaction. *Langmuir*, *13*(6), 1385–1387.

Singh, P. (2017). *Surface plasmon resonance: A boon for viral diagnostics*. Reference Module in Life Sciences.

Situ, C., Mooney, M. H., Elliott, C. T., & Buijs, J. (2010). Advances in surface plasmon resonance biosensor technology towards high-throughput, food-safety analysis. *TrAC Trends in Analytical Chemistry*, *29*(11), 1305–1315. https://doi.org/10.1016/j.trac.2010.09.003.

Soler, M., Huertas, C. S., & Lechuga, L. M. (2019). Label-free plasmonic biosensors for point-of-care diagnostics: A review. *Expert Review of Molecular Diagnostics*, *19*(1), 71–81. https://doi.org/10.1080/14737159.2019.1554435.

Sönnichsen, C., Reinhard, B. M., Liphardt, J., & Alivisatos, A. P. (2005). A molecular ruler based on plasmon coupling of single gold and silver nanoparticles. *Nature Biotechnology*, *23*(6).

Spoto, G., & Minunni, M. (2012). Surface plasmon resonance imaging: What next? *Journal of Physical Chemistry Letters*, *3*(18), 2682–2691. https://doi.org/10.1021/jz301053n.

Taitt, C. R., Anderson, G. P., & Ligler, F. S. (2005). Evanescent wave fluorescence biosensors. *Biosensors and Bioelectronics*, *20*(12), 2470–2487. https://doi.org/10.1016/j.bios.2004.10.026.

Taitt, C. R., Anderson, G. P., & Ligler, F. S. (2016). Evanescent wave fluorescence biosensors: Advances of the last decade. *Biosensors and Bioelectronics*, *76*, 103–112. https://doi.org/10.1016/j.bios.2015.07.040.

Tedeschi, L., Domenici, C., Ahluwalia, A., Baldini, F., & Mencaglia, A. (2003). Antibody immobilisation on fibre optic TIRF sensors. *Biosensors and Bioelectronics*, *19*(2), 85–93. https://doi.org/10.1016/S0956-5663(03)00173-8.

Thaxton, C. S., & Mirkin, C. A. (2005). Plasmon coupling measures up. *Nature Biotechnology*, *23*(6), 681–682. https://doi.org/10.1038/nbt0605-681.

Tian, Z. Q., Ren, B., & Wu, D. Y. (2002). Surface-enhanced Raman scattering: From noble to transition metals and from rough surfaces to ordered nanostructures. *Journal of Physical Chemistry B*, *106*(37), 9463–9483. https://doi.org/10.1021/jp0257449.

Turner, D. C., Chang, C., Fang, K., Brandow, S. L., & Murphy, D. B. (1995). Selective adhesion of functional microtubules to patterned silane surfaces. *Biophysical Journal*, *69*(6), 2782–2789. https://doi.org/10.1016/S0006-3495(95)80151-7.

Ulman, A. (2013). *An introduction to ultrathin organic films: From Langmuir-Blodgett to self-assembly*: (pp. 1–443). Elsevier Inc., Undefined, *https:/doi.org/10.1016/C2009-0-22306-3*.

Veríssimo, M. I., Gamelas, J. A., Fernandes, A. J., Evtuguin, D. V., & Gomes, M. T. S. (2020). A new formaldehyde optical sensor: Detecting milk adulteration. *Food Chemistry*, 126461. https://doi.org/10.1016/j.foodchem.2020.126461.

Wang, Y., Yang, Y., Liu, W., Ding, F., Zou, P., Wang, X., Zhao, Q., & Rao, H. (2019). A carbon dot-based ratiometric fluorometric and colorimetric method for determination of ascorbic acid and of the activity of ascorbic acid oxidase. *Microchimica Acta*, *186*(4), 246. https://doi.org/10.1007/s00604-019-3341-9.

Wang, X., Zhan, S., Huang, Z., & Hong, X. (2013). Review: Advances and applications of surface plasmon resonance biosensing instrumentation. *Instrumentation Science and Technology, 41*(6), 574–607. https://doi.org/10.1080/10739149.2013.807822.

Willets, K. A., & Van Duyne, R. P. (2007). Localized surface plasmon resonance spectroscopy and sensing. *Annual Review of Physical Chemistry, 58*, 267–297. https://doi.org/10.1146/annurev.physchem.58.032806.104607.

Wu, D. Y., Li, J. F., Ren, B., & Tian, Z. Q. (2008). Electrochemical surface-enhanced Raman spectroscopy of nanostructures. *Chemical Society Reviews, 37*(5), 1025–1041. https://doi.org/10.1039/b707872m.

Xie, X., Suleiman, A. A., & Guilbault, G. G. (1992). A fluorescence-based fiber optic biosensor for the flow-injection analysis of penicillin. *Biotechnology and Bioengineering, 39*(11), 1147–1150. https://doi.org/10.1002/bit.260391111.

Yue, D., Huang, Y., Zhang, J., Zhang, X., Cui, Y., Yang, Y., & Qian, G. (2018). A two-dimensional metal–organic framework as a fluorescent probe for ascorbic acid sensing. *European Journal of Inorganic Chemistry, 2018*(2), 173–177. https://doi.org/10.1002/ejic.201701079.

Zanchetta, G., Lanfranco, R., Giavazzi, F., Bellini, T., & Buscaglia, M. (2017). Emerging applications of label-free optical biosensors. *Nanophotonics, 6*(4), 627–645. https://doi.org/10.1515/nanoph-2016-0158.

Zhang, H., Song, D., Gao, S., Zhang, H., Zhang, J., & Sun, Y. (2013). Enhanced wavelength modulation SPR biosensor based on gold nanorods for immunoglobulin detection. *Talanta, 115*, 857–862. https://doi.org/10.1016/j.talanta.2013.06.059.

Zhong, Z., Gao, R., Chen, Q., & Jia, L. (2020). Dual-aptamers labeled polydopamine-polyethyleneimine copolymer dots assisted engineering a fluorescence biosensor for sensitive detection of *Pseudomonas aeruginosa* in food samples. *Spectrochimica Acta Part A: Molecular and Biomolecular Spectroscopy. 224*, https://doi.org/10.1016/j.saa.2019.117417.

Zhu, G., Agrawal, N., Singh, R., Kumar, S., Zhang, B., Saha, C., & Kumar, C. (2020). A novel periodically tapered structure-based gold nanoparticles and graphene oxide—Immobilized optical fiber sensor to detect ascorbic acid. *Optics & Laser Technology, 127*, 106156. https://doi.org/10.1016/j.optlastec.2020.106156.

Electrochemical biosensors: State of the art and future perspectives in food analysis

Introduction

Biosensor technology is used in the food industry as a new science that presents rapid, highly sensitive, and selectivity strategies for detecting residues in food products. The uses of nanotechnology in the food industry act as an alternative to conventional approaches for monitoring and maintaining food quality. Nanobiosensors, in combination with electronic processes, is a response to the specific issue. The use of these sensors to detect trace amounts of harmful chemical compounds, viruses, and bacteria in the food industry, agriculture, and the environment has made the advancement of quality control possible. Recently, electrochemical biosensors have focused primarily on clinical research on health, consistency, and sensitivity (Bhalla, Jolly, Formisano, & Estrela, 2016; Rotariu, Lagarde, Jaffrezic-Renault, & Bala, 2016). Interestingly, changes in the biosensor emphasis for food analysis have begun due to improved targeting accuracy, increasing demand for food safety and quality from stakeholders, and a significant decrease in analysis times when used conventional techniques (Kim, Singh, Bai, Leprun, & Bhunia, 2015). Electrochemical biosensor plays a crucial role in food analysis by adding nanoparticles to improve the specificity and selectivity that able to identify harmful pollutants, particularly pesticides, pathogenic microorganisms and antibiotic residues, food toxins, and foodborne organisms (Bunney et al., 2017). During the analysis, information on adulteration or counterfeit products is collected as well as the origin and manufacturing line of the food product to ensure the nutritional value of the product (Cao et al., 2012; Lavecchia, Tibuzzi, & Giardi, 2010).

Principle of electrochemical biosensor for food analysis

Electrochemical biosensors are usually designed using either two or three-electrode systems, namely, working electrode, reference electrode, and the counter electrode. Silver chloride is often used to develop reference electrodes that are maintained at a range from the reaction part that obtains and kept a stable potential during the reaction. By then, the working electrode is mainly as a transduction element in the biochemical reaction. The primary role of the counter electrode to provide a relationship between the surface of the electrode and electrolytic solution to supply current to the

167

Advanced Food Analysis Tools. https://doi.org/10.1016/B978-0-12-820591-4.00009-8

working electrode (Mishra, Barfidokht, Tehrani, & Mishra, 2018). The biosensor theory can be explained by the selective interaction between a target compound and the recognition factor, which will generate an electrical signal. Theoretically, the electrical signal refers to the concentration of the target analyte. Electrochemical biosensors can be categorized into a range of detection criteria, including amperometry, conductometry, electrochemical impedance spectroscopy, potentiometry, and voltammetry (Uniyal & Sharma, 2018).

Amperometry biosensor is focused on the analysis of the current created continuous redox potential signals that occur in the working electrode. Then, it is used to measure the reduced or oxidized species with the resulting current intensity. The potential difference between the reference and working electrode produce from the various concentration of the charged species that analyze in the potentiometry biosensor. The movement of ions to the cathode and anode electrodes that will produce conductance is then involved in the calculation of the conductometry biosensor. In voltammetry, the amperometric measurement of the electrode is used to determine the electroactive species concentration as a function of the voltage applied. In electrochemical impedance spectroscopy (EIS), the resistances and capacitances are determined by applying a small-amplitude sinusoidal AC excitation signal at a specific frequency. The obtained EIS plots will be used to quantify the analyte based on the magnitude of the impedance vector at a specific frequency (Uniyal & Sharma, 2018).

The recent development of the electrochemical biosensors for food analysis

Analysis biosensor detection system consists of components including sample analytes, receptors, transducers modified with nanomaterials, and detectors. The sample is shown in Fig. 9.1. The sample analyte is specific to the appropriate bioreceptor, with the biological response is transmitted to the detector. The transducer incorporated with specific nanomaterials able to enhance the system by employed either electrochemical, optical, and mass detection strategies (Srivastava et al., 2018). Enzymatic and nucleic acid-based biosensors are considered as advanced biosensing technology which has high or ultimate selectivity. Nucleic acid-based sensors include DNA as the recognition or binding entity formed by hybridization and can be divided into multiple groups, including an antibody or biosensor based on antigen and whole-cell sensors (Yang et al., 2016). These types of biosensors are often used to detect microorganisms and food toxins that mainly use of a single sensor platform. Nevertheless, there is a need for a smaller sensing device to provide portability, reasonable cost, and commercialization potential (Warriner, Reddy, Namvar, & Neethirajan, 2014).

Nanomaterials (nanoparticles, nanofibers) are incorporated into biosensors to meet the criteria of an ideal biosensor and driving the way for miniaturization (Shruthi, Amitha, & Mathew, 2014). Nanomaterials may increase the surface area and provide a strong bond to the bioreceptor to improved electrode response

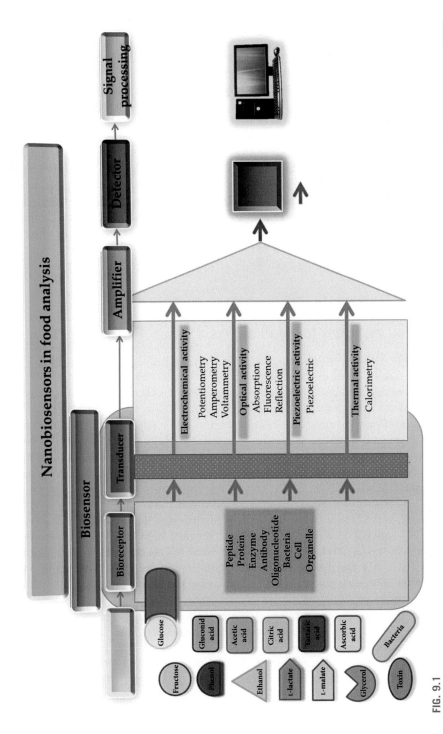

FIG. 9.1

Main components of nanomaterial-based electrochemical biosensor (Srivastava, Dev, & Karmakar, 2018).

characteristics. Nanomaterials also provide higher catalytic capacity, improved biocompatibility, and lower mass transfer resistance by increasing the volume ratio of surface to the area. In the same way, the larger surface area of the transducer will provide improved conductivity and sensitivity, as well as an increased ability to interact with lower detection limits. Nanomaterials such as carbon nanotubes can also be incorporated into the transducer to achieve higher electron transfer rates and improved transducer operation (Pashazadeh et al., 2017). Microfluidics has also received more attention in the production of electrochemical biosensors as throughput processing, sample reduction, and volume of reagents can be obtained. Moreover, microfluidics gives better sensitivity as well as providing a single platform for the extraction and identification process (Luka et al., 2015). Also, the continuous advancement of the electrochemical biosensor analytical characteristics leads to multiple analyte identification at the same time (Vigneshvar, Sudhakumari, Senthilkumaran, & Prakash, 2016). However, further research should be undertaken to ensure that the electrochemical biosensors can be used at any point in complex food matrices throughout the food supply chain, despite promising advances.

Potential analytes for food analysis
Pathogen

Growing cases of diseases caused by the ingestion of contaminated food attracted the attention of the researcher. The available conventional methods for detecting target pathogens such as *Salmonella, Escherichia coli, Listeria monocytogenes*, and *Clostridium botulinum* are often time-consuming. Usually, it takes several days to identify the microorganisms as cultivation methods fully and requires various biochemical testing. Considering that pathogenic bacteria frequently exist in complex food matrices with other nonpathogenic bacteria, a sensitive detection technique is required (Maalouf et al., 2007). Polymerase chain reaction (PCR) and enzyme-linked immunosorbent assay (ELISA) reduced detection time. However, several drawbacks are still encountered, including priming design, lack of the precise labeled secondary antibody as well as incompetent to separate viable and nonviable spores (Dwivedi & Jaykus, 2011). Therefore, a fast and more sensitive analytical approach, such as biosensor-based, is needed to identify the presence of harmful microorganisms at low concentrations within hours to ensure to inhibit the growth of target pathogens in food.

In recent years, the electrochemical biosensor has attracted more attention to the detection of foodborne pathogens because they are sensitive, low cost, and can be miniaturized. Generally, electrochemical biosensor takes within to identify the pathogenic bacteria with excellent reproducibility and repeatability system. Nonetheless, impedance-based biosensors are of primary interest, as high-sensitivity label-free detection can be obtained (Mishra et al., 2018). There are two designs commonly involve in the designing biosensor, namely, label-dependent and label-free methods—both strategies leading to the bioreceptor converting the biological recognition event into electrical signals. Label-based indirect detection of biological or physiochemical molecules, while label-dependent electrochemical biosensors are to induce an electrical shift for measurement.

Viswanathan, Rani, and Ho (2012) designed an electrochemical immunosensor to identify three foodborne pathogens simultaneously, namely, *E. coli* O157:H7, *Salmonella*, and *Campylobacter*. The combination of three separate antibodies to the microbes was immobilized with a practical multiwall carbon nanotube-polyamine on the surface of the screen-printed electrodes. Specific antibody-conjugated nanocrystals were used to release the various metal ions required to be further used in statistical analysis. Furthermore, Hassan, de la Escosura-Muñiz, and Merkoçi (2015) designed an amperometric biosensor to identify the presence of *E. coli* O157:H7 in minced beef and water by using a magnet sandwich assay between the AB-conjugated magnetic beads, second AB-conjugated gold nanoparticles (AuNPs), and target microorganism. The primary function of the AuNP label was to catalyze the hydrogen evolution reaction required to quantify the target *E. coli*.

Label-dependent design provides a practical and precise path for electron transfer, as well as increasing the rate of electron transfer, resulting in a low detection limit with a stronger specificity finding. The biosensor performance is generally improved since the target-label interaction can occur either in the solution or on the electrode surface. Nevertheless, the label-dependent design also has drawbacks, as the detection time-consuming, and the difficulty of the procedures will be faced (Xu, Wang, & Li, 2017). The application of label-free design in electrochemical biosensors has several advantages, including simple identification steps in a short time. As mentioned before, electrochemical biosensors based on label-free approaches can be done through the immobilization of receptors on the surface of electrodes. The label-free electrochemical biosensors can be combined into one test chip due to the precise identification of the target pathogen. However, label-free electrochemical biosensors require extra signal amplification since additional labels are removed as well as the incubation of target bacteria with bioreceptor-immobilized electrodes caused the label-free biosensor detection limit to be slightly higher than the label-dependent version (M. Xu et al., 2017).

According to Wang, Ye, and Ying (2012), membranes of natural microbes cells exhibit a capacitance that creates change in electrical parameters and directly induced by the bacterial cell attachment. Joung et al. (2013) designed an impedimetric immunosensor by utilizing a nanoporous membrane for the determination of *E. coli* O157:H7 in milk. The nanoporous alumina membrane reacts with hyaluronic acid to decrease the nonspecific binding and allows the immobilization of antibodies. The binding of microbes to the nanoporous membrane induces the blockage and increase of the ionic impedance of electrolytes. Lee et al. (2018) introduced one of the advanced methods for detecting a foodborne pathogen through the use of microfluidics integrated with patterned polyimide/polyester films for the amplification, mixing process, and identification strategies. The synthesis film help to reduce and integrate the functionalities into an individual integrated sensing chip within 10 min. The genes of foodborne pathogens can be simultaneously amplified by using the advanced film-based integrated biosensing chip that inserted an electrochemical signal into double-stranded DNA was successfully detect *Staphylococcus aureus* and *Escherichia coli*.

Pesticides

The prevalence of pesticide residues in food has increased food safety as pesticides accumulate in organs that may affect individual health (Alavanja, Hoppin, & Kamel, 2004). There are several types of traditional pesticide detection methods available, including gas chromatography, immunoassay, and capillary electrophoresis (Xu, Liu, & Lu, 2014). Nevertheless, the approaches have several drawbacks address, such as limited storage periods, extensive preparation, and the need for specialized equipment and professional skills (Lv et al., 2018). Arduini et al. (2019) designed a new three-dimensional origami paper integrated with the electrochemical biosensor system containing enzymes and substrates to identified paraoxon, 2,4-dichlorophenoxyacetic acid, and atrazine compound in the river water. Three separate pesticides were identified by the ability to inhibit butyrylcholinesterase, alkaline phosphatase, and tyrosinase, which shows that the number of pesticides strongly influences the degree of inhibition. The findings have shown that a three-dimensional origami paper-based biosensor provides fast, affordable, and reliable techniques for the detection of pesticides.

Yu, Wu, Zhao, Wei, and Lu (2015) determined the level of organophosphorus pesticides modifying carbon nanotubes (CNTs) and acetylcholinesterase (AChE) incorporated in biosensor tools, which functioned as an electronic bridge and signal amplifier and to monitor the efficacy of AChE immobilization. The hydrolysis of unbound acetylthiocholine chloride quantifies the organophosphorus. Tan et al. (2017) constructed electrochemical biosensor by using metal carbonyl conjugated AuNPs with bound organometallic osmium carbonyl construct electrochemical biosensor by using metal clusters that made the nanoparticles free from biomolecule interference. The activity of AChE to catalyze the hydrolysis of acetylthiocholine to thiocholine would be inhibited in the presence of glyphosate pesticides. Consequently, the color changes that appeared during the production of thiocholine induced by the aggregation of metal carbonyl conjugated AuNPs.

Heavy metals

Ikem and Egiebor (2005) identified heavy metals and semi-metals as metals with a density of more than 5 g/cm^3 and an atomic weight ranging from 563 to 3200. Heavy metals such as mercury, cadmium, and a few more, may cause toxic at concentrations higher than the allowable amount. Meanwhile, heavy metals such as iron, manganese, and copper will not harm to human beings when ingested at the level required for body metabolism. Food may be polluted with heavy metals as the contaminants are first consumed by phytoplankton, bacteria, fungi, and other tiny organisms living in the water. Instead, more abundant species can consume the bugs, which pass through the entire food supply chain (Tajkarimi et al., 2008). Therefore, in-situ identification of heavy metals in food must be achieved to minimize the impact of pollution. Electrochemical biosensors for the identification of heavy metals are extremely attractive as fast, low-cost, and sensitive analysis will be obtained compared to labor-intensive, and time-consuming conventional methods, including atomic absorption/emission spectroscopy and inductively, coupled plasma mass spectroscopy. Zhao, Jing, Xue, and Xu (2017) depicted the application of an electrochemical biosensor based on the catalytic hairpin assembly and synergistic amplification to detect the presence of plumbum ion (Pb2+). The Pt@Pd nanocages and electroactive toluidine blue were captured by the hybridization of DNA that caused in the formation of dendritic structure DNA. The structure enables the immobilization of manganese (III) mesotetrakis (4-*N*-methylpyridiniumyl)-porphyrin (MnTMPyP) for signal amplification in the system.

Furthermore, electrochemical biosensors in the detection of hydrogen peroxide can be improved by the use of appropriate hemoglobin immobilization strategies. Dos et al. (2019) demonstrated a combination of zein derived from corn seed with black carbon for hemoglobin immobilization. Zein was chosen for several reasons, in particular, because it is low cost and can be renewed, environmentally friendly, and stable in aqueous solutions (Corradini et al., 2014; Torres-Giner, Gimenez, & Lagaron, 2008). Hemoglobin should not be attached explicitly to electrode surfaces because excellent performance will not be achieved as hemoglobin has not been developed and will be partially denatured. Hence, efforts must be taken to overcome the limitations of hemoglobin by combining with carbon black that contains high sp2 carbon–carbon bonds to enhance the conductivity properties. Besides, the signal performance increased because of the large surface area and the conductive nature of the porous film containing black carbon and hemoglobin incorporated into the zine microsphere. Therefore, protein derived from renewable sources, such as zein, has been shown to act as a matrix for biomolecular immobilization when combined with a carbon content (Cammarota et al., 2013; Lo, Aldous, & Compton, 2012).

Veterinary drugs

Veterinary drugs are used for therapeutic and prophylactic purposes in animals to regulate infections of bacterial and prevent outbreaks of animal diseases (Lv et al., 2018). Antibiotics are an example of veterinary drugs used to enhance animal health and development. Nevertheless, the unnecessary use of antibiotics can lead to the development of bacterial resistance. Also, contaminants of such veterinary drugs and metabolites will remain and store in livestock products, for example, eggs, milk, and meat. The contamination of food may cause anaphylactic shock, allergies, irritation, and resistance to the pathogen (Baynes et al., 2016; Reig & Toldrá, 2008). Regulations have been established to ensure that byproducts of veterinary drugs are not exceeded to the maximum residual level permitted. The detection of veterinary drugs is, therefore, crucial to food safety and quality control. Govindasamy et al. (2017) developed hybrid material with molybdenum disulfide nanosheets (MoS_2) with functionalized multiwalled carbon nanotubes (f-MWCNTs) to detect the presence of chloramphenicol in milk, honey, and powdered milk. The hybrid nanomaterials prepared by using the hydrothermal process and provide high electro-chemical properties and excellent electrocatalytic ability to identify chloramphenicol in a low detection limit. The electrochemical biosensor developed shows a high degree of selectivity, even with interference from large excess species concentrations, with adequate repeatability, reproducibility, and stability.

A simple, low-cost, reliable, and good sensitive paper-based immunosensor fabricated by Wu et al. (2012).

Food toxins

Food toxins are mainly classified into mycotoxins, algal toxins, and plant/bacterial toxins. Dridi et al. (2017) defined food toxins as a wide range of natural substances that originate from fungi, algae, plants, or bacteria metabolism and may have adverse effects on human health at low doses. Contamination of food products can occur at any level of the food supply chain and has prompted most countries to lay down strict regulations to mitigate possible contamination. Mycotoxins are toxicants of low molecular weight produced by filamentous fungi, and complex chemical structures. The presence of mycotoxins in food has become a significant issue in the food industry that may cause genetic disorders and carcinogenic processes that can be found in different food types, particularly in agricultural products such as fruit and coffee, as well as in derivatives (Alshannaq & Yu, 2017; Marin, Ramos, Cano-Sancho, & Sanchis, 2013). Algal toxins, such as okadaic acid, patentoxins, and microcystin, is classified as secondary metabolites that are formed by phytoplankton, such as dinoflagellates and cyanobacteria. Contamination caused by algal toxins can occur rapidly due to the proliferation of phytoplankton toxin-producing species, or harmful algal blooms enter shellfish and fish (Dridi et al., 2017). Bacterial toxins divided into two groups, exotoxins, and endotoxin produced by gram-positive and gram-negative bacterial pathogens (Zhu et al., 2014). Modern portable biosensors integrated based electrochemical with nanomaterials be a promising alternative method for detecting toxins present in food products due to low detection limits and high selectivity and specificity for immediate food contamination detection (Vogiazi et al., 2019).

A biosensor includes a biological recognition element that acts responds explicitly to the objective of interest, as shown in Fig. 9.2. The biological reaction occurs at the interface of the sample solution and transducer. An electrode is used as a transducer which responsibility to convert the reaction into an electrical signal, voltage, or current. The electrochemical technique known as transduction collects, amplifies, and displays the signal by the signal processor. Bulbul, Hayat, and Andreescu (2015) depicted the construction of a novel electrochemical biosensor based on nonenzymatic nanocatalysts using nanoceria tag and graphene oxide to detect ochratoxin A in cereal samples. The use of different competitive mechanisms between the target labeled free and nanoceria is enabled to capture the target analyte using an

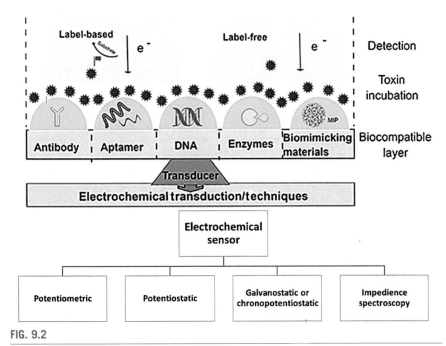

FIG. 9.2

Graphical components and operating concept of electrochemical biosensors used for toxins analysis.

immobilized aptamer, and the signal was produced by electro-oxidizing a generic redox species. Eissa, Ng, Siaj, and Zourob (2014) reported a highly specific and sensitive electrochemical biosensor by using an unlabeled DNA aptamer incorporated on a graphene electrode to detect microcystin-LR in fish samples. The fabrication of aptasensor was done based on the noncovalent bond used to assemble the DNA aptamer on graphene-modified screen-printed carbon electrodes, resulting in the reduction of $[Fe(CN)_6]^{4-/3-}$ and increased peak current when the target food toxin is present. Apart from low cost and high performance, the biosensor produced did not show any cross-reactivity to okadaic acid, microcystin-LA, and microcystin-YR.

Zhu, Shi, Feng, and Susan Zhou (2015) proposed a sandwich electrochemical impedance immunosensor to detect *Clostridium difficile* toxin A and toxin B. The signal was amplified using AuNPs conjugated with a single domain antibody based on the electron transfer resistance. In another study conducted by Luo, Liu, Xia, Xu, and Xie (2014) identified the *Clostridium difficile* toxin A using an aptamer selected through the systematic evolution of ligands and AuNPs synthesized by *Bacillus stearothermophilus*. The thiolated single-stranded DNA mounted on a Nafion-thionine-GNPS-modified screen-printed electrode via an Au-thiol interaction. Hybridization of the horseradish peroxidase (HRP)-labeled aptamer probe was done to complement the oligonucleotide of the capture probe to obtain an aptamer-DNA duplex. The developed sensors were based on the electrocatalytic characteristics of thionine due to the alteration of the electrode surface with HRP by aptamer-DNA duplex in the absence of TcdA, mediated by the generation of electrons through the enzymatic reaction of hydrogen peroxide via HRP catalysis.

Other chemical contaminants

Various electrochemical biosensors designed to detect the presence of additives in foods due to the misapplication of food additives that caused unfavorable health effects. Food additives such as Sudan I are a type of carcinogen widely used in chili powder due to its low cost of producing an attractive red color (Palanisamy, Kokulnathan, Chen, Velusamy, & Ramaraj, 2017).

Apart from food additives, the presence of carcinogens in food products has also become a significant food safety concern. Carcinogenic compounds may be produced during food processing, such as high-temperature cooking resulting in a group 2 carcinogen known as acrylamide (Hsu et al., 2016). Additionally, trimethylamine oxide decomposition into two forms of carcinogens, formaldehyde, and dimethylamine, may also occur during high-temperature cooking (Zhu, Jia, Li, Dong, & Li, 2013). Sani, Heng, Marugan, and Rajab (2018) developed an electrochemical DNA biosensor based on nanocomposites to detect carcinogens in Mackerel fish and cassava chips by immobilizing amine-terminated single-stranded DNA on silica nanospheres mounted on a screen-printed electrode using AuNPs. Carcinogens were identified based on three separate DNA sequences, which were useful DNA of 15-base guanine, 24-base guanine, and 24-base adenine thymine.

Electrochemical biosensors integrated with nanomaterials

Recently, there is an emerging trend in the integration of nanomaterials with biosensors that potentially enhance the sensitivity system, low-level detection, high stability, and rapid response rate. Nanomaterials play an essential role in biosensor enhancing transducer response properties and as matrices for receptors for immobilization. The selection of nanomaterials is based on the desired effects on the transducers (Kucherenko, Soldatkin, Kucherenko, Soldatkina, & Dzyadevych, 2019). According to Pérez-López and Merkoçi (2011), the use of nanomaterials in electrochemical biosensors that include a reduction in overpotentials of many analytically significant electrochemical reactions and reversibility of some redox reactions can provide many advantages. Fig. 9.2 depicted the main components and working concepts of electrochemical biosensors based on nanomaterials. Specifically, there are several examples of nanomaterials used in electrochemical biosensors, including carbon-based nanomaterials, metal and metal oxide nanoparticles, magnetic nanoparticles, and molecular imprinted polymers (Zeng, Zhu, Du, & Lin, 2016).

Carbon nanotubes

Carbon nanotubes can be divided into two main classes based on the amount of rolled layers consisting of single-walled carbon nanotubes (SWNTs) and multi-walled carbon nanotubes (MWNTs) (Zeng et al., 2016). SWNTs and MWNTs, mainly mechanical, electrical, and chemical, assists in the manufacture of electrodes in biosensors. The CNTs usually functionalized and activated by using carboxyl or amino groups or combinations with other materials such as metal nanoparticles to improve the solubility and biocompatibility of carbon nanotubes. MWNTs are multi-nested graphene sheets with large surface area, specific physical properties, flexible lengths, and reasonable prices with diameters of up to 100nm (Chen & Chatterjee, 2013). MWNTs, enhance biosensor efficiency by enabling the transfer of electrons between electroactive organisms and electrodes. Apart from that, MWNTs are often combined with metal nanoparticles to produce additional electrocatalytic sites as well as to improve electrode sensitivity and detection limits. Lin, Hong, and Chen (2013) demonstrated the use of carbon nanotubes to enhance the sensitivity and selectivity of the proposed biosensor during the food analysis. Nitrogen-doped graphene and nitrogen-doped carbon nanotubes or NGR-NCNT nanocomposites were electrodeposited to glassy carbon electrodes using potentiostat based on aqueous potassium chloride solution containing homogeneous NGR-NCNTs. The biosensor developed was used to detect the presence of toxic ractopamine and salbutamol in pig samples at the same time. It was proven that synergistic effects that result in better electrocatalytic properties to ractopamine and salbutamol were obtained by using a more compact structure of SMWNTs. Apart from this, the use of combined CNTs and molecular imprinted polymers (MIPs) has gained more interest in food research. The steric and hydrophobic and electrostatic interactions produced from MIPs and analytes reaction are known as antigen-like artificial antibody (Ag-Ab) interactions (Rotariu et al., 2016). The combination of CNTs and MIPs is one of the promising techniques, as MIPs have great potential to replace natural biorecognition and promote the sensitivity, selectivity, and stability of developed biosensors. Prasad, Jauhari, and Tiwari (2014) developed an MIP nanofilm-modified pencil graphite electrode dual prototype dispersing gold nanoparticles and CNT in the polymer layer to identify glyphosate and glufosinate simultaneously. The nanohybrids provide an excellent electron transfer capability for herbicide oxidation.

Graphene materials

Geim and Novoselov (2010) developed a true two-dimensional nanosheet known as graphene. The unique physicochemical characteristics have attracted researcher to use of graphene and its derivatives (graphene oxide and reduced graphene oxide). Noble metal nanoparticles are often incorporated with graphene to obtain a more comprehensive functional material with a desirable electrochemical activity. Zhu, Dietrich, Didier, Doyscher, and Märtlbauer (2014) demonstrated a simple green electrochemical model based on the electrostatic interaction to synthesize graphene-AuNRs nanocomposite (GN-AuNRs) to a glassy carbon electrode (GCE). The nanocomposite developed was used to assess the presence of methyl parathion (MP) in kiwi fruits. GN-AuNRs have several advantages since they are environmentally friendly and do not involve a chemical reduction of graphene oxide (GO). Similarly, the development of GN-AuNRs is natural, as it requires only the basis of electrostatic interaction that includes electrochemical reduction of GO-AuNRs to GN-AuNRs throughout the process. Based on square wave voltammetric (SWV) measurements, it has been shown that the biosensor has a high methyl parathion sensitivity due to increased conductivity, large surface area, functional adsorption capacity for more aromatic rings and high graphene catalytic capacity, and excellent electronic properties and AUNR's adsorption capacity. Wang et al. (2014) constructed a biosensor for the identification of clenbuterol in pork using a poly(sodium4-styrene sulfonate) (PSS) functionalized GR synthesis. The process includes a simple one-stage chemical reduction of exfoliated graphite oxides in the existence of PSS. The PSS-GR was used for the construction of the isopropanol-Nafion-PSS-GR composite film modified glass carbon electrode. Therefore, it can be inferred from the analysis that conductive polymer film-modified electrodes offer higher reproducibility with more convenient manufacturing compared to the monolayer electrodes. Electrodes with higher sensitivity and selectivity were also obtained.

Metal nanoparticles

The fabrication of the sensing interface in the biosensor is the frequent use in metal nanoparticles due to the unique properties such as excellent biocompatibility and catalysis. AuNPs are the most commonly used metal nanoparticles since the aggregation of AuNPs can result in color changes signaling the presence of the target analyte. Furthermore, AuNPs delivers excellent performance even without carbon-based nanomaterials. Improved functionalization of particles through different types of biomolecules can be achieved by using AuNPs as AuNPs provide high conductivity for massive surface area and surface energy, as well as by offering different surface functional groups. Zeng et al. (2016) illustrated the acetylcholinesterase (AChE) biosensors that use significant conductive AuNPs and other nanomaterials. The combination of AuNPs and cadmium telluride (CdTe) quantum dots via chitosan microspheres has been demonstrated in a study carried out by Du, Chen, Song, Li, and Chen (2008). The combined AChE had a high affinity to target analyte because AuNPs had a high ability to transfer electrons and a high-sensitivity analytical method for the detection of monocrotophos.

Besides, the combination resulted in better detection sensitivity, as the presence of synergistic effects in CdTe-GNP film increased the electron transfer and the electro-oxidation of thiocholine. The CdTe QDs-GNPs composite biosensor was therefore considered a promising technique in food analysis as a better response in terms of sensitivity compared to CdTe QDs or GNPs alone. Metal nanoparticles can be used for the detection of foodborne organisms, as demonstrated by (Li et al., 2013). The amperometric biosensor was designed to detect the presence of *Escherichia coli* O157:H7 by using fullerene, ferrocene, and thiolate chitosan nanolayer composites. The nanolayer provided active –SH functional groups as well as excellent biocompatibility. The antibodies were immobilized by a covalent reaction that occurred between biotin and avidin. As a result, it has been shown that a rapid and sensitive detection method can be obtained by using the biosensor created.

Magnetic nanoparticles

Magnetic particles are used in the design of a biosensor as nanomaterials can serve as supports and carriers during food analysis. The location and transport of magnetic nanoparticles can be monitored and controlled using a magnetic field and provide a large surface area as well as excellent biocompatibility (Zeng et al., 2016). Sun et al. (2015) developed an electrochemical-based immunosensor by applying a biocompatible quinone-rich polydopamine nanosphere modified glassy carbon electrode as the sensor framework for chlorpyrifos detection. Synthesis of the flake-like Fe_3O_4-coated CNTs was conducted to be used as the carrier for the multi-enzyme label, resulting in a high-performance food analytics biosensor. In another study, Han et al. (2014) developed an electrochemical magnetic molecular imprinted sensor focused on the self-assembly of Fe_3O_4@rGO composites directed by magnetic fields to detect azo dye amaranth. Modification of electrodes using the external magnetic field has provided many tangible benefits, such as rapid immobilization and orientation of magnetic composites, naturally formed nanostructure film to prevent severe aggregation, convenient thickness modulation, and the morphology of the modified film.

Conclusion and future perspectives

An electrochemical biosensor is suitable for food analysis throughout all stages of the supply chain due to the essential characteristics, which include the precision, flexibility, and adaptability of complicated food matrices, both in the present and shortly. It is undeniably clear that biosensors offer many advantages in food analysis compared to conventional techniques commonly used. Biosensors are expected to be used in digital technology to assist food producers, suppliers, authorities, and customers, in the real-time monitoring of foodstuffs, in particular dairy products and brewed products, which may aid in the decision-making process (Valderrama, Dudley, Doores, & Cutter, 2016; Zhang & Liu, 2016). Nonetheless, electrochemical biosensors need to strengthen their sensitivity, selectivity, sustainable cell behavior, and feasibility even under non-native conditions before their real-time application and commercialization purposes. It is also expected that biomimetic sensors such as electronic tongues and electronic noses will be used as well as low-specific sensor arrays capable of detecting numerous signals to provide a complete food analysis (Cetó, Voelcker, & Prieto-Simón, 2016). Meanwhile, the use of multiple biosensor forms is also a promising technique, for example, integration of electronic tongues with electronic noses lead to improved detection capabilities of a biomimetic system, as precisely as a biological system (Di Rosa, Leone, Cheli, & Chiofalo, 2017).

References

Alavanja, M. C. R., Hoppin, J. A., & Kamel, F. (2004). Health effects of chronic pesticide exposure: Cancer and neurotoxicity. *Annual Review of Public Health*, *25*, 155–197. https://doi.org/10.1146/annurev.publhealth.25.101802.123020.

Alshannaq, A., & Yu, J. H. (2017). Occurrence, toxicity, and analysis of major mycotoxins in food. *International Journal of Environmental Research and Public Health*. *14*(6) https://doi.org/10.3390/ijerph14060632.

Arduini, F., Cinti, S., Caratelli, V., Amendola, L., Palleschi, G., & Moscone, D. (2019). Origami multiple paper-based electrochemical biosensors for pesticide detection. *Biosensors and Bioelectronics*, *126*, 346–354. https://doi.org/10.1016/j.bios.2018.10.014.

Baynes, R. E., Dedonder, K., Kissell, L., Mzyk, D., Marmulak, T., Smith, G., ... Riviere, J. E. (2016). Health concerns and management of select veterinary drug residues. *Food and Chemical Toxicology*, *88*, 112–122. https://doi.org/10.1016/j.fct.2015.12.020.

Bhalla, N., Jolly, P., Formisano, N., & Estrela, P. (2016). Introduction to biosensors. *Essays in Biochemistry*, *60*(1), 1–8. https://doi.org/10.1042/EBC20150001.

Bulbul, G., Hayat, A., & Andreescu, S. (2015). A generic amplification strategy for electrochemical aptasensors using a non-enzymatic nanoceria tag. *Nanoscale*, *7*(31), 13230–13238. https://doi.org/10.1039/c5nr02628h.

Bunney, J., Williamson, S., Atkin, D., Jeanneret, M., Cozzolino, D., Chapman, J., ... Chandra, S. (2017). The use of electrochemical biosensors in food analysis. *Current Research in Nutrition and Food Science*, *5*(3), 183–195. https://doi.org/10.12944/CRNFSJ.5.3.02.

Cammarota, M., Lepore, M., Portaccio, M., Di Tuoro, D., Arduini, F., Moscone, D., & Mita, D. G. (2013). Laccase biosensor based on screen-printed electrode modified withthionine-carbon black nanocomposite, for bisphenol A detection. *Electrochimica Acta*, *109*, 340–347. https://doi.org/10.1016/j.electacta.2013.07.129.

Cao, M., Li, Z., Wang, J., Ge, W., Yue, T., Li, R., ... Yu, W. W. (2012). Food related applications of magnetic iron oxide nanoparticles: Enzyme immobilization, protein purification, and food analysis. *Trends in Food Science and Technology*, *27*(1), 47–56. https://doi.org/10.1016/j.tifs.2012.04.003.

Cetó, X., Voelcker, N. H., & Prieto-Simón, B. (2016). Bioelectronic tongues: New trends and applications in water and food analysis. *Biosensors and Bioelectronics*, *79*, 608–626. https://doi.org/10.1016/j.bios.2015.12.075.

Chen, A., & Chatterjee, S. (2013). Nanomaterials based electrochemical sensors for biomedical applications. *Chemical Society Reviews*, *42*(12), 5425–5438. https://doi.org/10.1039/c3cs35518g.

Corradini, E., Curti, P. S., Meniqueti, A. B., Martins, A. F., Rubira, A. F., & Muniz, E. C. (2014). Recent advances in food-packing, pharmaceutical and biomedical applications of zein and zein-based materials. *International Journal of Molecular Sciences*, *15*(12), 22438–22470. https://doi.org/10.3390/ijms151222438.

Di Rosa, A. R., Leone, F., Cheli, F., & Chiofalo, V. (2017). Fusion of electronic nose, electronic tongue and computer vision for animal source food authentication and quality assessment—A review. *Journal of Food Engineering*, *210*, 62–75. https://doi.org/10.1016/j.jfoodeng.2017.04.024.

Dos, T. S. P., de Oliveira, M. G. C., Santos, F. A., Raymundo-Pereira, P. A., Oliveira, J. O., & Janegitz, B. C. (2019). Use of zein microspheres to anchor carbon black and hemoglobin in electrochemical biosensors to detect hydrogen peroxide in cosmetic products, food and biological fluids. *Talanta, 194*, 737–744.

Dridi, F., Marrakchi, M., Gargouri, M., Saulnier, J., Jaffrezic-Renault, N., & Lagarde, F. (2017). *Nanomaterial-based electrochemical biosensors for food safety and quality assessment*: (pp. 167–204). *Nanobiosensors* Academic Press. https://doi.org/10.1016/B978-0-12-804301-1.00005-9.

Du, D., Chen, S., Song, D., Li, H., & Chen, X. (2008). Development of acetylcholinesterase biosensor based on CdTe quantum dots/gold nanoparticles modified chitosan microspheres interface. *Biosensors and Bioelectronics, 24*(3), 475–479. https://doi.org/10.1016/j.bios.2008.05.005.

Dwivedi, H. P., & Jaykus, L. A. (2011). Detection of pathogens in foods: The current state-of-the-art and future directions. *Critical Reviews in Microbiology, 37*(1), 40–63. https://doi.org/10.3109/1040841X.2010.506430.

Eissa, S., Ng, A., Siaj, M., & Zourob, M. (2014). Label-free voltammetric aptasensor for the sensitive detection of microcystin-LR using graphene-modified electrodes. *Analytical Chemistry, 86*(15), 7551–7557. https://doi.org/10.1021/ac501335k.

Geim, A. K., & Novoselov, K. S. (2010). The rise of graphene, nanoscience and technology: a collection of reviews from nature journals. *World Sci, 11–*19. https://doi.org/10.1142/9789814287005_0002.

Govindasamy, M., Chen, S. M., Mani, V., Devasenathipathy, R., Umamaheswari, R., Joseph Santhanaraj, K., & Sathiyan, A. (2017). Molybdenum disulfide nanosheets coated multiwalled carbon nanotubes composite for highly sensitive determination of chloramphenicol in food samples milk, honey and powdered milk. *Journal of Colloid and Interface Science, 485*, 129–136. https://doi.org/10.1016/j.jcis.2016.09.029.

Han, Q., Wang, X., Yang, Z., Zhu, W., Zhou, X., & Jiang, H. (2014). Fe3O4@rGO doped molecularly imprinted polymer membrane based on magnetic field directed self-assembly for the determination of amaranth. *Talanta, 123*, 101–108. https://doi.org/10.1016/j.talanta.2014.01.060.

Hassan, A. R. H. A. A., de la Escosura-Muñiz, A., & Merkoçi, A. (2015). Highly sensitive and rapid determination of Escherichia coli O157:H7 in minced beef and water using electrocatalytic gold nanoparticle tags. *Biosensors and Bioelectronics, 67*, 511–515. https://doi.org/10.1016/j.bios.2014.09.019.

Hsu, H. T., Chen, M. J., Tseng, T. P., Cheng, L. H., Huang, L. J., & Yeh, T. S. (2016). Kinetics for the distribution of acrylamide in French fries, fried oil and vapour during frying of potatoes. *Food Chemistry, 211*, 669–678. https://doi.org/10.1016/j.foodchem.2016.05.125.

Ikem, A., & Egiebor, N. O. (2005). Assessment of trace elements in canned fishes (mackerel, tuna, salmon, sardines and herrings) marketed in Georgia and Alabama (United States of America). *Journal of Food Composition and Analysis, 18*(8), 771–787. https://doi.org/10.1016/j.jfca.2004.11.002.

Joung, C. K., Kim, H. N., Lim, M. C., Jeon, T. J., Kim, H. Y., & Kim, Y. R. (2013). A nanoporous membrane-based impedimetric immunosensor for label-free detection of pathogenic bacteria in whole milk. *Biosensors and Bioelectronics, 44*(1), 210–215. https://doi.org/10.1016/j.bios.2013.01.024.

Kim, K. P., Singh, A. K., Bai, X., Leprun, L., & Bhunia, A. K. (2015). AK novel PCR assays complement laser biosensor-based method and facilitate *Listeria* species detection from food. *Sensors, 15*, 22672–22691.

Kucherenko, I. S., Soldatkin, O. O., Kucherenko, D. Y., Soldatkina, O. V., & Dzyadevych, S. V. (2019). Advances in nanomaterial application in enzyme-based electrochemical biosensors: A review. *Nanoscale Advances, 1*(12), 4560–4577. https://doi.org/10.1039/c9na00491b.

Lavecchia, T., Tibuzzi, A., & Giardi, M. T. (2010). Biosensors for functional food safety and analysis. *Advances in Experimental Medicine and Biology, 698*, 267–281. https://doi.org/10.1007/978-1-4419-7347-4_20.

Lee, T. J., Lim, S. Y., Shin, S. J., Kim, C. H., Jeong, S. W., Shin, S. Y., … Jung, G. Y. (2018). A film-based integrated chip for gene amplification and electrochemical detection of pathogens causing foodborne illnesses. *Analytica Chimica Acta, 1027*, 57–66. https://doi.org/10.1016/j.aca.2018.03.061.

Lin, K. C., Hong, C. P., & Chen, S. M. (2013). Simultaneous determination for toxic ractopamine and salbutamol in pork sample using hybrid carbon nanotubes. *Sensors and Actuators, B: Chemical, 177*, 428–436. https://doi.org/10.1016/j.snb.2012.11.052.

Li, Y., Fang, L., Cheng, P., Deng, J., Jiang, L., Huang, H., & Zheng, J. (2013). An electrochemical immunosensor for sensitive detection of Escherichia coli O157:H7 using C60 based biocompatible platform and enzyme functionalized Pt nanochains tracing tag. *Biosensors and Bioelectronics, 49*, 485–491. https://doi.org/10.1016/j.bios.2013.06.008.

Lo, T. W. B., Aldous, L., & Compton, R. G. (2012). The use of nano-carbon as an alternative to multi-walled carbon nanotubes in modified electrodes for adsorptive stripping voltammetry. *Sensors and Actuators, B: Chemical, 162*(1), 361–368. https://doi.org/10.1016/j.snb.2011.12.104.

Luka, G., Ahmadi, A., Najjaran, H., Alocilja, E., Derosa, M., Wolthers, K., … Hoorfar, M. (2015). Microfluidics integrated biosensors: A leading technology towards lab-on-A-chip and sensing applications. *Sensors (Switzerland), 15*(12), 30011–30031. https://doi.org/10.3390/s151229783.

Luo, P., Liu, Y., Xia, Y., Xu, H., & Xie, G. (2014). Aptamer biosensor for sensitive detection of toxin A of Clostridium difficile using gold nanoparticles synthesized by Bacillus stearothermophilus. *Biosensors and Bioelectronics, 54*, 217–221. https://doi.org/10.1016/j.bios.2013.11.013.

Lv, M., Liu, Y., Geng, J., Kou, X., Xin, Z., & Yang, D. (2018). Engineering nanomaterials-based biosensors for food safety detection. *Biosensors and Bioelectronics, 106*, 122–128. https://doi.org/10.1016/j.bios.2018.01.049.

Maalouf, R., Fournier-Wirth, C., Coste, J., Chebib, H., Saïkali, Y., Vittori, O., … Jaffrezic-Renault, N. (2007). Label-free detection of bacteria by electrochemical impedance spectroscopy: Comparison to surface plasmon resonance. *Analytical Chemistry, 79*(13), 4879–4886. https://doi.org/10.1021/ac070085n.

Marin, S., Ramos, A. J., Cano-Sancho, G., & Sanchis, V. (2013). Mycotoxins: Occurrence, toxicology, and exposure assessment. *Food and Chemical Toxicology, 60*, 218–237. https://doi.org/10.1016/j.fct.2013.07.047.

Mishra, G. K., Barfidokht, A., Tehrani, F., & Mishra, R. K. (2018). Food safety analysis using electrochemical biosensors. *Food. 7*(9)https://doi.org/10.3390/foods7090141.

Palanisamy, S., Kokulnathan, T., Chen, S. M., Velusamy, V., & Ramaraj, S. K. (2017). Voltammetric determination of Sudan I in food samples based on platinum nanoparticles decorated on graphene-β-cyclodextrin modified electrode. *Journal of Electroanalytical Chemistry, 794*, 64–70. https://doi.org/10.1016/j.jelechem.2017.03.041.

Pashazadeh, P., Mokhtarzadeh, A., Hasanzadeh, M., Hejazi, M., Hashemi, M., & de la Guardia, M. (2017). Nano-materials for use in sensing of salmonella infections: Recent advances. *Biosensors and Bioelectronics, 87*, 1050–1064. https://doi.org/10.1016/j.bios.2016.08.012.

Pérez-López, B., & Merkoçi, A. (2011). Nanomaterials based biosensors for food analysis applications. *Trends in Food Science and Technology, 22*(11), 625–639. https://doi.org/10.1016/j.tifs.2011.04.001.

Prasad, B. B., Jauhari, D., & Tiwari, M. P. (2014). Doubly imprinted polymer nanofilm-modified electrochemical sensor for ultra-trace simultaneous analysis of glyphosate and glufosinate. *Biosensors and Bioelectronics, 59*, 81–88. https://doi.org/10.1016/j.bios.2014.03.019.

Reig, M., & Toldrá, F. (2008). Veterinary drug residues in meat: Concerns and rapid methods for detection. *Meat Science, 78*(1–2), 60–67. https://doi.org/10.1016/j.meatsci.2007.07.029.

Rotariu, L., Lagarde, F., Jaffrezic-Renault, N., & Bala, C. (2016). Electrochemical biosensors for fast detection of food contaminants—Trends and perspective. *TrAC Trends in Analytical Chemistry, 79*, 80–87. https://doi.org/10.1016/j.trac.2015.12.017.

Sani, N. D. M., Heng, L. Y., Marugan, R. S. P. M., & Rajab, N. F. (2018). Electrochemical DNA biosensor for potential carcinogen detection in food sample. *Food Chemistry, 269*, 503–510. https://doi.org/10.1016/j.foodchem.2018.07.035.

Shruthi, G. S., Amitha, C. V., & Mathew, B. B. (2014). Biosensors: A modern day achievement. *Journal of Instrumentation Technology, 2*(1), 26–39.

Srivastava, A. K., Dev, A., & Karmakar, S. (2018). Nanosensors and nanobiosensors in food and agriculture. *Environmental Chemistry Letters, 16*(1), 161–182. https://doi.org/10.1007/s10311-017-0674-7.

Sun, Z., Wang, W., Wen, H., Gan, C., Lei, H., & Liu, Y. (2015). Sensitive electrochemical immunoassay for chlorpyrifos by using flake-like Fe3O4 modified carbon nanotubes as the enhanced multienzyme label. *Analytica Chimica Acta, 899*, 91–99. https://doi.org/10.1016/j.aca.2015.09.057.

Tajkarimi, M., Faghih, M. A., Poursoltani, H., Nejad, A. S., Motallebi, A. A., & Mahdavi, H. (2008). Lead residue levels in raw milk from different regions of Iran. *Food Control*, 495–498. https://doi.org/10.1016/j.foodcont.2007.05.015.

Tan, M. J., Hong, Z. Y., Chang, M. H., Liu, C. C., Cheng, H. F., Loh, X. J., Chen, C. H., Liao, C. D., & Kong, K. V. (2017). Metal carbonyl-gold nanoparticle conjugates for highly sensitive SERS detection of organophosphorus pesticides. *Biosensors and Bioelectronics, 96*, 167–172. https://doi.org/10.1016/j.bios.2017.05.005.

Torres-Giner, S., Gimenez, E., & Lagaron, J. M. (2008). Characterization of the morphology and thermal properties of Zein Prolamine nanostructures obtained by electrospinning. *Food Hydrocolloids, 22*(4), 601–614. https://doi.org/10.1016/j.foodhyd.2007.02.005.

Uniyal, S., & Sharma, R. K. (2018). Technological advancement in electrochemical biosensor based detection of organophosphate pesticide chlorpyrifos in the environment: A review of status and prospects. *Biosensors and Bioelectronics, 116*, 37–50. https://doi.org/10.1016/j.bios.2018.05.039.

Valderrama, W. B., Dudley, E. G., Doores, S., & Cutter, C. N. (2016). Commercially available rapid methods for detection of selected food-borne pathogens. *Critical Reviews in Food Science and Nutrition, 56*(9), 1519–1531. https://doi.org/10.1080/10408398.2013.775567.

Vigneshvar, S., Sudhakumari, C. C., Senthilkumaran, B., & Prakash, H. (2016). Recent advances in biosensor technology for potential applications—An overview. *Frontiers in Bioengineering and Biotechnology*. *4*, https://doi.org/10.3389/fbioe.2016.00011.

Viswanathan, S., Rani, C., & Ho, J. A. A. (2012). Electrochemical immunosensor for multiplexed detection of food-borne pathogens using nanocrystal bioconjugates and MWCNT screen-printed electrode. *Talanta, 94*, 315–319. https://doi.org/10.1016/j.talanta.2012.03.049.

Vogiazi, V., De La Cruz, A., Mishra, S., Shanov, V., Heineman, W. R., & Dionysiou, D. D. (2019). A comprehensive review: Development of electrochemical biosensors for detection of cyanotoxins in freshwater. *ACS Sensors, 4*(5), 1151–1173. https://doi.org/10.1021/acssensors.9b00376.

Wang, L., Yang, R., Chen, J., Li, J., Qu, L., & Harrington, P. B. (2014). Sensitive voltammetric sensor based on isopropanol-Nafion-PSS-GR nanocomposite modified glassy carbon electrode for determination of clenbuterol in pork. *Food Chemistry, 164*, 113–118. https://doi.org/10.1016/j.foodchem.2014.04.052.

Wang, Y., Ye, Z., & Ying, Y. (2012). New trends in impedimetric biosensors for the detection of foodborne pathogenic bacteria. *Sensors, 12*(3), 3449–3471. https://doi.org/10.3390/s120303449.

Warriner, K., Reddy, S. M., Namvar, A., & Neethirajan, S. (2014). Developments in nanoparticles for use in biosensors to assess food safety and quality. *Trends in Food Science and Technology, 40*(2), 183–199. https://doi.org/10.1016/j.tifs.2014.07.008.

Wu, X., Kuang, H., Hao, C., Xing, C., Wang, L., & Xu, C. (2012). Paper supported immunosensor for detection of antibiotics. *Biosensors and Bioelectronics, 33*(1), 309–312. https://doi.org/10.1016/j.bios.2012.01.017.

Xu, M. L., Liu, J. B., & Lu, J. (2014). Determination and control of pesticide residues in beverages: A review of extraction techniques, chromatography, and rapid detection methods. *Applied Spectroscopy Reviews, 49*(2), 97–120. https://doi.org/10.1080/05704928.2013.803978.

Xu, M., Wang, R., & Li, Y. (2017). Electrochemical biosensors for rapid detection of Escherichia coli O157:H7. *Talanta, 162*, 511–522. https://doi.org/10.1016/j.talanta.2016.10.050.

Yang, T., Huang, H., Zhu, F., Lin, Q., Zhang, L., & Liu, J. (2016). Recent progresses in nanobiosensing for food safety analysis. *Sensors (Switzerland). 16*(7)https://doi.org/10.3390/s16071118.

Yu, G., Wu, W., Zhao, Q., Wei, X., & Lu, Q. (2015). Efficient immobilization of acetylcholinesterase onto amino functionalized carbon nanotubes for the fabrication of high sensitive organophosphorus pesticides biosensors. *Biosensors and Bioelectronics, 68*, 288–294. https://doi.org/10.1016/j.bios.2015.01.005.

Zeng, Y., Zhu, Z., Du, D., & Lin, Y. (2016). Nanomaterial-based electrochemical biosensors for food safety. *Journal of Electroanalytical Chemistry, 781*, 147–154. https://doi.org/10.1016/j.jelechem.2016.10.030.

Zhang, D., & Liu, Q. (2016). Biosensors and bioelectronics on smartphone for portable biochemical detection. *Biosensors and Bioelectronics, 75*, 273–284. https://doi.org/10.1016/j.bios.2015.08.037.

Zhao, J., Jing, P., Xue, S., & Xu, W. (2017). Dendritic structure DNA for specific metal ion biosensor based on catalytic hairpin assembly and a sensitive synergistic amplification strategy. *Biosensors and Bioelectronics, 87*, 157–163. https://doi.org/10.1016/j.bios.2016.08.032.

Zhu, J., Jia, J., Li, X., Dong, L., & Li, J. (2013). ESR studies on the thermal decomposition of trimethylamine oxide to formaldehyde and dimethylamine in jumbo squid (Dosidicus gigas) extract. *Food Chemistry, 141*(4), 3881–3888. https://doi.org/10.1016/j.foodchem.2013.06.083.

Zhu, K., Dietrich, R., Didier, A., Doyscher, D., & Märtlbauer, E. (2014). Recent developments in antibody-based assays for the detection of bacterial toxins. *Toxins, 6*(4), 1325–1348. https://doi.org/10.3390/toxins6041325.

Zhu, W., Liu, W., Li, T., Yue, X., Liu, T., Zhang, W., … Wang, J. (2014). Facile green synthesis of graphene-Au nanorod nanoassembly for on-line extraction and sensitive stripping analysis of methyl parathion. *Electrochimica Acta*, *146*, 419–428. https://doi.org/10.1016/j.electacta.2014.09.085.

Zhu, Z., Shi, L., Feng, H., & Susan Zhou, H. (2015). Single domain antibody coated gold nanoparticles as enhancer for Clostridium difficile toxin detection by electrochemical impedance immunosensors. *Bioelectrochemistry*, *101*, 153–158. https://doi.org/10.1016/j.bioelechem.2014.10.003.

Nanotechnology-based on microfluidic devices lab-on-a-chip for food analysis

10

Introduction

With growing populations and the global industrial revolution, the food industry has drawn particular attention and constant expectations in terms of safety, efficiency, sustainability, protection, and smart packaging, as well as high prices for individual consumers and the food industry. Consumers are the ones who need to acknowledge their food's nutritional quality and, most importantly, the wellbeing. These situations require the development and use of urgent, efficient, secure, field-deployable, and highly sensitive substances in food (Weng & Neethirajan, 2017). The existence of low-abundance components such as preservatives, allergens, contaminants (pesticides, heavy metals), and some other additives in the food matrix with varying reactivity and actions presents serious challenges in the analysis of foods. On the other hand, the quality of food is of serious concern to both individual consumers and the food industry, which is in desperate need of healthy foods rich in nutrients and preventive disease. In such a growing and rapidly developing world, ensuring food safety and quality involved the demand for inexpensive, simple, compact, effective, reliable, and easy-to-use analytical instruments (Al Mughairy & Al-Lawati, 2020). The growing concern about health risks associated with a food allergy, food poisoning, and foodborne disease has guided the development of regulations on food safety over time and the advancement of reliable food analysis techniques. Nevertheless, allergens, pesticides, heavy metals, additives, and other chemicals also physical pollutants that come into contact through manufacturing processes and agricultural products can also have an impact on food safety and quality (Busa et al., 2016; Sasaki et al., 2002)

Many analytical techniques have been developed such as, chromatographic based, spectroscopic, biological immune, and enzyme-based, and microbiological assays in food analysis. Besides, these methods demonstrate exceptional feasibility in integrated with different types of detection systems. Despite the high sensitivity of the methods mentioned, yet some of the methods are time-consuming, costly, need complex pretreatment, and experienced operators. The high use of solvents, the inherent properties of flow-based systems, also represented a limitation that forces

Advanced Food Analysis Tools. https://doi.org/10.1016/B978-0-12-820591-4.00010-4

scientists to replace them with miniature systems such as microfluidics. In this sense, in many other fields of science and research, including agriculture and the food industry, microfluid chemical analysis has enormous potential which will encourage and eventually revolutionize the whole process of food analysis (Weng & Neethirajan, 2017). The idea of integrating optics, fluids, electronics, and biosensors into very small channels is state-of-the-art technology. Use extremely small amounts of fluid (micro-to-pico-liter) from solvents and chemicals such as high throughput, a high degree of control, reduced waste generation, etc. On the other hand, it is clear that fewer resources have many virtues (Tsao, 2016).

In many chemical analyses, this can eventually be understood as a valid substitute for a large number of conventional standard analytical bench-top procedures. In addition, microfluidics will fulfill the value of the "green approach" in chemical analysis (Gupta, Ramesh, Ahmed, & Kakkar, 2016). Over time the concept of microfluidic has improved, for example, microfluidics was cited as the platforms that provided solutions to move into confined microchannels (Mark, Haeberle, Roth, Von Stetten, & Zengerle, 2010). Moreover, with the rapid development of microfluidics, numerous new platforms have been implemented, such as paper and fabric, which have been modified to include other platforms as well (Alahmad, Tungkijananansin, Kaneta, & Varanusupakul, 2018; Busa et al., 2016; Sriram et al., 2017). In addition, the chip-based analysis is designed for aqueous phase analytes mainly by convection of molecules, while only a few drops of diffusion added to the mixing process are required for paper/cloth systems and the process is relatively slow (Liu, Zhang, Li, & Zhang, 2016). The use of solvent, which is the greatest virtue of all microfluidics, requires only a few drops of microfluidic reagents based on paper/cloth, while the chip-based analysis absorbs a few milliliters. As regards handling and disposal, microfluidics in paper/cloth is more labor-intensive and laborious than chip systems (Sriram et al., 2017). The additional drying processes for individual reagents on the paper/cloth can be considered as a principal downside for this type of analysis (Hua, Li, Wang, & Lu, 2018). One of the main advantages of microfluidic paper/cloth is the usefulness of using solid-phase components such as nanoparticles and extraction beads, which are more practical for this type of platform than other microfluidic systems.

Microfluidics is a system that measured at least 10^{-6} to 10^{-8} volumes of liquids using tens to hundreds of micrometers or scale channels. There are four classes in the microfluidics area, which are molecular analysis, biomolecular, biodefence, and microelectronics. Microfluidics is classified as multidisciplinary fields including chemistry, biochemistry, engineering physics, and biotechnology. Microfluidics chip, often recognized as a laboratory-on- a-chip combining sample pretreatment, stability response, separation, detection and other microchip systems that can replace many of the functions of conventional biochemistry laboratories (McDonald et al., 2000; Xu, Zhu, Colon, Huh, & Balhoff, 2017). This chapter specifically focuses on important developments in the use of microfluidic devices in food analysis based on the systems, biorecognition, and various nanomaterials and methods of manufacturing will be explored and inspected.

Microfluidic devices

Microfluidic systems provide an exciting alternative to analytical research, enabling reductions in the use of mobile phases, solutions and chemical residue production, analytical costs, and operational simplification. However, there is a problem that is often not addressed which is costly and difficult to use outside the laboratory as electrochemical microfluidic systems require a commercial. As microfluidic instruments typically are strident outfits for noninvasive research fields and irrespective of the type of technology used in microfluidics. Ultimately, the monitoring system must understand and evaluate the capabilities of these analytical techniques employed and to be able to interpret the analytical results of those analyses. In addition, Microfluidic detection systems can typically be categorized into three categories: optical (Gai, Li, & Yeung, 2011), electrochemical (Li et al., 2018), and mass spectrometric (MS). The first detection system in the microfluidic research is based on optical means due to its ease of coupling, extended applications, rapid response, and high sensitivity of the optical detection. This broad class includes conventional absorption (Jackman, Floyd, Ghodssi, Schmidt, & Jensen, 2001), surface-enhanced Raman scattering (SERS) (Chen & Choo, 2008), fluorescence (Chabinyc et al., 2001), chemiluminescence (He, Zhang, Huang, & Hu, 2007), surface plasmon resonance (Hassani & Skorobogatiy, 2006), and spectroscopies. The intensive development of various microfluidic optical detection systems allows us to easily deduce two features of the spatial detection route which are off-chip and on-chip techniques. For off-chip, the free space optical detection system used is chemiluminescence, fluorescence, and absorption. In comparison, strong and lightweight on-chip implementations such as the planar microwaveguide, microlens, and optofluidic laser are examples of on-chip strategies. The performance of miniaturized systems is limited by the ability of analytes to identify residual amounts. Significant efforts are being made to allow the use of other effective analytical methods, such as UV–Vis spectroscopy, fluorescence, electrochemistry, and chemiluminescence (Gai et al., 2011; Krishnan, Namasivayam, Lin, Pal, & Burns, 2001).

Basic principles of microfluidic

Microfluidic is the science and technology of devices that use tens- to-hundred-micrometer channels that can move or control small volumes of fluids from liter to microliter (Whitesides, 2006). It is a new multidisciplinary field that includes chemistry, fluidic mechanics, biology, nanomaterials, nanotechnology, and engineering known as the lab-on-a-chip (LOC) or micro-complete analysis system (mTAS), due to its miniaturization and integration characteristics (Nge, Rogers, & Woolley, 2013). Microfluidics can perform in multiple functions such as mixing, pretreatment, reaction, separation, and detection on a chip of only a few square centimeters or even tinier. There are five main components of microfluidics which are micropump, micromixer, microvalve, and detector as shown in Fig. 10.1.

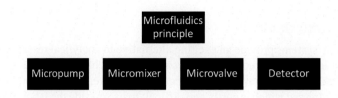

FIG. 10.1

The basic main components of the microfluidics device.

Micropump

Micropump is one of the most critical components in a microfluidic device by controlling the flow rate which enhanced the accuracy and reliability of the analytical results. It performs various functions including sample reagent distribution, mixing, reaction, analysis, or discharge (Zhou, Zhang, Li, & Wang, 2016). Fluid monitoring can be classified as mechanical micropumps (moving parts) and nonmechanical micropumps (without moving parts). Continuous flow pumps are used more frequently because of their more convenient production and efficient flow control (Gutmann, Cantillo, & Kappe, 2015; Li, Xing, & Zhang, 2009). Depending on the operating principle, the flow control of the pumps can be divided into the capillary flow, pressure-driven flow, and electrokinetic flow. Due to its simplicity and efficiency, capillary flow is a common mechanism for fluid transport in microfluidic systems. Based on capillary flow, microfluidic paper-based devices have been widely reported and have become the first microfluidic system to have a significant market share (Elizalde, Urteaga, & Berli, 2015; Noh & Phillips, 2010; Songok & Toivakka, 2016). Pressure-driven flow is based on pressure gradients used by liquid transport pumps to enable the continuous processing of multiple samples, which is of key importance for online monitoring (Desmet et al., 2002; Hardy, Uechi, Zhen, & Pirouz Kavehpour, 2009; Li, Zhao, & Liu, 2013). Basic research facilities are less suitable for on-site experiments because the most common way to induce pressure-driven flows is through the use of syringe pumps, which are well designed and easy to implement but are quite extensive, costly, and not ideal for miniaturization. Electrokinetic flow is a common process in miniaturized analytical systems for fluid actuation. Electrokinetic flow, in response to an external electrical field, deals with the combined movement of liquids (electroosmosis) and molecules or particles (electrophoresis) in a continuous flow system (Cabrera & Yager, 2001; Krishnamoorthy, Bedekar, Feng, & Sundaram, 2007).

Micromixer

The design of novel micromixers is necessary to improve the mixing ability and is essential for system performance and integration. Microfluidic mixers can either be classed as passive or active. Passive micromixers do not require external energy, whereby the mixing efficiency is usually improved by specially designed microchannel configurations to either optimize surface area or multiple species contact time, or both (Lee, Chang, Wang, & Fu, 2011; Lee, Yamada, & Seki, 2005; Nichols, Ferullo, & Baeumner, 2006). In comparison, active micromixers need an external energy force to speed up the sample species diffusion cycle. Effective mixing is typically applied through the integration of a mechanical transducer (acoustic or ultrasonic) (Renaudin, Chabot, Grondin, Aimez, & Charette, 2010; Watanabe, Hasegawa, & Abe, 2018), dielectrophoretic (Salmanzadeh, Shafiee, Davalos, & Stremler, 2011), magnetic (Zhu & Nguyen, 2012), thermal (Vreeland & Locascio, 2003) or electro-hydrodynamic force (El Moctar, Aubry, & Batton, 2003; Samiei, De Leon Derby, Den Berg, & Hoorfar, 2017) into a microfluidic device using microfabrication technology.

Microvalve

Microvalve plays a key role in making fully integrated microfluidic analytical systems, as well as determine the flow direction or mode of movement of pumped liquids. Similarly, both active and passive microvalves are subdivided and both types are powered by mechanical and nonmechanical forces. For example, the Passive capillary valve techniques control the fluid flow by the microchannel's geometry or surface wetting properties (Balsam, Bruck, & Rasooly, 2015; Mark et al., 2009), which is useful for passive microfluidic systems because of their autonomous and spontaneous valve capacity. Besides, the virtual valves are used for sample injection and transport in microchip capillary electrophoresis (CE) systems (Braschler et al., 2007; Lai, Xu, & Allbritton, 2011), where fluid control depends solely on the geometry of the microchannel intersection and the operating parameters applied, such as the activation potential and length.

Detector

Incredibly sensitive detectors are becoming more important due to small sample volumes in microfluidic analytical instruments. The transducers are broadly similar to those used in traditional laboratories, with both attempts being made to incorporate them into the microfluidic analytical system and to adjust them in a way that is compatible with small volumes of fluid. Electrochemical and optical sensing techniques are the most common transducers in microfluidic devices. The integration of electrochemical detection techniques such as potentiometry (Chango, Palacio, & Cerdà, 2018; Yoon et al., 2017), amperometry (Gonzalez-Rivera & Osma, 2015; Olcer et al., 2014; Ölcer et al., 2015), conductometry (Díaz-González et al., 2015) in microfluidic system platforms is very successful due to their ease of miniaturization and high sensitivity. Fluorescence-based detection is the most popular approach in the optical analysis system category, due to the simplicity of combining the excitation and detection sources of fluorescence with the sensor, as well as its ability to detect fluorescence in low-volume samples. The dependence of the signal on the length of the optical path or sample turbidity is difficult for on-chip applications. Mass spectrometry is seen as an effective alternative to these detection methods, but the main problem is the on-chip integration of the detection system.

Types of microfluid systems
Continuous-flow microfluids

The continuous-flow microfluidic systems work through consistent manipulation and flow of unphasic fluids through sealed off microchannels. Fluids are usually controlled by hydrodynamic pumps and are fully controlled by micron channels caused by glass, silicon, metals, ceramics, or plastics types (Dressler, Maceiczyk, Chang, & Demello, 2014). There are two standard liquid treatment procedures in continuous flow microfluidics that mix and separate a mixture of reagents needed for a wide range of biological and chemical assays because of interactions involving biological methods including protein folding and enzyme reactions needed to be initiated (Nguyen, 2012). The separation process serves as an essential function in sample preparation for analytical chemistry and biological application (Sajeesh & Sen, 2014). The use of microfluidic continuous flow for mixing and separating tends to be internally inconsistent, but limited because of parabolic flow profiles in biological sciences, is inherent and analyte molecules are in close contact with channel walls that can cause precipitation, fouling, or contamination (Kumar et al., 2012). According to Nguyen, Hejazian, Ooi, and Kashaninejad (2017) the dominant laminar and low-Reynolds-number flow regime has led interruptions in mixing and separation methods, suggesting a wider need for long mixing and separation.

Droplet-based microfluids

Droplet-based microfluidic systems operate on the motion of isolated droplets in microchannels using streams of immiscible fluids. There are two types of microfluidic-based droplet systems such as the optical and segmented-flow microfluidics systems. The sample or reagent phase is disrupted in the segmented flow system by the immiscible carrier phase that causes the sample or reagent to be separated into discrete droplets. The droplet flows do not affect several of the constraints encountered in continuous flows, such as the residence time distribution. This is because the droplets in the immiscible carrier phase move apart from each other and the channel walls (Dressler et al., 2014). There are a number of available methods that are ready for use in droplet manipulation, such as mixing, splitting, merging, and incubation. One of the most effective means is to insert multiple laminar streams of aqueous reagents into an immiscible carrier fluid, thereby generating rapid flow instability in the formation of droplets (Tice, Song, Lyon, & Ismagilov, 2003). According to Huebner et al. (2007) the devices provide for new high-throughput technology capable of generating microdroplets, parallelization, integration, effective tools analysis, and also suitable for applications where isolated reaction sites are required to prevent cross-contamination. Droplet microfluidics has been broadly used for biological detection, including exosomes (Liu et al., 2018), biomarkers of cancer (Zhou, 2018), extracellular secretion (Shen et al., 2018) and so forth. Droplet-based technology was also an innovative and strong analytical approach for microbe research with the aid of microfluidic methods (Dagkesamanskaya et al., 2018).

Highly distributed single-cell aqueous phase in a carrier oil, in which microbes can expand and proliferate independently with ultra-high-density to microcolonies in such microdroplets, providing benefits in single-cell analysis applications (Mongersun, Smeenk, Pratx, Asuri, & Abbyad, 2016). As an independent microreactor, each droplet consumes only a few pico-liters to a few nanoliter reagents. Several studies have shown that bacteria can be cultured and detected on microfluidic devices based on droplets (Gao, Jin, Zhou, & Jiang, 2019; Zhu et al., 2018; Zhu et al., 2019). Bian et al. (2015) explained that droplet-based optical PCR was a novel approach for high sensitivity and rapid analysis from bacterial extract for Salmonella detection and directly lysed thermally in droplets (Jang et al., 2017). Moreover, the digital PCR can typically be constrained by the type of sample available and cannot differentiate viable salmonella, which significantly increases the complexity and cost of bacteria detection.

Digital microfluids

The optical microfluidics system practices of discrete samples of liquid, or droplets, to support the purpose as discreetly as continuous microfluidics. The devices used in the digital microfluidic system are most likely compatible with conventional microfluidics, excluding the additional droplet formation and transport circuits. According to Link et al. (2006), Electronic actuation is preferred instead of using micropumps and other micromechanical components, because miniaturization of the electrode and easy incorporation into a single device reduces the necessary size. Silicon, its other derivatives such as PDMS (poly-dimethylsiloxane) and glass are selected materials used in the fabrication of digital microfluidic devices due to their chemical inertness (Choi, Ng, Fobel, & Wheeler, 2012). There are numerous methods employed in the Digital microfluidics system when performing various operations such as electrowetting, dielectrophoresis (DEP), Opto-electro-wetting (OEW), thermo-capillary effect, and surface acoustic waves. The application of digital microfluidics may involve a variety of disciplines, such as biology, chemistry, chemical engineering, and the increasing use of this technology (Sukhatme & Agarwal, 2012).

Two standard Electronic microfluidic system configurations are either a single plate (open) and two-plate (closed). The two-plate configuration is the droplets slot between two substrates that were covered with the electrode. Typically the upper plate comprises a continuous ground electrode formed by a conductive indium tin oxide (ITO), which is a transparent layer while the lower layer provided a variety of actuating electrodes. Droplets remain on a single substratum for a one-plate set-up that contains both the upper and lower layers (Choi et al., 2012).

Whitesides (2006) stated that the digital microfluidics method reduced the volume of the sample to nanoliter or pico-liter which the smaller the volume of the reagent, the faster the result achieved. In a digital microfluidics system, the minimal flow volume is set by the sensitivity of the detector, which means that the flow is not measured by the sensitivity of the flow sensor since there is no flow sensor in the digital microfluidics system.

Biorecognition/bioreceptor site used in microfluid lab-on-a-chip

Antibodies

The antibody, or also known as immunoglobin, is a protein generated by the plasma membrane that is used primarily by the immune system to fight or protect against pathogenic bacteria and viruses. The principle of antibody-based sensors also referred to as immunosensors is based on the antibody–antigen reaction specificity which will result in a change in the transducer signal. Four immunosensor modes are primary, competitive, sandwich and binding inhibition mode is focused on the inhibition of binding between an unlabeled surface-immobilized antibody and a labeled secondary antibody in the appearance of a surface-binding analyte (Borisov & Wolfbeis, 2008). Nonetheless, batch-to-batch variation, the potential for cross-reaction between specific target types, costly and diminished antibodies to chemical and physical stability are a few drawbacks that use antibodies as biorecognition. Such problems led scientists to investigate yet another alternative to ligands of biorecognition (Sapsford, Bradburne, Delehanty, & Medintz, 2008). Wang et al. (2015) reported that the LIF microsystem had been integrated into the multichannel microfluidic chip to detect the *Salmonella typhimurium* in meat pork samples. They found that the detection limit was 37 CFU/mL and that the sensitivity of the assay improved with the use of CdSe/ZnS QDs as fluorescent detectors but still using the same systems.

Aptamer

The aptamer is characterized as an amino acid polymer or a single-strand nucleic acid with high specificity, accuracy, and affinity to a target analyte that needs to be assessed for which small molecules can be found in whole cells (Ellington & Szostak, 1990; Nimjee, Rusconi, & Sullenger, 2005). The aptamer can bind to their various ligands with a steady dissociation of the spectrum from micromolar to pico-molar. Using a wide range of analytes, such as pathogen detection, secondary metabolite product (toxin), proteins, and whole cells, the aptamer can also be assigned for analysis (Luka et al., 2015). Typically, the aptamer is immobilized on reliable support that can be freely eliminated, but the aptamer can still respond freely with its substratum or unique analyte. The use of aptamers in microfluidic chips is due to its benefits, such as acting as a biological recognition factor over antibodies, long-term stabilities, inexpensive and provide quick synthesis (Ciobanu, Taylor, Wilburn, & Cliffel, 2008). The aptamer may be modified with labels that have little influence on the binding site's performance, its stability, or binding properties against analytes (Luka et al., 2015). The in-vitro selection method called Exponential Enrichment Systematic Evolution of Ligands (SELEX) may be used to produce synthetic oligonucleotide aptamer. Such aptamers serve as biomimetic biorecognition layers for use in the identification of a wide range of analytes, such as amino acids, antibiotics, co-factors, drugs, metal ions, nucleic acids, and organic dyes (Ellington & Szostak, 1992).

Enzymes

The enzyme is a protein-based molecule that acts as a catalyst. The enzymes catalyze the chemical reaction by speeding up the chemical reaction, which remains unchanged or used up during the process. Based on (Hilvert, 2000), enzymes can catalyze a chemical reaction at a rate ranging from 105 to 1017, which is higher than uncatalyzed reactions. The principle behind this approach is the oxidation–reduction or redox reaction in which the enzyme functions as a biosensor (Luka et al., 2015). On top of that, the reaction will be performed under specific conditions, including low temperature and ion pressure, neutral pH to avoid disruption of function and enzyme properties to significantly improve the life span of the biosensor (Rocchitta et al., 2016). Each enzyme is specialized to the biomolecules in which the produced product is quantified using a transducer (Srinivasan & Tung, 2015). Additionally, enzymes could generate other products such as ions, protons, heat, light, and electrons in which these products can be measured. However, a reduction in the production of enzyme products due to analyte will hinder the enzyme in the biorecognition layer. Nucleophilic groups, such as amino acids, carboxyl, sulfhydryl, hydroxyl, phenolic, and thiol groups, are present in amino acids with enzymes that are not part of the covalent bonding active site. Covalent bonds facilitated the binding of enzymes by water-insoluble binding agents to protect matrices (Subrahmanyam, Piletsky, & Turner, 2002).

Material for microfluid device fabrication
Inorganic material
Silicon
Silicon was the very first substance used in the microfluid chip for its resistance to organic solvents, easy metal handling, high thermoconductivity, and electroosmotic functional mobility. Since the silicon has a high elastic modulus, turning silicon into active fluid components such as valves and pumps is indeed not easy. Silicon is an opaque substance that is transparent to infrared, not visible light, making it difficult to detect traditional fluorescence or fluid imaging. This problem can be solved by

mixing it with transparent materials such as polymer or glass to develop a hybrid system due to silicone surface chemistry, the silanol group has well-developed chemistry, so that the modification can be made quickly to mitigate nonspecific adsorption or to boost cell growth, for example, through chemical modification. The silicone-based system can be produced using a wet or dry etching or an additive process like deposition of metal or chemical vapor.

Glass

The glass was chosen for the construction of a microfluidic silicon chip as it is optically transparent and does not allow the electrical motion of the glass, which is known as an amorphous material. Glass is well-suited material for biological samples. in addition, it is also a material that is not gas-permeable and has comparatively low nonspecific adsorption. Because the glass is not gas-permeable, this material cannot be used for long-term cell culture because gas can pass through glass chips which usually contain channels and chambers. CE is a major application of glass chips. This application is less expensive, or, in other words, cheaper than CE standards. In addition, this approach is more compatible with parallel processing and also offers valve-free injection by directly using an electroosmotic flow which can isolate the analyte in a few seconds. Other than typical glass chip applications, there are also other applications such as droplet forming on-chip reactions, solvent extraction, and in-situ processing.

Polymers

Elastomer

Elastomers comprise of cross-linked polymer chains that can normally be intertwined, stretched or compressed when the external force is applied, but when the external force is removed, the original shape is restored.

Polydimethylsiloxane (PDMS)

Polydimethylsiloxane (PDMS) is the most common elastomer in microfluidics due to its reasonable cost, rapid manufacturing, and ease of use. The PDMS chip can be sealed reversibly and conformally to another piece of PDMS, glass, or other material by traditional machining or photolithography. According to Araci and Quake (2012) PDMS has a weak elastic modulus (300–500 kPa) and gas permeability, which makes PDMS ideal for manufacturing valves and pumps. Roman, Hlaus, Bass, Seelhammer, and Culbertson (2005) stated that it is more influenced by nonspecific adsorption and pervasion by hydrophobic molecules, despite its inherent hydrophobic nature. Chemical alteration of PDMS may fix problems such as plasma exposure that hydrophilizes the exposed PDMS surface, but the surface that has developed hydrophilic properties is not stable and will return to its original shape after a short period of time (Bodas & Khan-Malek, 2006; Hillborg, Tomczak, Olàh, Schönherr, & Vancso, 2004). One of the implications of PDMS existence hydrophobic surface is its susceptibility to the absorption and dissolution of hydrophobic molecules when interacting with nonpolar solvents. Adsorption of biomolecules on canal walls is also a common issue for PDMS-manufactured microfluidic devices that caused limited application in aqueous solutions.

Thermoset polyester (TPE)

Thermoset polyester (TPE) is hydrophobic material and requires surface modification to allow water to flow through the microfluidic channels either through buffer additives or through chemical reactions. The thermoset pieces cannot be reshaped back once it is formed due to the healing step needs an irreversible chemical reaction. TPE is called optically transparent, because it is extremely translucent over the visible range yet absisorbs UV light (Kim, Demello, Chang, Hong, & O'Hare, 2011). According to Roy, Galas, and Veres (2011), it is proved that the similar TPE valves to those made from PMS can be produced as well. On the other hand, TPE still can dissolve in a chlorinated solvent even it stabilizes when exposed to various other solvents. Besides, Thermoset has greater power, enabling the manufacture of high-aspect-ratio and free-standing structures.

Paper

Microfluidic systems integrated with paper and textiles have shown great potential applications in resource-limited diagnostic environments, environmental control, and food safety surveillance (Ma, Nilghaz, Choi, Liu, & Lu, 2018). Microfluidic systems can incorporate switches, separators, and mixers in a variety of ways on a single platform, offering low-cost miniaturized designs, requiring little handling experience, being environmentally friendly, and detecting a variety of chemicals. Nonetheless, certain measures in the preparation of samples for microfluid analysis, such as the filtration and concentration of samples and reagents, are not well known. Paper-based microfluidic devices have an excellent ability to control small volumes of an aqueous solution, which may be a downside when a small number of reagents are used to collect low levels of different analytes. Thereby, filtering and concentration of analytes and reagents are important for the better functioning of microfluidic paper-based devices, regardless of the nature of the sample (Gomes & Sales, 2015; Nilghaz & Lu, 2019). Since chemical hazards in food are toxic to consumers, the maximum residue limit for most chemical contaminants in food is usually one part per million or less, the use of paper-based microfluidic devices for food safety monitoring is still in its infancy (Delatour, Racault, Bessaire, & Desmarchelier, 2018). Besides, paper-based microfluidic devices are more suitable compared to conventional techniques as it offers an alternative low-cost, widely available, simple fabrication methods and highly sensitive platform to monitor food safety in the field (Zhang, Zuo, & Ye, 2015). For paper-based microfluidic devices, further on-chip pretreatment of reagents and analytes is needed to reach a low detection limit needed by the food industry.

Paper is an excellent microfluidic material made from cellulose and has a matrix that is highly porous and good for absorbing or removing liquids. Paper is a cheap substratum that can be found all over the world and can be modified by chemical use through changes in composition/formulation or surface chemistry. Paper can be disposed of through burning or natural degradation methods that can reduce chemical waste to the environment (Martinez, Phillips, Whitesides, & Carrilho, 2010; Pelton, 2009). According to Busa et al. (2016) the selection for the type of paper material is important for manufacturing processes, such as cutting, inkjet printing, wax patterning, wax pencil drawing, wax printing, screen printing, contact stamping, and photolithography. In their research, Jokerst et al. (2012) documented the development of an μPAD to detect *Escherichia coli* O157: H7, *Listeria monocytogenes* and *S. typhimurium* in ready-to-eat (RTE) meat samples. However, this method clearly required less time compared to a standard gold method, which requires several days for bacterial detection and enumeration. The paper-based analytical instruments lack high resolution and have high sensitivity compared to silicon, glass, or plastic-based devices. Even though with these limitations, paper-based analytical devices are useful to the point-of-need supervising that demands inexpensive analysis for continuous testing, especially in less developed industries of a country where sophisticated instrumentation and any relating or using the analysis/scientific approach are limited.

The antibiotic residues in food samples can be detected through the sensitive and rapid method by using the filtration behavior of paper combined with aggregation and precipitation of chemical reactive (Nilghaz & Lu, 2019). By using this concept, the presence of oxytetracycline and norfloxacin residues in pork was successfully detected using metal complexation on microfluidic paper-based analytical devices (μPADs). The base substrate (top layer of the device) was produced by printing letter channels of the words "oxytetracycline" and "norfloxacin" before functionalization with copper (II) sulfate pentahydrate in 0.5 M sodium hydroxide and iron (III) nitrate nanohydrate in 5 mM ammonia solution for the detection of oxytetracycline and norfloxacin. A transition metal hydroxide is formed when a reaction triggers a solid on paper and allows the antibiotic residue to binding to metal ions through coordination chemistry. The metal ion-antibiotic complex for both oxytetracycline and norfloxacin in pork could form on the filter paper and produce a noticeable color change with a detection limit of 1 ppm. This filtration and concentration technique in conjunction with a simple text-reporting method helps end-users to achieve a low detection limit as well as a quick understanding of findings in food safety monitoring.

Hydrogel

Hydrogels are three-dimensional networks of hydrophilic polymer chains that extend in an aqueous medium where the water can be predominantly material. The hydrogel is highly porous, with a controllable pore size that allowed the diffusion of small molecules or bioparticles (Ren, Zhou, & Wu, 2013). The consistency of the material used with the cell is an important factor in performing experiments based on cell culture. In general, the hydrogel is not harmful or toxic to living tissue (biocompatible), and different hydrogel have different affinities with animal cells (Tibbitt & Anseth, 2009) as well as an excellent matrix for the study of cellular biology. Choi et al. (2007)

mentioned the majority of animal-derived hydrogel used are collagen and matrigel as they promote excellent cell adhesion and proliferation. However, based on research by Huang et al. (2011), alginate and agarose from plant-derived hydrogels and synthetic ones like polyacrylamide or polyethylene glycol (PEG) may be used as an alternative to hydrogel derived from animals. This alternative hydrogels have high flexibility and enriched adaptability of the formulation but appear to lack for cell adhesion.

Some documented bonding techniques are the melting of a thin layer of the bonding surface by heating or chemical before connecting and using a second linking agent at the interface. Besides, there are two strategies for the creation of microchannels had been adopted (Huang et al., 2011). Firstly, the direct writing method involving direct laser writing (LDW) and gelation of gel solution from a moving nozzle, which can create arbitrary low-speed 3D structures. The other method involves a two-step process, which is a channel generation followed by channel sealing. However, hydrogel also tends to have limitations that only supports the lower resolution (micrometer scale) in microfabrication compared to other polymers (nanometer scale), and the hydrogel with encapsulated cells may not be well suitable to some micromanufacturing processes.

Hybrid and composite materials
Cyclic olefin copolymer (COC)
Cyclic olefin polymer (COP) is an amorphous material that belongs to a class of polymer-based on the monomer and ethane cyclic olefin. There is a variety of commercially available brand names for COP material. They usually referred to it as cyclic olefin copolymer (COC), since they made up more than one monomer form. COC is a new polymer underclass optical thermoplastic with new properties compared to existing thermoplastics used, such as PC and PMMA. COC is a thermoplastic copolymer composed of ethylene and norbornene using a metallocene catalyst. COC is a material that has low moisture absorption, high water barrier, high heat deflection temperature, high optical transmission, high chemical resistance, as well as commonly used in microfluidics (Khanarian, 2001).

However, COC also has several disadvantages compared to the other plastics, such as brittleness and low heat diffusivity may lead to limited use in some applications. The gadget made up of COC is not suitable for research, including a medicinal product, due to its hydrophobic nature, which makes it vulnerable to uncontrolled nonspecific adsorption of proteins and cell bonds when exposed to living tissues or liquids. In some cases, unspecific protein/cell adsorption may be detrimental to the design of performance, such as in vivo biosensors and cardiovascular stent surfaces. The surface of the COC chip surface was modified by (Jena & Yue, 2012) using a UV-photography technique incorporating MPC monomers with neutral phospholipids to reduce adsorption (protein or another hydrophobic compound).

Paper/polymer hybrid device

Microfluid immunoassay instruments have some uncommon characteristics, such as a wide area-to-volume ratio, reduced sample requirement, and fast assay procedure (Mohammed & Desmulliez, 2011), which may reduce the analysis time from hours to minutes. Paper/polymer hybrid microfluidic microplates such as PMMA and PDMS are designed to solve the issue of conventional ELISA such as short incubation time, high use volume of expensive reagents, and well-equipped laboratories. Paper-hybrid devices are based on the concept of microfluidic chips and allow the movement of the biomolecule to be controlled and provide high flow control efficiency. Porous paper is equipped with living samples, which provide 3D material for the storage, protection, and reaction of the reagent. Paper-based microfluidic devices have provided a new low-cost platform for various applications related to health care and food safety analysis in low-resource settings (Li, Nie, Cheng, Goodale, & Whitesides, 2010; Nie et al., 2010). Deiss, Funes-Huacca, Bal, Tjhung, and Derda (2014), used a paper/PDMS hybrid microfluidic system to cultivate bacteria and detect their resistance to antibiotics. They noticed that the antibiotic susceptibility test (AST) in a paper-based portable device showed similar results on performance, reproducibility, and predictive capacity to the Kirby–Bauer AST in agar Petri dishes.

Fabrication method

Photolithography

Photolithography or optical lithography is a method used in microfabrication to give a thin layer pattern or a bulk of a substrate or material. By using the light, either blue or ultraviolet (UV) light the geometric design will be transmitted from a photomask to a light-sensitive polymer called a photoresist, that exposed and formed 3D images on the substratum. The selective development eliminates the resistance depending on its exposure state and then assigns etching, plating, sputtering, evaporation or other processes involved in microelectronics to the remaining photoresist pattern on the surface. Mack (2008) claimed that the processing stage of the traditional optical lithography process can commonly be sequencing from the preparation of substrates, photoresis spin coat, postapply bake, exposure, postexposure bake, creation, and postbake. The principle of photolithography is quite similar to traditional photography in which the light-sensitive thin film is altered by the use of light through a chemical reaction which can create an image through the subsequent process of development. In the processes of photography, the absorption of multiphoton by silver compounds was involved, while the positive photoresists included the shattering of an organic compound through the absorption of single-photon in photolithography (Dill, 1975).

Two physical effects that restrict the optical UV lithography are light diffraction and light scattering, resulting in structure weakening. The photoresist can be used in both negative and positive processes. From previous research by (Dill, 1975), the positive photoresist is usually a type of photoresist consisting of three-component materials, which are a base resin (film-making properties), a photoactive compound, and volatile solvents in the manufacture of liquid material for application. Positive photoresist tends to occur when the photochemical reaction during the exposure of a resistant rupture or split of the primary and side polymer chain, which weakens the polymer resulting in exposed resistant solubilization. In negative photoresist, the random cross-linking of leading chains or pendant side chains during the photochemical reaction toughened the polymer, making it less soluble (Martinez-Duarte & Madou, 2011).

Soft lithography

Soft lithography is a group nonlithographic method that uses a soft elastomeric stamp (usually PDMS) for micro- and nanofabrication. Generally, the key element for soft lithography is an elastomeric block with patterned relief structures on its surface. According to Xia and Whitesides (1998), there are currently several soft lithography techniques are available including micro-contact printing (μCP), replica molding (REM), micro-transfer molding (μTM), capillary micro-molding (MIMIC), and solvent-assisted micro-molding (SAMIM). REM is the first soft lithography technique which widely used as central elements in microfluidics with elastomer PDMS to imprint patterned relief structures on the surface of the master mold (Folch, 2016). Besides, Micro-contact printing (μCP) is the only method that created different wettability to the surfaces with ordered domains while Micro-transfer molding (μTM) is the only technique of soft lithography that allows the 3D structure to be made.

Soft lithography procedures show that every elastomeric stamp or mold is an important element for the allocation of substrate shapes and flexible organic molecules that are widely used in the manufacture of microelectronic systems. Rogers and Nuzzo (2005) stated that the soft lithography method can be divided into two parts, namely the fabrication of elastomeric elements and the use of elastomeric elements to design features in geometries defined by the relief elements themselves. Soft lithography methods can be applied directly and used by a wide range of users since they are easy to learn and low cost of capital. Apart from that, this approach can also solve the limitation of diffraction by photolithography projection and enable for quasi-three-dimensional structures. In addition, this method often creates patterns and structures on nonplanar surfaces and can be used with a wide range of materials and surface chemicals.

Nevertheless, this method also has its limitations to be overcome before soft lithography can interact with photolithography in the main application of microfabrication. First, the pattern in the stamp or mold may be modified by the deformation of the elastomer used, including pairing, sagging, swelling, and shrinking, followed by the demonstration of the materials that must be compatible with current integrated circuit processes. This method created a higher level of defect compared to photolithography. The micro-contact printing works well with a limited range only, but REM, µTM, and SAMIM have left a thin polymer film on the surface.

Nanoimprinting

Nanoimprint lithography (NIL) is a method of manufacturing micro or nanometer-scale design and is also known as new nonconventional lithography. The term might be new but the imprinting concept is still old to replicate. Hot Embossing Lithography (HEL)/Thermal Nanoimprint Lithography (T-NIL) and UV-based Nanoimprint Lithography (UV-NIL) are two important fundamentals for NIL process. From the previous study by (Chou, Krauss, & Renstrom, 1996), there are two necessary steps or concepts in nanoprint lithograph, one of them is by imprinted the surface with a nanostructure mold to create thickness in the resistor and then remove the mold by press the surface. The second step is the use of an anisotropic etching process, such as reactive ion etching to eliminate the residual resist in the compressed zone. In addition, Nanoimprint lithography uses direct contact between the mold and thermoplastics or UV-curable resistance to produce pattern without costly and complicated optics and light sources to shape the image.

According to Lan and Ding (2010), there are various substrates that can be used for NIL, including silicon wafers, glass plates, flexible polymer film, polyethylene terephthalate (PET) polymer film, and even nonplanar substrates. Besides, compared to the other lithography techniques, NIL is capable of producing large-scale and complex three-dimensional (3D) micro/nanostructures with low cost and high throughput. Nanoimprint lithography is not really restricted to the impact of wave diffraction, scattering, and interference in a resist and backscattering from a substrate (Chou et al., 1996)

Advantages and limitations of microfluidics for food analysis

Microfluidic systems are highly beneficial in food research as they are compact, allowing on-site analysis, disposability, and low construction costs. In addition, the future integration of multiple processes facilitates the automation of assays and increases the analytical efficiency and efficient use of unskilled operators. Microfluidic chips have a large capacity for high throughput analysis through the ability to multiplex and parallelize various assays. New micromanufacturing methods and multiplexing technologies are important for the development of low-cost, compact, and high-performance microfluidic analytical instruments.

The constraint on the use of microfluidic devices in the food industry is the need for specialized equipment, the lack of portability, the high cost of production, and the complexity. In addition, manufacturing processes typically involve time-consuming, thermal, and mass transfer functions within microfluidic channels and their effect on overall functionality, which is an obstacle to new concepts in microfluidic systems. Microfluidics technology needs to be improved, as it is an important enabling technology that effectively incorporates various areas of research for a wide range of scientific and commercial applications. In addition, new technologies and systems must operate at a higher level of accuracy and throughput than current automated macroscale equipment to be used on-site.

Conclusion

Food analysis today needs to develop lightweight, reliable, cost-effective, and high-sensitivity analytical tools for safety and quality control to meet regulatory and consumer requirements. Microfluidic analytical systems become a powerful tool as an alternative to traditional laboratories, due to their potential use in high-performance food safety and quality sectors. It can conduct laboratory processes across small volumes of analytes, leading to a reduction in the use of reagents, reduced energy consumption, immediate analysis of multiple analytes on a single platform, and the most important real-time detection. In the future, the combination of the microfluidic chip or LOC with nanomaterial and new biomolecules, biosensing, will give compact, fast, cost-effective, and high-sensitivity analytical tools for food analysis.

Furthermore, the future LOC will provide a high degree of portability and multi-complex capabilities, reliability, and robustness of the 3D platform and miniaturized electronic system, configure a highly capable microfluidic system inside and outside the laboratory, which could further increase the scope of analytical chemistry to both scientists and untrained staff. Even though some commercial probes are available in the markets for certain chemicals and species, but in-situ, compact multiplexing technologies, accurate and fully automated systems are still needed for many applications. It is still difficult to replace many microfluidic elements such as pumps, detection, and imaging devices. On the other hand, the incorporation of sample pretreatment, separation, and detection routines into a single chip requires massive efforts due to the complexity of the food matrix. Overall, the significance of miniaturized systems and their application developments are expected to attract growing interest in food analysis.

References

Al Mughairy, B., & Al-Lawati, H. A. J. (2020). Recent analytical advancements in microfluidics using chemiluminescence detection systems for food analysis. *TrAC Trends in Analytical Chemistry. 124*, https://doi.org/10.1016/j.trac.2019.115802.

Alahmad, W., Tungkijanansin, N., Kaneta, T., & Varanusupakul, P. (2018). A colorimetric paper-based analytical device coupled with hollow fiber membrane liquid phase microextraction (HF-LPME) for highly sensitive detection of hexavalent chromium in water samples. *Talanta, 190*, 78–84. https://doi.org/10.1016/j.talanta.2018.07.056.

Araci, I. E., & Quake, S. R. (2012). Microfluidic very large scale integration (mVLSI) with integrated micromechanical valves. *Lab on a Chip, 12*(16), 2803–2806. https://doi.org/10.1039/c2lc40258k.

Balsam, J., Bruck, H. A., & Rasooly, A. (2015). *Two-layer lab-on-a-chip (LOC) with passive capillary valves for mHealth medical diagnostics*: (pp. 247–258). *Mobile health technologies* New York, NY: Humana Press. https://doi.org/10.1007/978-1-4939-2172-0_17.

Bian, X., Jing, F., Li, G., Fan, X., Jia, C., Zhou, H., … Zhao, J. (2015). A microfluidic droplet digital PCR for simultaneous detection of pathogenic Escherichia coli O157 and Listeria monocytogenes. *Biosensors and Bioelectronics*, *74*, 770–777. https://doi.org/10.1016/j.bios.2015.07.016.

Bodas, D., & Khan-Malek, C. (2006). Formation of more stable hydrophilic surfaces of PDMS by plasma and chemical treatments. *Microelectronic Engineering*, *83*(4–9), 1277–1279. https://doi.org/10.1016/j.mee.2006.01.195.

Borisov, S. M., & Wolfbeis, O. S. (2008). Optical biosensors. *Chemical Reviews*, *108*(2), 423–461. https://doi.org/10.1021/cr068105t.

Braschler, T., Theytaz, J., Zvitov-Marabi, R., Lintel, H. V., Loche, G., Kunze, A., … Renaud, P. (2007). A virtual valve for smooth contamination-free flow switching. *Lab on a Chip*, *7*(9), 1111–1113. https://doi.org/10.1039/b708360b.

Busa, L. S. A., Mohammadi, S., Maeki, M., Ishida, A., Tani, H., & Tokeshi, M. (2016). Advances in microfluidic paper-based analytical devices for food and water analysis. *Micromachines*, *7*(5), 86. https://doi.org/10.3390/mi7050086.

Cabrera, C. R., & Yager, P. (2001). Continuous concentration of bacteria in a microfluidic flow cell using electrokinetic techniques. *Electrophoresis*. https://doi.org/10.1002/1522-2683(200101)22:2<355::AID-ELPS355>3.0.CO;2-C United States.

Chabinyc, M. L., Chiu, D. T., McDonald, J. C., Stroock, A. D., Christian, J. F., Karger, A. M., & Whitesides, G. M. (2001). An integrated fluorescence detection system in poly (dimethylsiloxane) for microfluidic applications. *Analytical Chemistry*, *73*(18), 4491–4498. https://doi.org/10.1021/ac010423z.

Chango, G., Palacio, E., & Cerdà, V. (2018). Potentiometric chip-based multipumping flow system for the simultaneous determination of fluoride, chloride, pH, and redox potential in water samples. *Talanta*, *186*, 554–560. https://doi.org/10.1016/j.talanta.2018.04.087.

Chen, L., & Choo, J. (2008). Recent advances in surface-enhanced Raman scattering detection technology for microfluidic chips. *Electrophoresis*, *29*(9), 1815–1828. https://doi.org/10.1002/elps.200700554.

Choi, N. W., Cabodi, M., Held, B., Gleghorn, J. P., Bonassar, L. J., & Stroock, A. D. (2007). Microfluidic scaffolds for tissue engineering. *Nature Materials*, *6*(11), 908–915. https://doi.org/10.1038/nmat2022.

Choi, K., Ng, A. H. C., Fobel, R., & Wheeler, A. R. (2012). Digital microfluidics. *Annual Review of Analytical Chemistry*, *5*, 413–440. https://doi.org/10.1146/annurev-anchem-062011-143028.

Chou, S. Y., Krauss, P. R., & Renstrom, P. J. (1996). Nanoimprint lithography. *Journal of Vacuum Science and Technology B: Microelectronics and Nanometer Structures*, *14*(6), 4129–4133.

Ciobanu, M., Taylor, D. E., Wilburn, J. P., & Cliffel, D. E. (2008). Glucose and lactate biosensors for scanning electrochemical microscopy imaging of single live cells. *Analytical Chemistry*, *80*(8), 2717–2727. https://doi.org/10.1021/ac7021184.

Dagkesamanskaya, A., Langer, K., Tauzin, A. S., Rouzeau, C., Lestrade, D., Potocki-Veronese, G., Boitard, L., Bibette, J., Baudry, J., Pompon, D., & Anton-Leberre, V. (2018). Use of photoswitchable fluorescent proteins for droplet-based microfluidic screening. *Journal of Microbiological Methods*, *147*, 59–65. https://doi.org/10.1016/j.mimet.2018.03.001.

Deiss, F., Funes-Huacca, M. E., Bal, J., Tjhung, K. F., & Derda, R. (2014). Antimicrobial susceptibility assays in paper-based portable culture devices. *Lab on a Chip*, *14*(1), 167–171. https://doi.org/10.1039/c3lc50887k.

Delatour, T., Racault, L., Bessaire, T., & Desmarchelier, A. (2018). Screening of veterinary drug residues in food by LC-MS/MS. Background and challenges. *Food Additives and Contaminants: Part A, Chemistry, Analysis, Control, Exposure and Risk Assessment*, *35*(4), 632–645. https://doi.org/10.1080/19440049.2018.1426890.

Desmet, G., Vervoort, N., Clicq, D., Huau, A., Gzil, P., & Baron, G. V. (2002). Shear-flow-based chromatographic separations as an alternative to pressure-driven liquid chromatography. *Journal of Chromatography A*. https://doi.org/10.1016/S0021-9673(01)01511-4 Belgium.

Díaz-González, M., Salvador, J. P., Bonilla, D., Marco, M. P., Fernández-Sánchez, C., & Baldi, A. (2015). A microfluidic device for the automated electrical readout of low-density glass-slide microarrays. *Biosensors and Bioelectronics*, *74*, 698–704.

Dill, F. H. (1975). Optical lithography. *IEEE Transactions on Electron Devices*, *22*(7), 440–444. https://doi.org/10.1109/T-ED.1975.18158.

Dressler, O. J., Maceiczyk, R. M., Chang, S. I., & Demello, A. J. (2014). Droplet-based microfluidics: Enabling impact on drug discovery. *Journal of Biomolecular Screening*, *19*(4), 483–496. https://doi.org/10.1177/1087057113510401.

Elizalde, E., Urteaga, R., & Berli, C. L. A. (2015). Rational design of capillary-driven flows for paper-based microfluidics. *Lab on a Chip*, *15*(10), 2173–2180. https://doi.org/10.1039/c4lc01487a.

Ellington, A. D., & Szostak, J. W. (1990). In vitro selection of RNA molecules that bind specific ligands. *Nature*, *346*(6287), 818–822. https://doi.org/10.1038/346818a0.

Ellington, A. D., & Szostak, J. W. (1992). Selection in vitro of single-stranded DNA molecules that fold into specific ligand-binding structures. *Nature*, *355*(6363), 850–852. https://doi.org/10.1038/355850a0.

El Moctar, A. O., Aubry, N., & Batton, J. (2003). Electro-hydrodynamic micro-fluidic mixer. *Lab on a Chip*, *3*(4), 273–280. https://doi.org/10.1039/B306868B.

Folch, A. (2016). *Introduction to bioMEMS*. CRC Press.

Gai, H., Li, Y., & Yeung, E. S. (2011). Optical detection systems on microfluidic chips. *Topics in Current Chemistry*, *304*, 171–201. https://doi.org/10.1007/128_2011_144.

Gao, D., Jin, F., Zhou, M., & Jiang, Y. (2019). Recent advances in single cell manipulation and biochemical analysis on microfluidics. *Analyst*, *144*(3), 766–781. https://doi.org/10.1039/c8an01186a.

Gomes, H. I. A. S., & Sales, M. G. F. (2015). Development of paper-based color test-strip for drug detection in aquatic environment: Application to oxytetracycline. *Biosensors and Bioelectronics*, *65*, 54–61. https://doi.org/10.1016/j.bios.2014.10.006.

Gonzalez-Rivera, J. C., & Osma, J. F. (2015). Fabrication of an amperometric flow-injection microfluidic biosensor based on laccase for in situ determination of phenolic compounds. *BioMed Research International*. *2015*, https://doi.org/10.1155/2015/845261.

Gupta, S., Ramesh, K., Ahmed, S., & Kakkar, V. (2016). Lab-on-chip technology: A review on design trends and future scope in biomedical applications. *International Journal of Bio-Science and Bio-Technology*, *8*(5), 311–322. https://doi.org/10.14257/ijbsbt.2016.8.5.28.

Gutmann, B., Cantillo, D., & Kappe, C. O. (2015). Continuous-flow technology—A tool for the safe manufacturing of active pharmaceutical ingredients. *Angewandte Chemie, International Edition*, *54*(23), 6688–6728. https://doi.org/10.1002/anie.201409318.

Hardy, B. S., Uechi, K., Zhen, J., & Pirouz Kavehpour, H. (2009). The deformation of flexible PDMS microchannels under a pressure driven flow. *Lab on a Chip*, *9*(7), 935–938. https://doi.org/10.1039/b813061b.

Hassani, A., & Skorobogatiy, M. (2006). Design of the microstructured optical fiber-based surface plasmon resonance sensors with enhanced microfluidics. *Optics Express*, *14*(24), 11616–11621. https://doi.org/10.1364/OE.14.011616.

He, D., Zhang, Z., Huang, Y., & Hu, Y. (2007). Chemiluminescence microflow injection analysis system on a chip for the determination of nitrite in food. *Food Chemistry*, *101*(2), 667–672. https://doi.org/10.1016/j.foodchem.2006.02.024.

Hillborg, H., Tomczak, N., Olàh, A., Schönherr, H., & Vancso, G. J. (2004). Nanoscale hydrophobic recovery: A chemical force microscopy study of UV/ozone-treated cross-linked poly(dimethylsiloxane). *Langmuir*, *20*(3), 785–794. https://doi.org/10.1021/la035552k.

Hilvert, D. (2000). Critical analysis of antibody catalysis. *Annual Review of Biochemistry*, *69*, 751–793. https://doi.org/10.1146/annurev.biochem.69.1.751.

Hua, M. Z., Li, S., Wang, S., & Lu, X. (2018). Detecting chemical hazards in foods using microfluidic paper-based analytical devices (µPADs): The real-world application. *Micromachines*. *9*(1)https://doi.org/10.3390/mi9010032.

Huang, G. Y., Zhou, L. H., Zhang, Q. C., Chen, Y. M., Sun, W., Xu, F., & Lu, T. J. (2011). Microfluidic hydrogels for tissue engineering. *Biofabrication*. *3*(1). https://doi.org/10.1088/1758-5082/3/1/012001.

Huebner, A., Srisa-Art, M., Holt, D., Abell, C., Hollfelder, F., DeMello, A. J., & Edel, J. B. (2007). Quantitative detection of protein expression in single cells using droplet microfluidics. *Chemical Communications*, *12*, 1218–1220. https://doi.org/10.1039/b618570c.

Jackman, R. J., Floyd, T. M., Ghodssi, R., Schmidt, M. A., & Jensen, K. F. (2001). Microfluidic systems with on-line UV detection fabricated in photodefinable epoxy. *Journal of Micromechanics and Microengineering*, *11*(3), 263–269. https://doi.org/10.1088/0960-1317/11/3/316.

Jang, M., Jeong, S. W., Bae, N. H., Song, Y., Lee, T. J., Lee, M. K., … Lee, K. G. (2017). Droplet-based digital PCR system for detection of single-cell level of foodborne pathogens. *BioChip Journal*, *11*(4), 329–337. https://doi.org/10.1007/s13206-017-1410-x.

Jena, R. K., & Yue, C. Y. (2012). Cyclic olefin copolymer based microfluidic devices for biochip applications: Ultraviolet surface grafting using 2-methacryloyloxyethyl phosphorylcholine. *Biomicrofluidics*. *6*(1). https://doi.org/10.1063/1.3682098.

Jokerst, J. C., Adkins, J. A., Bisha, B., Mentele, M. M., Goodridge, L. D., & Henry, C. S. (2012). Development of a paper-based analytical device for colorimetric detection of select foodborne pathogens. *Analytical Chemistry*, *84*(6), 2900–2907. https://doi.org/10.1021/ac203466y.

Khanarian, G. (2001). Optical properties of cyclic olefin copolymers. *Optical Engineering*, *40*(6), 1024–1030. https://doi.org/10.1117/1.1369411.

Kim, J. Y., Demello, A. J., Chang, S. I., Hong, J., & O'Hare, D. (2011). Thermoset polyester droplet-based microfluidic devices for high frequency generation. *Lab on a Chip*, *11*(23), 4108–4112. https://doi.org/10.1039/c1lc20603f.

Krishnamoorthy, S., Bedekar, A. S., Feng, J., & Sundaram, S. (2007). Simulation-based analysis of fluid flow and electrokinetic phenomena in microfluidic devices. *Clinics in Laboratory Medicine*, *27*(1), 41–59. https://doi.org/10.1016/j.cll.2006.12.014.

Krishnan, M., Namasivayam, V., Lin, R., Pal, R., & Burns, M. A. (2001). Microfabricated reaction and separation systems. *Current Opinion in Biotechnology*, *12*(1), 92–98. https://doi.org/10.1016/S0958-1669(00)00166-X.

Kumar, K., Nightingale, A. M., Krishnadasan, S. H., Kamaly, N., Wylenzinska-Arridge, M., Zeissler, K., ... Demello, J. C. (2012). Direct synthesis of dextran-coated superparamagnetic iron oxide nanoparticles in a capillary-based droplet reactor. *Journal of Materials Chemistry, 22*(11), 4704–4708. https://doi.org/10.1039/c2jm30257h.

Lai, H. H., Xu, W., & Allbritton, N. L. (2011). Use of a virtual wall valve in polydimethylsiloxane microfluidic devices for bioanalytical applications. *Biomicrofluidics, 5*(2).

Lan, H., & Ding, Y. (2010). *Nanoimprint lithography*: (pp. 457–494). InTech.

Lee, C. Y., Chang, C. L., Wang, Y. N., & Fu, L. M. (2011). Microfluidic mixing: A review. *International Journal of Molecular Sciences, 12*(5), 3263–3287. https://doi.org/10.3390/ijms12053263.

Lee, N. Y., Yamada, M., & Seki, M. (2005). Development of a passive micromixer based on repeated fluid twisting and flattening, and its application to DNA purification. *Analytical and Bioanalytical Chemistry*. https://doi.org/10.1007/s00216-005-0073-y Japan.

Li, X. J., Nie, Z. H., Cheng, C. M., Goodale, A. B., & Whitesides, G. M. (2010). Paper-based electrochemical ELISA. In: *14th International Conference on Miniaturized Systems for Chemistry and Life Sciences 2010, MicroTAS 2010. United States.*

Li, Y., Xing, D., & Zhang, C. (2009). Rapid detection of genetically modified organisms on a continuous-flow polymerase chain reaction microfluidics. *Analytical Biochemistry, 385* (1), 42–49. https://doi.org/10.1016/j.ab.2008.10.028.

Li, S., Zhang, C., Wang, S., Liu, Q., Feng, H., Ma, X., & Guo, J. (2018). Electrochemical microfluidics techniques for heavy metal ion detection. *Analyst, 143*(18), 4230–4246. https://doi.org/10.1039/c8an01067f.

Li, X., Zhao, S., & Liu, Y. M. (2013). Evaluation of a microchip electrophoresis-mass spectrometry platform deploying a pressure-driven make-up flow. *Journal of Chromatography A, 1285*, 159–164. https://doi.org/10.1016/j.chroma.2013.02.031.

Link, D. R., Grasland-Mongrain, E., Duri, A., Sarrazin, F., Cheng, Z., Cristobal, G., ... Weitz, D. A. (2006). Electric control of droplets in microfluidic devices. *Angewandte Chemie, International Edition, 45*(16), 2556–2560. https://doi.org/10.1002/anie.200503540.

Liu, C., Xu, X., Li, B., Situ, B., Pan, W., Hu, Y., ... Zheng, L. (2018). Single-exosome-counting immunoassays for cancer diagnostics. *Nano Letters, 18*(7), 4226–4232. https://doi.org/10.1021/acs.nanolett.8b01184.

Liu, R., Zhang, P., Li, H., & Zhang, C. (2016). Lab-on-cloth integrated with gravity/capillary flow chemiluminescence (GCF-CL): Towards simple, inexpensive, portable, flow system for measuring trivalent chromium in water. *Sensors and Actuators, B: Chemical, 236*, 35–43. https://doi.org/10.1016/j.snb.2016.05.088.

Luka, G., Ahmadi, A., Najjaran, H., Alocilja, E., Derosa, M., Wolthers, K., ... Hoorfar, M. (2015). Microfluidics integrated biosensors: A leading technology towards lab-on-A-chip and sensing applications. *Sensors (Switzerland), 15*(12), 30011–30031. https://doi.org/10.3390/s151229783.

Ma, L., Nilghaz, A., Choi, J. R., Liu, X., & Lu, X. (2018). Rapid detection of clenbuterol in milk using microfluidic paper-based ELISA. *Food Chemistry, 246*, 437–441. https://doi.org/10.1016/j.foodchem.2017.12.022.

Mack, C. (2008). *Fundamental principles of optical lithography: The science of microfabrication*. John Wiley & Sons.

Mark, D., Haeberle, S., Roth, G., Von Stetten, F., & Zengerle, R. (2010). Microfluidic lab-on-a-chip platforms: Requirements, characteristics and applications. *Chemical Society Reviews, 39*(3), 1153–1182. https://doi.org/10.1039/b820557b.

Mark, D., Metz, T., Haeberle, S., Lutz, S., Ducrée, J., Zengerle, R., & Von Stetten, F. (2009). Centrifugo-pneumatic valve for metering of highly wetting liquids on centrifugal microfluidic platforms. *Lab on a Chip*, *9*(24), 3599–3603. https://doi.org/10.1039/b914415c.

Martinez, A. W., Phillips, S. T., Whitesides, G. M., & Carrilho, E. (2010). Diagnostics for the developing world: Microfluidic paper-based analytical devices. *Analytical Chemistry*. https://doi.org/10.1021/ac9013989.

Martinez-Duarte, R., & Madou, M. (2011). SU-8 photolithography and its impact on microfluidics. *Microfluidics and Nanofluidics Handbook*, (2006), 231–268.

McDonald, J. C., Duffy, D. C., Anderson, J. R., Chiu, D. T., Wu, H., Schueller, O. J. A., & Whitesides, G. M. (2000). Fabrication of microfluidic systems in poly(dimethylsiloxane). *Electrophoresis*, *21*(1), 27–40. https://doi.org/10.1002/(SICI)1522-2683(20000101) 21:1<27::AID-ELPS27>3.0.CO;2-C.

Mohammed, M. I., & Desmulliez, M. P. Y. (2011). Lab-on-a-chip based immunosensor principles and technologies for the detection of cardiac biomarkers: A review. *Lab on a Chip*, *11*(4), 569–595. https://doi.org/10.1039/c0lc00204f.

Mongersun, A., Smeenk, I., Pratx, G., Asuri, P., & Abbyad, P. (2016). Droplet microfluidic platform for the determination of single-cell lactate release. *Analytical Chemistry*, *88* (6), 3257–3263. https://doi.org/10.1021/acs.analchem.5b04681.

Nge, P. N., Rogers, C. I., & Woolley, A. T. (2013). Advances in microfluidic materials, functions, integration, and applications. *Chemical Reviews*, *113*(4), 2550–2583. https://doi.org/ 10.1021/cr300337x.

Nguyen, N. T. (2012). Micro-magnetofluidics: Interactions between magnetism and fluid flow on the microscale. *Microfluidics and Nanofluidics*, *12*(1-4), 1–16. https://doi.org/10.1007/ s10404-011-0903-5.

Nguyen, N. T., Hejazian, M., Ooi, C. H., & Kashaninejad, N. (2017). Recent advances and future perspectives on microfluidic liquid handling. *Micromachines*. *8*(6)https://doi.org/ 10.3390/mi8060186.

Nichols, K. P., Ferullo, J. R., & Baeumner, A. J. (2006). Recirculating, passive micromixer with a novel sawtooth structure. *Lab on a Chip*, *6*(2), 242–246. https://doi.org/10.1039/ b509034b.

Nie, Z., Nijhuis, C. A., Gong, J., Chen, X., Kumachev, A., Martinez, A. W., … Whitesides, G. M. (2010). Electrochemical sensing in paper-based microfluidic devices. *Lab on a Chip*, *10*(4), 477–483. https://doi.org/10.1039/b917150a.

Nilghaz, A., & Lu, X. (2019). Detection of antibiotic residues in pork using paper-based microfluidic device coupled with filtration and concentration. *Analytica Chimica Acta*, *1046*, 163–169. https://doi.org/10.1016/j.aca.2018.09.041.

Nimjee, S. M., Rusconi, C. P., & Sullenger, B. A. (2005). Aptamers: An emerging class of therapeutics. *Annual Review of Medicine*, *56*, 555–583. https://doi.org/10.1146/annurev. med.56.062904.144915.

Noh, H., & Phillips, S. T. (2010). Metering the capillary-driven flow of fluids in paper-based microfluidic devices. *Analytical Chemistry*, *82*(10), 4181–4187. https://doi.org/10.1021/ ac100431y.

Ölcer, Z., Esen, E., Ersoy, A., Budak, S., Sever Kaya, D., Yağmur Gök, M., … Uludag, Y. (2015). Microfluidics and nanoparticles based amperometric biosensor for the detection of cyanobacteria (Planktothrix agardhii NIVA-CYA 116) DNA. *Biosensors and Bioelectronics*, *70*, 426–432. https://doi.org/10.1016/j.bios.2015.03.052.

Olcer, Z., Esen, E., Muhammad, T., Ersoy, A., Budak, S., & Uludag, Y. (2014). Fast and sensitive detection of mycotoxins in wheat using microfluidics based real-time electrochemical profiling. *Biosensors and Bioelectronics*, *62*, 163–169. https://doi.org/10.1016/j.bios.2014.06.025.

Pelton, R. (2009). Bioactive paper provides a low-cost platform for diagnostics. *TrAC Trends in Analytical Chemistry*, *28*(8), 925–942. https://doi.org/10.1016/j.trac.2009.05.005.

Ren, K., Zhou, J., & Wu, H. (2013). Materials for microfluidic chip fabrication. *Accounts of Chemical Research*, *46*(11), 2396–2406. https://doi.org/10.1021/ar300314s.

Renaudin, A., Chabot, V., Grondin, E., Aimez, V., & Charette, P. G. (2010). Integrated active mixing and biosensing using surface acoustic waves (SAW) and surface plasmon resonance (SPR) on a common substrate. *Lab on a Chip*, *10*(1), 111–115. https://doi.org/10.1039/b911953a.

Rocchitta, G., Spanu, A., Babudieri, S., Latte, G., Madeddu, G., Galleri, G., Nuvoli, S., Bagella, P., Demartis, M. I., Fiore, V., & Manetti, R. (2016). Enzyme biosensors for biomedical applications: Strategies for safeguarding analytical performances in biological fluids. *Sensors*, *16*(6), 780. https://doi.org/10.3390/s16060780.

Rogers, J. A., & Nuzzo, R. G. (2005). Recent progress in soft lithography. *Materials Today*, *8*(2), 50–56. https://doi.org/10.1016/S1369-7021(05)00702-9.

Roman, G. T., Hlaus, T., Bass, K. J., Seelhammer, T. G., & Culbertson, C. T. (2005). Sol-gel modified poly(dimethylsiloxane) microfluidic devices with high electroosmotic mobilities and hydrophilic channel wall characteristics. *Analytical Chemistry*, *77*(5), 1414–1422. https://doi.org/10.1021/ac048811z.

Roy, E., Galas, J. C., & Veres, T. (2011). Thermoplastic elastomers for microfluidics: Towards a high-throughput fabrication method of multilayered microfluidic devices. *Lab on a Chip*, *11*(18), 3193–3196. https://doi.org/10.1039/c1lc20251k.

Sajeesh, P., & Sen, A. K. (2014). Particle separation and sorting in microfluidic devices: A review. *Microfluidics and Nanofluidics*, *17*(1), 1–52. https://doi.org/10.1007/s10404-013-1291-9.

Salmanzadeh, A., Shafiee, H., Davalos, R. V., & Stremler, M. A. (2011). Microfluidic mixing using contactless dielectrophoresis. *Electrophoresis*, *32*(18), 2569–2578. https://doi.org/10.1002/elps.201100171.

Samiei, E., De Leon Derby, M. D., Den Berg, A. V., & Hoorfar, M. (2017). An electrohydrodynamic technique for rapid mixing in stationary droplets on digital microfluidic platforms. *Lab on a Chip*, *17*(2), 227–234. https://doi.org/10.1039/C6LC00997B.

Sapsford, K. E., Bradburne, C., Delehanty, J. B., & Medintz, I. L. (2008). Sensors for detecting biological agents. *Materials Today*, *11*(3), 38–49. https://doi.org/10.1016/S1369-7021(08)70018-X.

Sasaki, Y. F., Kawaguchi, S., Kamaya, A., Ohshita, M., Kabasawa, K., Iwama, K., … Tsuda, S. (2002). The comet assay with 8 mouse organs: Results with 39 currently used food additives. *Mutation Research, Genetic Toxicology and Environmental Mutagenesis*, *519*(1–2), 103–119. https://doi.org/10.1016/S1383-5718(02)00128-6.

Shen, R., Liu, P., Zhang, Y., Yu, Z., Chen, X., Zhou, L., … Liu, J. (2018). Sensitive detection of single-cell secreted H_2O_2 by integrating a microfluidic droplet sensor and Au nanoclusters. *Analytical Chemistry*, *90*(7), 4478–4484. https://doi.org/10.1021/acs.analchem.7b04798.

Songok, J., & Toivakka, M. (2016). Enhancing capillary-driven flow for paper-based microfluidic channels. *ACS Applied Materials and Interfaces*, *8*(44), 30523–30530. https://doi.org/10.1021/acsami.6b08117.

Srinivasan, B., & Tung, S. (2015). Development and applications of portable biosensors. *Journal of Laboratory Automation*, *20*(4), 365–389. https://doi.org/10.1177/2211068215581349.

Sriram, G., Bhat, M. P., Patil, P., Uthappa, U. T., Jung, H. Y., Altalhi, T., Kumeria, T., Aminabhavi, T. M., Pai, R. K., & Kurkuri, M. D. (2017). Paper-based microfluidic analytical devices for colorimetric detection of toxic ions: A review. *TrAC Trends in Analytical Chemistry*, *93*, 212–227. https://doi.org/10.1016/j.trac.2017.06.005.

Subrahmanyam, S., Piletsky, S. A., & Turner, A. P. F. (2002). Application of natural receptors in sensors and assays. *Analytical Chemistry*, *74*(16), 3942–3951. https://doi.org/10.1021/ac025673+.

Sukhatme, S., & Agarwal, A. (2012). Digital microfluidics: Techniques, their applications and advantages. *Journal Bioengineer & Biomedical Science*. 8, https://doi.org/10.4172/2155-9538.S8-001.

Tibbitt, M. W., & Anseth, K. S. (2009). Hydrogels as extracellular matrix mimics for 3D cell culture. *Biotechnology and Bioengineering*, *103*(4), 655–663. https://doi.org/10.1002/bit.22361.

Tice, J. D., Song, H., Lyon, A. D., & Ismagilov, R. F. (2003). Formation of droplets and mixing in multiphase microfluidics at low values of the reynolds and the capillary numbers. *Langmuir*, *19*(22), 9127–9133. https://doi.org/10.1021/la030090w.

Tsao, C. W. (2016). Polymer microfluidics: Simple, low-cost fabrication process bridging academic lab research to commercialized production. *Micromachines*. 7(12)https://doi.org/10.3390/mi7120225.

Vreeland, W. N., & Locascio, L. E. (2003). Using bioinspired thermally triggered liposomes for high-efficiency mixing and reagent delivery in microfluidic devices. *Analytical Chemistry*, *75*(24), 6906–6911. https://doi.org/10.1021/ac034850j.

Wang, R., Ni, Y., Xu, Y., Jiang, Y., Dong, C., & Chuan, N. (2015). Immuno-capture and in situ detection of Salmonella typhimurium on a novel microfluidic chip. *Analytica Chimica Acta*, *853*(1), 710–717. https://doi.org/10.1016/j.aca.2014.10.042.

Watanabe, A., Hasegawa, K., & Abe, Y. (2018). Contactless fluid manipulation in air: Droplet coalescence and active mixing by acoustic levitation. *Scientific Reports*. 8(1). https://doi.org/10.1038/s41598-018-28451-5.

Weng, X., & Neethirajan, S. (2017). Ensuring food safety: Quality monitoring using microfluidics. *Trends in Food Science and Technology*, *65*, 10–22. https://doi.org/10.1016/j.tifs.2017.04.015.

Whitesides, G. M. (2006). The origins and the future of microfluidics. *Nature*, *442*(7101).

Xia, Y., & Whitesides, G. M. (1998). Soft lithography. *Angewandte Chemie International Edition*, *37*(5), 550–575.

Xu, K., Zhu, P., Colon, T., Huh, C., & Balhoff, M. (2017). A microfluidic investigation of the synergistic effect of nanoparticles and surfactants in macro-emulsion-based enhanced oil recovery. *SPE Journal*, *22*(2), 459–469. https://doi.org/10.2118/179691-PA.

Yoon, J. H., Kim, K. H., Bae, N. H., Sim, G. S., Oh, Y. J., Lee, S. J., … Choi, B. G. (2017). Fabrication of newspaper-based potentiometric platforms for flexible and disposable ion sensors. *Journal of Colloid and Interface Science*, *508*, 167–173. https://doi.org/10.1016/j.jcis.2017.08.036.

Zhang, Y., Zuo, P., & Ye, B. C. (2015). A low-cost and simple paper-based microfluidic device for simultaneous multiplex determination of different types of chemical contaminants in food. *Biosensors and Bioelectronics*, *68*, 14–19. https://doi.org/10.1016/j.bios.2014.12.042.

Zhou, W. (2018). Development of immunomagnetic droplet-based digital immuno-PCR for the quantification of prostate specific antigen. *Analytical Methods*, *10*(29), 3690–3695. https://doi.org/10.1039/c8ay00921j.

Zhou, C., Zhang, H., Li, Z., & Wang, W. (2016). Chemistry pumps: A review of chemically powered micropumps. *Lab on a Chip*, *16*(10), 1797–1811. https://doi.org/10.1039/c6lc00032k.

Zhu, G. P., & Nguyen, N. T. (2012). Rapid magnetofluidic mixing in a uniform magnetic field. *Lab on a Chip*, *12*(22), 4772–4780. https://doi.org/10.1039/c2lc40818j.

Zhu, X. D., Shi, X., Wang, S. W., Chu, J., Zhu, W. H., Ye, B. C., … Wang, Y. H. (2019). High-throughput screening of high lactic acid-producing Bacillus coagulans by droplet microfluidic based flow cytometry with fluorescence activated cell sorting. *RSC Advances*, *9*(8), 4507–4513. https://doi.org/10.1039/C8RA09684H.

Zhu, X., Shi, X., Chu, J., Ye, B., Zuo, P., & Wang, Y. (2018). Quantitative analysis of the growth of individual Bacillus coagulans cells by microdroplet technology. *Bioresources and Bioprocessing*, *5*(1), 1–8. https://doi.org/10.1186/s40643-018-0229-1.

Application of nanomaterials-based sensor for food analysis

Introduction

As a global problem, the problem of food safety has drawn public concern both within food manufacturing as well as among consumers. Food safety is generally defined as a practice aimed at ensuring consumer safety in food' from farm to fork.' Food safety is a recommendation to minimize occurrences of foodborne illness. Food safety materials cover an extensive range of physical, chemical, and microbial exposures and other related contaminants or toxins Wilcock, Pun, Khanona, & Aung, 2004. Food adulteration can be defined as pests, environmental contaminants, additives, agrochemical traces, hazards, etc. (Feng & Sun, 2012). In recent years, the recurrent phenomenon of food safety dilemmas has affected human beings, and the issue of food safety is now the primary concern of the people. At this point, scientific methods have a vital role to play in food quality and safety.

Food analysis and safety confirmation currently depend on conventional chromatography, such as liquid chromatography (Badoud, Ernest, Hammel, & Huertas-Pérez, 2018; Trevisan, Owen, Calatayud-Vernich, Breuer, & Picó, 2017) or gas chromatography (Jeong et al., 2017; Cordero, Schmarr, Reichenbach, & Bicchi, 2018), to achieve high precision and sensitivity. Nevertheless, the main bottlenecks that restrict their use in on-site testing are complicated procedures, bulky and costly tools. It appears that the responsiveness and portability of the tools can not correspond simultaneously. Hence, scientist focus on other prospective approaches, for example, molecular imprinting Technology (MIT) (Yin et al., 2018), fluorometric technique (Abd-Elghany & Sallam, 2015), electrochemical method Gómez-López, Gila, & Allende, 2017 and Raman spectroscopy (Wang, Wu, et al., 2017). Unfortunately, the same problem still exists. Furthermore, the direct identification of food pathogens or micro-organisms by chromatography, electrochemistry, and Raman spectroscopy is difficult. Scientists are making efforts to develop detection methods that are easier and more effective, recognizing the shortcomings of bulky devices.

Nanotechnology advancement has facilitated the transformation of conventional branches of science and technology, specifically the discovery of intelligent and active packaging and nanosensors. There are various novel nanomaterials developed to optimize production and control the quality and safety of the food. A novel strategy for monitoring food analysis has been developed for nanotechnology in the field of biosensors. A biosensor is a tool employed to identify biological components using an electrochemical signal probe. Samples, receivers, electrical interfaces,

213

Advanced Food Analysis Tools. https://doi.org/10.1016/B978-0-12-820591-4.00011-6

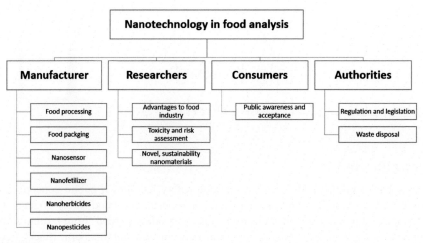

FIG. 11.1

Schematic of food nanotechnology from scientific research to the product on the market and to the consumer's plate. Scientific research is a one-way production that provides guidance both to food producers for the production of commodities and to regulatory and legislative agencies.

transducers, and signal processors are components inside the biosensor. The biosensor will measure linearity, sensitivity, selectivity, and response time when analytics are detected in food products. Nanotechnology integration with a biosensor exhibits a rapid, convenient, comfortable, eco-friendly, highly sensitive and accurate detection approach compared to other analytical techniques including enzyme-linked immunosorbent assay (ELISA), polymerase chain reaction (PCR), gas chromatography–mass spectrometry, high-performance liquid chromatography, and spectrophotometry. The use of nanomaterials such as carbon nanotubes (CNTs), quantum dots (QDTs), graphene, magnetic nanoparticles (NPs), gold NPs (AuNPs), nanowires, nanotubes, and nanofibers with integrated electrochemical biosensors will increase the performance of biosensors in food analysis and achieve better results. Food nanotechnology for the product on the market requires a great deal of research and effort, basic features of nanotoxicity, regulation, or know-how on food nanotechnology, public knowledge, and acceptance, all of which are strictly interrelated, as shown in the Fig. 11.1. This chapter will examine the application of nanomaterials biosensors to various food analyzes.

Nanotechnology-based biosensors

Presently, many food pollutants and residues are growing, which has contributed to high demand for analysis of possible food pollution, such as toxin, pesticide, pathogens, and illegal food additives (Dominguez et al., 2017). The mixture of contaminants in food that present serious health risks. The new techniques have, therefore, been used to detect pollutants in food, such as chromatographic methods and mass spectrometry methods. The introduction of a novel method or advanced method, such as biosensor technology, is essential for the determination of various analytes (Díaz, Ibáñez, Sancho, & Hernández, 2012). Nanotechnology explains that the smaller size of materials was down to a nanometer. The decrease in the size of nanometer-scale materials that redesign the biological, physical, and chemical properties that create new applications from 10 to 9 m (Ozin & Arsenault, 2015; Ponce, Ayala-Zavala, Marcovich, Vázquez, & Ansorena, 2018). The combination of a large area with a smaller particle size gives NPs unique characteristics and vast potential for food processing and manufacturing (Chau, Wu, & Yen, 2007). Additionally, the mixture of nanotechnology and biosensor is converted into nanotechnology-based biosensors or nanosensors. Nanobiosensors are devices constructed from nanomaterials that can be used to assess nanoscale events. Such nanomaterials include CNTs, NPs, nanotubes, QDTs, nanotubes, graphene, and other biological nanomaterials (Pandit, Dasgupta, Dewan, & Prince, 2016). A number of biosensing devices that used nanostructures or NPs in research studies around the world have been investigated due to the advantages of food processing (Fig. 11.2). This provides an opportunity to tackle food safety-related issues (Lv et al., 2018).

Trends in nanobiosensors technology

In this age of technology, the food industry is demanding fast, high-sensitivity, and low-cost food analysis techniques, such as the determination of foodborne pathogens or the analysis of biological compounds in food. The market is not only in the area of food science but also in another field, such as medicine. They used nano biosensor technology to detect and track diseases in medicine. The development of highly sensitive biosensors is one of the challenges in engineering and science in the 21st century (Sagadevan & Periasamy, 2014). The sensitivity and specificity of the nano biosensor need to be improved in order to meet the requirements of different fields. Advances in nanotechnology have been potential for progress in food analysis. The ability to identify pathogens and harmful chemicals in food can provide researchers and the food industry with detailed knowledge to detect the presence of pollutants. Traditional methods, such as chromatography and mass spectrometry, are time-consuming, require a high concentration of the sample, and may produce false results (Bellan, Wu, & Langer, 2011). Nevertheless, the use of nanobiosensors now makes a useful contribution to the chemical-proof and processing environments of food products. This is because nano biosensors are inexpensive, more comfortable to operate, and produce accurate results in a short time (Patra, Mahato, & Kumar, 2019). As a result, nanobiosensors become promising tools for food analysis due to rapid, low cost, high sensitivity, and small amounts of samples required for the broadest range of biomaterial identification.

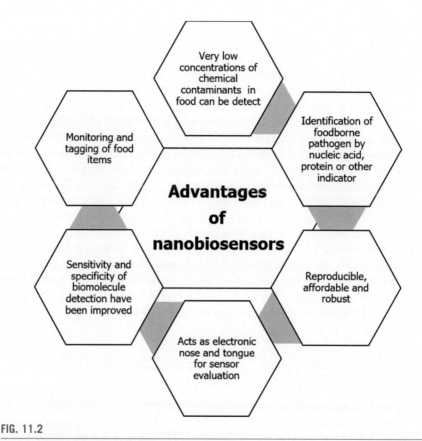

FIG. 11.2

The advantages of nanobiosensors.

Furthermore, the new state-of-the-art biosensor technologies are based on sample PCR and ELISA technique used as an alternative in food analysis (Bellan et al., 2011). ELISA has been a powerful tool for food safety and verification due to its strengths, such as flexibility, high sensitivity, and efficiency of operation. Indeed, the relatively low sensitivity and precision are the main constraints of the conventional ELISA, which have limited the application in food analysis (Wu et al., 2019). In a distinctive arrangement, ELISA shows immobilization probes with specific binding to the analyte molecules known as the ELISA sandwich. Sandwich ELISA is one of the most accurate ELISA protocols (Cerda-Kipper, Montiel, & Hosseini, 2018). The protocol is the detection of an antibody that binds to analytes captured by the conjugated enzyme. Each bound of the enzyme is then referred to as the presence of the analyte (Bellan et al., 2011). Hence, the development of successful approaches to minimizing difficulties is of utmost concern. There is a lot of advancement has been done to improve the efficiency, sensitivity, and reliability of the modern ELISA to date. Luckily, the nanomaterial-based ELISA (nano-ELISA) significantly improved ELISA and obtained better performance. While PCR is a technique for amplifying copies of DNA sequences due to the presence of analyte molecules that replicate millions of copies of DNA sequences (Joshi & Deshpande, 2010), both of these techniques may increase the error of analysis so that appropriate sample preparation is required and the sample should be handled intensively. Moreover, the sensitivity of the analysis using these methods was not sufficient to detect the desired amounts of analyte. A full scale of new biosensors based on nanomaterials is, therefore, being developed to address the challenges of new methods of food analysis.

Nanomaterials for biosensing devices

Recently, nanomaterials are rapidly developing and commonly used in the catalysis, structural components, nanoelectronics, biosensors, data storage, and biomaterials sectors (Cao, 2004; Dominguez et al., 2017). Nanomaterials act as a transducer in the part of the biosensor. Nanowires, NPs, and nanotubes are examples of nanomaterials and are an exciting tool due to the full surface area, which has different and unique characteristics and specific chemical and physical properties (Pandit et al., 2016). NPs of less than 100nm are made up of NPs at one dimension. Newly developed nanomaterial-based biosensing devices can determine minute amounts of analyte due to the unique characteristics of nanomaterials with nanoscale dimensions. The classification of nanomaterials is based on size and dimensions. Three types of nanomaterials are zero-dimensional (0D), one-dimensional (1D), two-dimensional (2D), and three-dimensional (3D) (Malhotra & Ali, 2018a). All 0D nanomaterials exist in nanoscale dimensions, such as NPs such as silver, palladium, QDTs, platinum, and gold. NPs have a spherical size, shape of polygon and cube, and a diameter of 1 to 50nm. 1D nanomaterial has a number of dimensions ranging from 1 to 100nm, and the other two are in macroscale. The examples of 1D nanomaterials are QDTs, metal oxides such as ZnO, TiO_2, and CeO_2, nanotubes, metals such as Au, Si, and Ag, nanorods, and nanofibers. Next, 2D nanomaterials have nanoscale for two dimensions and macroscale for one dimension. Types of 2D nanomaterials include nanosheets, nanothin films, nanowalls, or thin-film multilayers, which in square microns. Ultimately, all 3D nanomaterials reside in the macroscale dimension. The example of 3D nanomaterials is bulk materials made from separate blocks and has a nanometer-scale of 1 to 100nm (Malhotra & Ali, 2018a).

Carbon nanotubes (CNTs)

CNTs have been widely used in biosensors over the last decade. Not only biosensing tools but also diagnostics, cell monitoring, and labeling, tissue engineering, drug delivery, and delivery of biomolecules. CNT-based biosensors have been used to detect high sensitivity of food analytes, the monitoring environment, the analysis of medicines, and the analysis of food safety (Pandit et al., 2016). CNTs exist in a hollow cylindrical form and small in dimension, having a micrometer scale in length and a nanometer scale in diameter (Qiu & Yang, 2017). The CNTs consist of the rolling of the graphene layer. Chiral, armchair, and zigzag are CNTs. CNTs can be divided into single-walled CNTs and multiwalled CNTs (MWCNTs). The single-walled CNTs are made of 2D graphene sheets formed into a cylindrical shape. It has a 2-nm diameter and a 100-μm length with 1D nanowire characteristics. Meanwhile, MWCNTs consist of multiple layers of graphene sheets. (Malhotra & Ali, 2018a) CNTs are excellent as thermal conductors due to their unique characteristics, which have high chemical stability and the efficiency of mechanical and electrical properties. CNTs are used in biosensors for fuel cells, drug delivery, capacitors, secondary batteries and nano molecules filtration, cancer biomarker detection, neurochemical detection, and other biomolecules detection (Harris & Harris, 2009; Pandit et al., 2016).

Nanoparticles

NPs have also been widely used in various biosensor development due to their unique characteristics and high sensitivity. When molecules or analytes are attached to the surface of the NPs, they will change color. Changes in the properties of NPs varied their shape and size for different applications (Pandit et al., 2016). NPs are the most important class of nanomaterials because they have less than 100 nm in one dimension and can be in 0D, 1D, 2D, and 3D shapes (Laurent et al., 2008; Tiwari, Tiwari, & Kim, 2012). NPs are complex molecules because they are made up of three layers. The first layer is the surface layer, which contains different surfactants, small molecules, polymers, and metal ions. Next, the shell layer that has different chemical properties from the core layer. Finally, the layer which acts as the central point for NPs (Shin, Cho, Kannan, Lee, & Kim, 2016). NPs may be categorized as carbon-based, metal-based, ceramic, semiconductor, polymeric, and lipid-based.

CNTs and fullerenes are examples of carbon NPs. Fullerenes are 0D nanomaterials and are made up of carbon atoms in spherical and other shapes. The structure of fullerenes is similar to that of graphite, which has graphene sheets (Malhotra and Ali, 2018b). Metal NPs are made up of precursor metals which have a unique optical property. Metal NPs are, therefore, often used in many fields of research. Noble metals such as silver, copper, and gold are examples of NP metals. AuNPs are currently the most widely used NPs in biosensor applications due to their nontoxic element, have an inert core, and help to obtain useful quality scanning electron microscopy (SEM) images (Dreaden, Alkilany, Huang, Murphy, & El-Sayed, 2012; Khan, Abdalla, & Qurashi, 2017). Inorganic, nonmetallic NPs are the characteristics of ceramic NPs produced by sequential cooling and heating during the synthesis process. Ceramics NPs may also occur in porous, amorphous, hollow, dense, and polycrystalline forms (Sigmund et al., 2006). Semiconductor NPs consist of metal and nonmetal properties and are available in a variety of applications (Ali et al., 2017; Khan, Saeed, & Khan, 2019). Polymer NPs are organic materials and exist in the structure of nanocapsules and nanospheres (Mansha, Khan, Ullah, &

Qurashi, 2017). Lipid-based NPs are spherical and have a diameter of between 10 and 1000 nm. They also have a solid core made of lipids and a soluble lipophilic compound in the matrix. Core lipid-based NPs can be stabilized by emulsifiers and surfactants (Rawat, Jain, & Singh, 2011).

Quantum dots (QDs)

In the 21st century, QDs became a new tool for researchers due to their unusual optical and physical properties, which made them an effective luminescent medium. QDs are inorganic semiconductor nanomaterials that can be found in the shape of nanocrystals with a range of 1 to 10 nm in diameter. Ligands will improve the stability of QDs by introducing aqueous buffer solutions (Ghasemi, Peymani, & Afifi, 2009; Xu and Zheng, 2019). QDs are often used in optical biosensors for chemical analysis, ion detection, and molecular biology. Plus, they have also been used in food science for the identification of viruses, proteins, and pathogens (Bonilla, Bozkurt, Ansari, Sozer, & Kokini, 2016). QDs are ideal for optical analysis in the food industry due to their cost-effective, quick detection, large absorption wavelength, and high sensitivity (Pandit et al., 2016).

Graphene

Graphene is a 2D nanomaterial most commonly used in biosensor technology due to its excellent properties, including high room temperature, high elasticity, high thermal conductivity, and robust mechanical properties. It is a transparent material that has low production costs and is not harmful to the environment (Pandit et al., 2016). Graphene is an sp^2-hybridized carbon layer with a 0.142-nm bond length and was the first 2D crystalline substance recorded in 2004. It is a building block of quasi 1D CNTs, 3D graphite, and quasi 0D buckyballs (Malhotra & Ali, 2018a; Neto, Guinea, Peres, Novoselov, & Geim, 2009). The use of graphene in biosensors make the biosensors able to determine and quantify various of the virus, pathogen, heavy metal ion, and diseases. Food analysis researchers often use Graphene-based biosensors because this detection method is sensitive, quick, and straightforward (Peña-Bahamonde, Nguyen, Fanourakis, & Rodrigues, 2018).

Fullerenes

Fullerenes are 0D nanomaterials with 60 atoms and draw researchers 'attention due to their wide range of applications (Ju-Nam & Lead, 2008). These are made of hollow spherical shapes, also known as buckyball and other forms. Fullerenes are similar to graphite, which consists of graphene sheets and become pentagonal or hexagonal rings. Fullerenes have a range of sizes between 30 and 3000 carbon atoms. C_{24}, C_{28}, C_{32}, C_{36}, C_{50}, C_{60} and C_{70} are different types of fullerenes. C_{60} was the most stable fullerene produced by 20 hexagons and 12 pentagons with sp^2-bonded carbon atoms (Malhotra & Ali, 2018a). C_{60} fullerene has a wide range of antimicrobial activity and acts as an antifouling agent for ceramic membranes. C_{60} reduces the number of bacteria and inactive many of *Escherichia coli* cells (Chae et al., 2009; Lyon, Brown, & Alvarez, 2008).

Application of biosensor-based nanomaterials in food analysis

Nanotechnologies and biosensors are combined and applied in various food analysis. Since the past decades, the combination of nanomaterials with different types of biosensors has been continuously growing. Nanobiosensors have many functions and highly versatile for food analysis due to their unique characteristics of nanomaterials, which produce fast, low cost, user-friendly, and high sensitivity nano biosensors for food analysis applications. The application of nanomaterials biosensor in food analysis, including detection of pathogen and toxin, detection of pesticide residue, detection of heavy metals, detection of illegal additives, and detection of drugs. The summary of the application of nanomaterials-based biosensor in various food analysis is available in Table 11.1.

Pathogens and toxin

Even though food packaging currently has vacuum and pasteurization treatment to improve the shelf life of food, still pathogenic bacteria can affect food. *Escherichia coli*, *Listeria,* and *Salmonella* are the most common foodborne pathogens found in food products (Akyol, 2018). Previously, Wilson et al. (2019) used iron oxide (Fe_3O_4) magnetic NPs with a sensor to detect *E. coli, Staphylococcus aureus, and Salmonella typhimurium* in apple juice. This nanosensor serves as a cost-effective and fast screening method with a detection limit of *E. coli* in apple juice of $3.5 \, CFU \, mL^{-1}$. Zhong et al. (2019) used cadmium sulfide quantum dots (Cs-QDTs) with electrochemical immunobiosensor for sensitive detection of *E. coli* in milk samples. This integration nanomaterial with a sensor successfully detected *E. coli* with a detection limit as $3 \, CFU \, mL^{-1}$. Zou et al. (2019) used AuNPs coupled with nanoconjugates of polypyrrole-reduced graphene oxide (PPy-rGO) in biosensor for detection of *E. coli* in milk. This sensor has stable, high reproducibility and high selectivity with a low limit of detection of $10 \, CFU \, mL^{-1}$. Zheng et al. (2019) used AuNPs aggregates with microfluidic colorimetric biosensors for the fast detection of *E. coli* in chicken. This biosensor gives good sensitivity with a detection limit of $50 \, CFU \, mL^{-1}$. Zhou et al. (2018) assist silver NPs (AgNPs) with rGO composites in fiber optic surface plasmon resonance (FOSPR) sensor to detect E. coli in juice, including apple juice, vegetable juice, and orange juice. This SPR sensor poses excellent specificity with the limit of detection of $5.0 \times 10^2 \, CFU \, mL^{-1}$. Suaifan et al. (2017) used specific magnetic NPs with colorimetric biosensors to detect *E. coli* in food products. This biosensor has high applicability with a detection limit of $12 \, CFU \, mL^{-1}$.

Table 11.1 Application of nanomaterials biosensor in various food analysis.

Food analysis	Nanomaterials	Analytes	Food sample	LOD	Reference
Detection of pathogens	Fe₃O₄ MNPs	*E. coli*	Apple juice	$3.5\,CFU\,mL^{-1}$	Wilson et al. (2019)
	Cs-QDTs	*E. coli*	Milk	$3.5\,CFU\,mL^{-1}$	Zhong et al. (2019)
	AuNPs/PPy-rGO	*E. coli*	Milk	$10\,CFU\,mL^{-1}$	Zou, Liang, She, and Kraatz (2019)
	AuNPs	*E. coli*	Chicken	$50\,CFU\,mL^{-1}$	Zheng et al. (2019)
	AgNPs/rGO	*E. coli*	Apple juice, orange juice, vegetable juice	$5.0 \times 102\,CFU\,mL^{-1}$	Zhou et al. (2018)
	MNPs	*E. coli*	Ground beef, turkey sausage, milk, lettuce	$12\,CFU\,mL^{-1}$	Suaifan, Alhogail, and Zourob (2017)
	FNCs	*Salmonella*	Chicken	$14\,CFU\,mL^{-1}$	Zhang et al. (2019)
	MNPs	*Salmonella*	Chicken	$1.6 \times 101\,CFU\,mL^{-1}$	Guo et al. (2019)
	AuNPs	*Salmonella*	Pork meat	$4\,CFU\,mL^{-1}$	Ma, Xu, Xia, and Wang (2018)
	Fe3O4 NPC	*Salmonella*	Milk	$105\,CFU\,mL^{-1}$	Zou et al. (2018)
	rGO-CHI	*Salmonella*	Raw chicken meat	$10–1\,CFU\,mL^{-1}$	Dinshaw et al. (2017)
	AuNPs	*Salmonella*	Milk	$103\,CFU\,mL^{-1}$	Wang, Zhao, Chen, Wang, and Liu (2016)
	AuNPs	*Listeria*	Milk	$3.7 \times 106\,CFU\,mL^{-1}$	Wang, Liu, et al. (2017)
	Fe3O4 NPC	*Listeria*	Sterile milk	$5.4 \times 103\,CFU\,mL^{-1}$	Zhang et al. (2016)
	AuNPs	*Shigella*	Smoked salmon	$80\,CFU\,mL^{-1}$	Feng, Shen, Wu, Dai, and Wang (2019)
Detection of toxins	CS-f-graphene	Ochratoxin A	Grape juice	$1\,fg\,mL^{-1}$	Kaur et al. (2019)
	AuNPs	Ochratoxin A	Wine	$0.001\,ppb$	Chen et al. (2018)
	Fe3O4/oMWCNTs	Aflatoxin B1	Peanut, maize, wheat, rice	$0.02\,ng\,mL^{-1}$	Wang et al. (2019)
	Fe3O4 MNPs, pg-CNNSs	Aflatoxin B1	Maize	$0.002\,ng\,mL^{-1}$	Xie et al. (2019)

Continued

Table 11.1 Application of nanomaterials biosensor in various food analysis. *Continued*

Food analysis	Nanomaterials	Analytes	Food sample	LOD	Reference
Detection of pesticides residue	QDTs/AuNPs	Aflatoxin B1	Rice, peanut	3.4 nM	Sabet, Hosseini, Khabbaz, Dadmehr, and Ganjali (2017)
	AuAg nanochains	Thiram	Apple	0.03 ppm	Jiao et al. (2019)
	AgNPs	Diazinon	Bean, potato, grape, apple	7 ng mL^{-1}	Shrivas et al. (2019)
	Ag/NC	Thiram, Thiabendazole	Apple, cabbage	0.5 ng/cm^2, 5 ng/cm^2	Chen, Huang, Kong, and Lin (2019)
	Au/Ag NPs	Profenofos. Oxamyl. Thiacloprid	Peach	6.1 mg kg^{-1}, 0.1 mg kg^{-1}	Yaseen, Pu, and Sun (2019)
	AuNPs	Dimethoate	Lemon, tangerine	0.004 ppm	Hung, Lee, Hu, and Chiu (2018)
	rGO	Carbaryl	Tomato	1.9 nmol L^{-1}	da Silva, Vanzela, Defavari, and Cesarino (2018)
	NbC/Mo nanocomposite	Fenitrothion	Grape, cranberry	0.15 nM	Govindasamy et al. (2018)
	GO	Carbaryl	Cabbage, spinach	0.15 ng mL^{-1}	Li, Shi, Han, Xiao, and Zhou (2017)
	CuNWs and GR MWCNTs	Methyl parathion Malathion	Garlic Lettuce	50 nM 1 fM	Chen et al. (2016) Kaur, Thakur, and Prabhakar (2016)
	Fe3O4 MNPs/ GR	Chlorpyrifos	Cabbage, spinach	0.02 µg L^{-1}	Wang et al. (2016)

Table 11.1 Application of nanomaterials biosensor in various food analysis. *Continued*

Food analysis	Nanomaterials	Analytes	Food sample	LOD	Reference
Detection of heavy metals	AgNPs	Hg+	dried *XXXhyllanthus acidus*	$8.3 \times 10^{-7}\,mol\,L^{-1}$	Sk et al. (2019)
	MnFe2O4 Nas	Hg+	Tuna fish	0.14 nM	Kogularasu et al. (2018)
	AuNPs-PGE	Hg+	Fish	0.004 aM	Hasanjani and Zarei (2019)
	GO	Cd2+ Pb2+	Raw milk	0.58 nM, 1.08 nM	Priya, Dhanalakshmi, Thennarasu, and Thinakaran (2018)
Detection of illegal additives	AgNPs	Melamine	Raw milk	0.01 ppm	Rajput (2018)
	CA-NSs	Melamine	Raw milk	1.04 ± 0.05 pM	Rahman and Ahmed (2018)
	PBNPs	Clenbuterol	Bacon, pork kidney, pork	$1.0\,ng\,mL^{-1}$	Zhao et al. (2018)
	UCNPs	Sudan I-IV	Chili powder	$2.83\,ng\,mL^{-1}$	Fang et al. (2016)
Detection of veterinary drugs	AuNPs nanoprobes	Chloramphenicol	Milk	$0.13\,pg\,mL^{-1}$	Huang et al. (2019)
	MWCNTs AuNPs	Sulfapyridine	Milk	$8.8\,ng\,mL^{-1}$	Moreno, Adnane, Salghi, Zougagh, and Ríos (2019)
	Pt-Au NWs	Penicillin Tetracycline	Chicken, beef	$41.2\,\mu A/\mu M\,cm^2$, $26.4\,A/\mu M\,cm^2$	Li, Liu, Sarpong, and Gu (2019)
	PEDOT MnO2 nanocomposite	Sulfamethazine	Milk, honey	$0.16\,\mu M$	Su and Cheng (2018)
	MoS2-f-MWCNTs	Chloramphenicol	Milk, honey, powdered milk	$0.015\,\mu M$	Govindasamy et al. (2017)
	AuNPs	Chloramphenicol	Milk, honey, shrimp	0.1 nM	Sharma, Akshath, Bhatt, Thakur, and Raghavarao (2017)
	AuNPs	Kanamycin	Milk	321 pM	Ramezani, Danesh, Lavaee, Abnous, and Taghdisi (2016)

Furthermore, Zhang et al. (2019) used Fe nanoclusters (FNCs) with biosensor for the fast detection of *Salmonella* in chicken. This sensor proposed a broad linear range and a low detection limit of $14\,CFU\,mL^{-1}$. Guo et al. (2019) used magnetic NP with biosensor for sensitive detection of *Salmonella* in chicken. The mean recovery was 99.8% and with a limit of detection of $1.6 \times 10^1\,CFU\,mL^{-1}$. Ma et al. (2018) used AuNP-based SERS aptasensor for the detection of *Salmonella* in pork meat with a detection limit of $4\,CFU\,mL^{-1}$. Zou et al. (2018) used Fe^3O^4 NP cluster-based biosensor for the rapid identification of *Salmonella* in milk. This biosensor was fast and sensitive for the detection of pathogens in food with a detection limit of $10^5\,CFU\,mL^{-1}$. Dinshaw et al. (2017) used rGO chitosan-based aptasensor to detect *Salmonella* in raw chicken meat. This sensor was particular for food analysis and had the lowest detection limit of $10^{-1}\,CFU\,mL^{-1}$. Wang et al. (2016) used the AuNP-based sensor for multiple detections of *Salmonella* in milk and have a limit of detection of $10^3\,CFU\,mL^{-1}$.

Similarly, Wang, Liu, et al. (2017) used a AuNP-based immunosensor for quantification of *Listeria* in milk within 13 h. This assay was efficient and had a limit of detection of $3.7 \times 10^6\,CFU\,mL^{-1}$. Zhang et al. (2016) used Fe_3O_4 NP cluster-based aptasensor to identify *Listeria* in sterile milk samples. It stated that this method was accurate and rapid, with a detection limit of $5.4 \times 10^3\,CFU\,mL^{-1}$. Besides that, *Shigella* also found as the most popular pathogenic bacteria present in foodstuff in China. Recently, Feng et al. (2019) used AuNPs to fabricated colorimetric aptasensor for the detection of *Shigella* in smoked salmon. This colorimetric aptasensor was convenient and straightforward, with a detection limit of $80\,CFU\,mL^{-1}$.

Other than that, toxins can also be found in foods. Some of the toxins are naturally produced in food, such as mycotoxins. A mycotoxin is usually found in bananas, cereals, peanuts, and vegetables such as Aflatoxin A and Ochratoxin A. As a result, several nanomaterial-based biosensors have been used for food analysis to detect pathogens and toxins in various food items. Kaur et al. (2019) assist graphene doped chitosan (CS-f-graphene) electrochemical aptasensor-based nanocomposites for the quantification of ochratoxin A in grape juice samples. This advanced sensor has been characterized by field emission-scanning electron microscopy (FE-SEM) and Fourier transform infrared spectroscopy (FTIR). The graphene has increased the surface area of the electrode, and sensor performance has been improved with a detection limit of $1\,fg\,mL^{-1}$. Chen et al. (2018) used AuNP conjugated with DNA combined to ultrasensitive electrochemical aptasensor for the determination of Ochratoxin A in wine samples. This AuNP conjugates implied excellent attention for food analysis applications. The low detection limit of 0.001 ppb was obtained. Afterward, Wang et al. (2019) used magnetic oxidized MWCNTs (Fe^3O^4/oMWCNTs) combined with DNAzyme aptasensor for rapid detection of aflatoxin B1 in peanut, maize, wheat, and rice. This biosensor produced high sensitivity with the limit of detection of $0.02\,ng\,mL^{-1}$. Xie et al. (2019) used Fe_3O_4 magnetic NPs with g-C_3N_4 nanosheets in immunosensor for the determination of aflatoxin B1 in maize. This simple detection method has reduced the assay time with a detection limit of $0.002\,ng\,mL^{-1}$.

Sabet et al. (2017) developed aptasensor based on QDTs and AuNPs for the detection of aflatoxin B1 in rice and peanut. This nano biosensor has a detection limit of 3.4 nM.

Pesticides residue

Biosensors based on nanomaterials have been applied in food analysis to identify pesticide residuals in food products. Generally, the pesticide is widely used to manage pests infection, for example, diseases of plants, weeds, and insects (Winter, 2017). However, residues of pesticides present in crops may affect the consumers' health. Thus, the use of nanomaterial-based biosensors can help in the rapid detection of pesticide residues in food. Previously, Jiao et al. (2019) built an AuAg nanochain based on a surface-enhanced Raman spectroscopy biosensor for the detection of pesticide residues (thiram) on the apple surface. An efficient SERS nanosensor has been developed for interconnecting AuAg nano chains with bimetallic particles. The lowest concentration of thiram on apple surfaces of the SERS nano biosensor was 0.03 ppm. Shrivas et al. (2019) developed an AgNP-based chemical sensor for the identification of diazinon pesticide in beans, potato, grapes, and apples. The detection of this type of pesticide is based on color changes of yellow, AgNPs to pinkish-red. These AgNPs were excellent for the quantitative detection of diazinon pesticide in vegetables with a detection limit of 7 ng mL^{-1}. Meanwhile, Chen, Huang, et al. (2019) designed jelly-like Ag nanocellulose film-based SERS biosensor for fast determination of pesticide on apples and cabbages. The texture jelly-like Ag nanocellulose substrate enables useful contacts to fruits and vegetable samples. This nanosensor achieves rapid pesticide SERS detection with a limit of detection of 0.5 ng/cm^2, and 5 ng/cm^2 for both types of pesticides have been found, which are thiram and thiabendazole. Yaseen et al. (2019) fabricated AuNPs coated with silver-based on SERS biosensor for determination of different types of insecticide residues in peach fruits such as profenofos, oxamyl, and thiacloprid. This biosensor has good accuracy and simultaneous detection.

da Silva et al. (2018) developed rGO-based biosensor with acetylcholinesterase enzyme for detection of carbaryl pesticides in tomato. The identification of carbaryl pesticides was succeeded with a detection limit of 1.9 nmol L^{-1}. Next, Hung et al. (2018) fabricated fluorescence biosensor based on Rhodamine B with AuNPs for the determination of dimethoate pesticide in fruit samples. The AuNPs have increased the fluorescence intensity with 86–116% recovery of biosensor performance with a detection limit of 0.004 ppm. Govindasamy et al. (2018) established an electrochemical biosensor based on the hybridization of niobium carbide (NbC) with molybdenum (Mo) NPs for detection of fenitrothion pesticides in fruit samples. These functional nanomaterials have successfully detected fenitrothion in grapes and cranberry with a detection limit of 0.15 nM.

Li et al. (2017) developed an electrochemical biosensor based on immobilization of graphene oxide (GO) with acetylcholinesterase for the determination of carbaryl pesticide in cabbages and spinach. The GO network was efficient in promoting the rate of electron transfer and enables the entree of substrates into active centers. This biosensor has excellent working performance with a detection limit of $0.15\,ng\,mL^{-1}$. Chen et al. (2016) fabricated the electrochemical biosensor based on a nanocomposite of graphene with copper nanowires for the detection of methyl parathion pesticides in garlic samples. This biosensor has high stability and reproducibility with a limit of detection of 50 nM. After that, Kaur et al. (2016) conducted an amperometric biosensor based on MWCNTs, which deposited on the surface of fluorine-doped tin oxide for the assays of malathion pesticides in lettuces samples. The biosensor recoveries performance was 96% to 98% with a detection limit of 1 fM. Meanwhile, Wang et al. (2016) developed a sensitive electrochemical biosensor based on Fe_3O_4 magnetic NP composite with graphene for the determination of chlorpyrifos pesticide residues in vegetables. The nanocomposite film has improved the biosensor properties and has a limit of detection of $0.02\ 0.02\,\mu g\,L^{-1}$.

Heavy metals

The nanomaterials-based biosensor also applied in the detection of hazardous heavy metals in food products. Cadmium (Cd^{2+}), mercury (Hg^+), and lead (Pb^{2+}) are the most common heavy metals ions found in food. A various analytical method has been used, such as GC–MS and HPLC, although these methods were time-consuming and low sensitivity. Hence, nano biosensor has been developed due to excellent nanomaterials properties for rapid food analysis. In recent years, Sk et al. (2019) reported the colorimetric biosensor based on AgNPs for discriminatory sensing of mercury ions in dried *Phyllanthus acidus* fruit. AgNPs showed a reversible response toward Hg^+ ion. It has been proven that this method was environmentally friendly and easy to use with a limit of detection of $8.3 \times 10^{-7}\,mol\,L^{-1}$. Subsequently, Kogularasu et al. (2018) fabricated manganese ferrite ($MnFe_2O_4$) nanoagglomerates (NAs) based biosensor for determination of mercury ions in tuna fish. The unique structure of this nano biosensor obtained detection limit of mercury ions was 0.14 nM.

Meanwhile, Hasanjani and Zarei (2019) described a novel electrochemical biosensor based on DNA with poly-L-methionine-AuNPs and pencil graphite electrode for detection of mercury ions in fish samples. This method showed better selectivity toward mercury ions with a detection limit of 0.004 aM. Priya et al. (2018) fabricated a novel electrochemical biosensor using GO composite with k-carrageenan and L-cysteine for sensing the cadmium ions and lead ions in raw milk. The nanocomposite biosensor showed a good result with outstanding linearity and low detection limit.

Illegal additives

Biosensors based on nanomaterials have also been developed for the detection of illegal additives in various food products. Illegal chemicals have adverse effects on the health of the user. Sudan, melamine, and clenbuterol are the most common additives that have been illegally added to food. The development of nanomaterials biosensors, therefore, has many advantages for the food industry. Lately, Rajput (2018) constructed sensitive colorimetric biosensors based on AgNPs for the determination of melamine in milk. Interaction of Ag^+ ions with melamine compound resulting in a low detection limit of 0.01 ppm. Rahman and Ahmed (2018) developed an electrochemical biosensor based on Cadmium doped antimony oxide nanostructures (CA-NSs) to the level of melamine measured in milk samples. This developed biosensor represents good sensitivity and broad scales with a detection limit of 1.04 ± 0.05 pM. Zhao et al. (2018) organized a food analysis using biosensor based on Prussian blue nanoparticles (PBNPs) for efficient determination of clenbuterol in bacon, pork kidney, and pork. Small amounts of analytes were needed for the detection, which results in clearly visible results. These PBNPs have improved the sensor sensitivity compare to AuNPs with detection of $1.0 \, \text{ng} \, \text{mL}^{-1}$. Following this, Fang et al. (2016) reported a novel nano biosensor based on hexadecyl trimethyl ammonium bromide (CTAB) fluorescence stabilized by upconversion nanoparticles (UCNPs) for the determination of Sudan dyes in chili powder samples.

Veterinary drugs

Apart from all the applications of nanomaterials biosensors in the food analysis referred to above, nanobiosensors can also be used to detect residues of veterinary drugs in livestock products such as milk, eggs, and meat. Veterinary medicines are commonly used to monitor and prevent animal diseases from bacterial infections. However, residues of veterinary medicines will accumulate in livestock products. Currently, Huang et al. (2019) developed a colorimetric sensor based on a gold nanoprobe for the sensing of chloramphenicol drugs in milk samples. The AuNPs were functionalized with a DNAzyme, which exhibits an excellent amplification signal of the nanoprobe and better sensing performance with a low limit of detection of $0.13 \, \text{pg} \, \text{mL}^{-1}$. Moreno et al. (2019) fabricated a SERS sensor based on a combination of AuNPs and MWCNTs for the determination of sulfapyridine drugs in milk. This nanostructured hybrid SERS biosensor detecting the veterinary drugs in milk with a detection limit of $8.8 \, \text{ng} \, \text{mL}^{-1}$. Subsequently, Li et al. (2019) reported a novel electrochemical biosensor based on nanowire hybridization of AuNPs with platinum NPs for the detection of penicillin and tetracycline in chicken and beef. The Pt—Au nanowires have been prepared and are simultaneously responsible for the actual sample tests.

Su et al. (2019) developed a novel electrochemical sensor based on polymer nanocomposite-modified screen-printed carbon electrode for the detection of sulfamethazine drugs in milk and honey samples. This nanocomposite electrode has a broad linear range and satisfying recovery of sensor performance with a detection limit of 0.16 μM. Govindasamy et al. (2017) designed an electrochemical sensor based on Mo disulfide nanosheets coated with MWCNTs for highly sensitive sensing of chloramphenicol drugs in milk, honey, and powdered milk. After that, Sharma et al. (2017) developed a convenient enzyme biosensor based on AuNPs for the determination of chloramphenicol drugs in milk. Honey and shrimp samples.

Coenzyme A was used for the stabilization of AuNPs. Similarly, Ramezani et al. (2016) also used AuNPs in fluorescent aptasensors for the rapid detection of kanamycin in milk. This aptasensor has been shown to be highly selective toward a kanamycin drug with a detection limit of 321 pM.

Conclusions

With advances in biosensors, nanotechnologies, and efficient analytical tools, various traditional food-based nanomaterials have been developed, resulting in excellent selectivity, high sensitivity, low cost, selectivity, and no time-consuming nanobiosensors. The integration of the biosensor with nanomaterial technology has resulted in a new sensor platform for monitoring and immobilization of biomolecules in food analysis. Nanotechnology is dominant in the development of a variety of biosensors based on nanomaterials. Nonetheless, some progress needs to be made when designing a novel nanomaterial used in the field of biosensors. New nanostructures and nanomaterials, such as PBNPs, need to be explored for use in the biosensor. Although a wide range of nanomaterial-based biosensors has been produced over the past decades, the potential target of a small amount of analyte detection and low-cost devices in the laboratory has not yet been achieved. Many of the food, university, and food science industries have still used conventional devices at expensive, such as HPLC and GC–MS. Research programs must, therefore, be undertaken in each university around the world to discover lower-cost and higher-quality biosensors among students.

References

Abd-Elghany, S. M., & Sallam, K. I. (2015). Rapid determination of total aflatoxins and ochratoxins A in meat products by immuno-affinity fluorimetry. *Food Chemistry*, *179*, 253–256. https://doi.org/10.1016/j.foodchem.2015.01.140.

Akyol, I. (2018). Development and application of RTi-PCR method for common food pathogen presence and quantity in beef, sheep and chicken meat. *Meat Science*, *137*, 9–15. https://doi.org/10.1016/j.meatsci.2017.11.001.

Ali, S., Khan, I., Khan, S. A., Sohail, M., Ahmed, R., ur Rehman, A., & Morsy, M. A. (2017). Electrocatalytic performance of Ni@ Pt core–shell nanoparticles supported on carbon nanotubes for methanol oxidation reaction. *Journal of Electroanalytical Chemistry*, *795*, 17–25. https://doi.org/10.1016/j.jelechem.2017.04.040.

Badoud, F., Ernest, M., Hammel, Y. A., & Huertas-Pérez, J. F. (2018). Artifact-controlled quantification of folpet and phthalimide in food by liquid chromatography-high resolution mass spectrometry. *Food Control*, *91*, 412–420. https://doi.org/10.1016/j.foodcont.2018.04.012.

Bellan, L. M., Wu, D., & Langer, R. S. (2011). Current trends in nanobiosensor technology. *Wiley Interdisciplinary Reviews: Nanomedicine and Nanobiotechnology*, *3*(3), 229–246. https://doi.org/10.1002/wnan.136.

Bonilla, J. C., Bozkurt, F., Ansari, S., Sozer, N., & Kokini, J. L. (2016). Applications of quantum dots in food science and biology. *Trends in Food Science and Technology, 53*, 75–89. https://doi.org/10.1016/j.tifs.2016.04.006.

Cao, G. (2004). *Nanostructures and nanomaterials: Synthesis, properties and applications.* Singapore: World Scientific.

Cerda-Kipper, A. S., Montiel, B. E., & Hosseini, S. (2018). Radioimmunoassay and enzyme-linked immunosorbent assay. In *Reference module in chemistry, molecular sciences and chemical engineering* (pp. 1–21). Elsevier.

Chae, S. R., Wang, S., Hendren, Z. D., Wiesner, M. R., Watanabe, Y., & Gunsch, C. K. (2009). Effects of fullerene nanoparticles on Escherichia coli K12 respiratory activity in aqueous suspension and potential use for membrane biofouling control. *Journal of Membrane Science, 329*(1–2), 68–74. https://doi.org/10.1016/j.memsci.2008.12.023.

Chau, C. F., Wu, S. H., & Yen, G. C. (2007). The development of regulations for food nanotechnology. *Trends in Food Science and Technology, 18*(5), 269–280. https://doi.org/10.1016/j.tifs.2007.01.007.

Chen, M., Hou, C., Huo, D., Dong, L., Yang, M., & Fa, H. (2016). A novel electrochemical biosensor based on graphene and Cu nanowires hybrid nanocomposites. *Nano, 11*(11) 1650128.

Chen, J., Huang, M., Kong, L., & Lin, M. (2019). Jellylike flexible nanocellulose SERS substrate for rapid in-situ non-invasive pesticide detection in fruits/vegetables. *Carbohydrate Polymers, 205*, 596–600. https://doi.org/10.1016/j.carbpol.2018.10.059.

Chen, W., Yan, C., Cheng, L., Yao, L., Xue, F., & Xu, J. (2018). An ultrasensitive signal-on electrochemical aptasensor for ochratoxin A determination based on DNA controlled layer-by-layer assembly of dual gold nanoparticle conjugates. *Biosensors and Bioelectronics, 117*, 845–851. https://doi.org/10.1016/j.bios.2018.07.012.

Cordero, C., Schmarr, H. G., Reichenbach, S. E., & Bicchi, C. (2018). Current developments in analyzing food volatiles by multidimensional gas chromatographic techniques. *Journal of Agricultural and Food Chemistry, 66*(10), 2226–2236. https://doi.org/10.1021/acs.jafc.6b04997.

da Silva, M. K. L., Vanzela, H. C., Defavari, L. M., & Cesarino, I. (2018). Determination of carbamate pesticide in food using a biosensor based on reduced graphene oxide and acetylcholinesterase enzyme. *Sensors and Actuators, B: Chemical, 277*, 555–561. https://doi.org/10.1016/j.snb.2018.09.051.

Díaz, R., Ibáñez, M., Sancho, J. V., & Hernández, F. (2012). Target and non-target screening strategies for organic contaminants, residues and illicit substances in food, environmental and human biological samples by UHPLC-QTOF-MS. *Analytical Methods, 4*(1), 196–209. https://doi.org/10.1039/c1ay05385j.

Dinshaw, I. J., Muniandy, S., Teh, S. J., Ibrahim, F., Leo, B. F., & Thong, K. L. (2017). Development of an aptasensor using reduced graphene oxide chitosan complex to detect Salmonella. *Journal of Electroanalytical Chemistry, 806*, 88–96. https://doi.org/10.1016/j.jelechem.2017.10.054.

Dominguez, R. B., Hayat, A., Alonso, G. A., Gutiérrez, J. M., Muñoz, R., & Marty, J. L. (2017). Nanomaterial-based biosensors for food contaminant assessment. In *Nanobiosensors* (pp. 805–839). Chicago: Academic Press. https://doi.org/10.1016/B978-0-12-804301-1.00019-9.

Dreaden, E. C., Alkilany, A. M., Huang, X., Murphy, C. J., & El-Sayed, M. A. (2012). The golden age: Gold nanoparticles for biomedicine. *Chemical Society Reviews, 41*(7), 2740–2779. https://doi.org/10.1039/c1cs15237h.

Fang, A., Long, Q., Wu, Q., Li, H., Zhang, Y., & Yao, S. (2016). Upconversion nanosensor for sensitive fluorescence detection of Sudan I-IV based on inner filter effect. *Talanta, 148*, 129–134. https://doi.org/10.1016/j.talanta.2015.10.048.

Feng, J., Shen, Q., Wu, J., Dai, Z., & Wang, Y. (2019). Naked-eyes detection of Shigella flexneri in food samples based on a novel gold nanoparticle-based colorimetric aptasensor. *Food Control, 98*, 333–341. https://doi.org/10.1016/j.foodcont.2018.11.048.

Feng, Y. Z., & Sun, D. W. (2012). Application of hyperspectral imaging in food safety inspection and control: A review. *Critical Reviews in Food Science and Nutrition, 52*(11), 1039–1058. https://doi.org/10.1080/10408398.2011.651542.

Ghasemi, Y., Peymani, P., & Afifi, S. (2009). Quantum dot: Magic nanoparticle for imaging, detection and targeting. *Acta Bio-Medica de L'Ateneo Parmense, 80*(2), 156–165. Retrieved from http://www.actabiomedica.it/data/2009/2_2009/ghasemi.pdf.

Gómez-López, V. M., Gil, M. I., & Allende, A. (2017). A novel electrochemical device as a disinfection system to maintain water quality during washing of ready to eat fresh produce. *Food Control, 71*, 242–247. https://doi.org/10.1016/j.foodcont.2016.07.001.

Govindasamy, M., Chen, S. M., Mani, V., Devasenathipathy, R., Umamaheswari, R., Joseph Santhanaraj, K., & Sathiyan, A. (2017). Molybdenum disulfide nanosheets coated multi-walled carbon nanotubes composite for highly sensitive determination of chloramphenicol in food samples milk, honey and powdered milk. *Journal of Colloid and Interface Science, 485*, 129–136. https://doi.org/10.1016/j.jcis.2016.09.029.

Govindasamy, M., Rajaji, U., Chen, S. M., Kumaravel, S., Chen, T. W., Al-Hemaid, F. M. A., … Elshikh, M. S. (2018). Detection of pesticide residues (fenitrothion) in fruit samples based on niobium carbide@molybdenum nanocomposite: An electrocatalytic approach. *Analytica Chimica Acta, 1030*, 52–60. https://doi.org/10.1016/j.aca.2018.05.044.

Guo, R., Wang, S., Huang, F., Chen, Q., Li, Y., Liao, M., & Lin, J. (2019). Rapid detection of Salmonella Typhimurium using magnetic nanoparticle immunoseparation, nanocluster signal amplification and smartphone image analysis. *Sensors and Actuators, B: Chemical, 284*, 134–139. https://doi.org/10.1016/j.snb.2018.12.110.

Harris, P. J., & Harris, P. J. F. (2009). *Carbon nanotube science: Synthesis, properties and applications.* Cambridge University Press.

Hasanjani, H. R. A., & Zarei, K. (2019). An electrochemical sensor for attomolar determination of mercury (II) using DNA/poly-L-methionine-gold nanoparticles/pencil graphite electrode. *Biosensors and Bioelectronics, 128*, 1–8. https://doi.org/10.1016/j.bios.2018.12.039.

Huang, W., Zhang, H., Lai, G., Liu, S., Li, B., & Yu, A. (2019). Sensitive and rapid aptasensing of chloramphenicol by colorimetric signal transduction with a DNAzyme-functionalized gold nanoprobe. *Food Chemistry, 270*, 287–292. https://doi.org/10.1016/j.foodchem.2018.07.127.

Hung, S. H., Lee, J. Y., Hu, C. C., & Chiu, T. C. (2018). Gold-nanoparticle-based fluorescent "turn-on" sensor for selective and sensitive detection of dimethoate. *Food Chemistry, 260*, 61–65. https://doi.org/10.1016/j.foodchem.2018.03.149.

Jeong, E. J., Lee, S. H., Kim, B. T., Lee, G., Yun, S. S., Lim, H. S., & Kim, Y. S. (2017). An analysis method for determining residual hexane in health functional food products using static headspace gas chromatography. *Food Science and Biotechnology, 26*(2), 363–368. https://doi.org/10.1007/s10068-017-0049-7.

Jiao, A., Dong, X., Zhang, H., Xu, L., Tian, Y., Liu, X., & Chen, M. (2019). Construction of pure worm-like AuAg nanochains for ultrasensitive SERS detection of pesticide residues on apple surfaces. *Spectrochimica Acta Part A, Molecular and Biomolecular Spectroscopy, 209*, 241–247. https://doi.org/10.1016/j.saa.2018.10.051.

Joshi, M., & Deshpande, J. D. (2010). Polymerase chain reaction: Methods, principles and application. *International Journal of Biomedical Research*, *2*(1), 81–97.

Ju-Nam, Y., & Lead, J. R. (2008). Manufactured nanoparticles: An overview of their chemistry, interactions and potential environmental implications. *Science of the Total Environment*, *400*(1–3), 396–414. https://doi.org/10.1016/j.scitotenv.2008.06.042.

Kaur, N., Bharti, A., Batra, S., Rana, S., Rana, S., Bhalla, A., & Prabhakar, N. (2019). An electrochemical aptasensor based on graphene doped chitosan nanocomposites for determination of Ochratoxin A. *Microchemical Journal*, *144*, 102–109. https://doi.org/10.1016/j.microc.2018.08.064.

Kaur, N., Thakur, H., & Prabhakar, N. (2016). Conducting polymer and multi-walled carbon nanotubes nanocomposites based amperometric biosensor for detection of organophosphate. *Journal of Electroanalytical Chemistry*, *775*, 121–128. https://doi.org/10.1016/j.jelechem.2016.05.037.

Khan, I., Abdalla, A., & Qurashi, A. (2017). Synthesis of hierarchical WO3 and Bi2O3/WO3 nanocomposite for solar-driven water splitting applications. *International Journal of Hydrogen Energy*, *42*(5), 3431–3439. https://doi.org/10.1016/j.ijhydene.2016.11.105.

Khan, I., Saeed, K., & Khan, I. (2019). Nanoparticles: Properties, applications and toxicities. *Arabian Journal of Chemistry*, *12*(7), 908–931. https://doi.org/10.1016/j.arabjc.2017.05.011.

Kogularasu, S., Akilarasan, M., Chen, S. M., Elaiyappillai, E., Johnson, P. M., Chen, T. W., … Elshikh, M. S. (2018). A comparative study on conventionally prepared MnFe2O4 nanospheres and template-synthesized novel MnFe2O4 nano-agglomerates as the electrodes for biosensing of mercury contaminations and supercapacitor applications. *Electrochimica Acta*, *290*, 533–543. https://doi.org/10.1016/j.electacta.2018.09.028.

Laurent, S., Forge, D., Port, M., Roch, A., Robic, C., Vander Elst, L., & Muller, R. N. (2008). Magnetic iron oxide nanoparticles: Synthesis, stabilization, vectorization, physicochemical characterizations, and biological applications. *Chemical Reviews*, *108*(6), 2064–2110. https://doi.org/10.1021/cr068445e.

Li, Z., Liu, C., Sarpong, V., & Gu, Z. (2019). Multisegment nanowire/nanoparticle hybrid arrays as electrochemical biosensors for simultaneous detection of antibiotics. *Biosensors and Bioelectronics*, *126*, 632–639. https://doi.org/10.1016/j.bios.2018.10.025.

Li, Y., Shi, L., Han, G., Xiao, Y., & Zhou, W. (2017). Electrochemical biosensing of carbaryl based on acetylcholinesterase immobilized onto electrochemically inducing porous graphene oxide network. *Sensors and Actuators, B: Chemical*, *238*, 945–953. https://doi.org/10.1016/j.snb.2016.07.152.

Lv, M., Liu, Y., Geng, J., Kou, X., Xin, Z., & Yang, D. (2018). Engineering nanomaterials-based biosensors for food safety detection. *Biosensors and Bioelectronics*, *106*, 122–128. https://doi.org/10.1016/j.bios.2018.01.049.

Lyon, D. Y., Brown, D. A., & Alvarez, P. J. J. (2008). Implications and potential applications of bactericidal fullerene water suspensions: Effect of nc60 concentration, exposure conditions and shelf life. *Water Science and Technology*, *57*(10), 1533–1538. https://doi.org/10.2166/wst.2008.282.

Ma, X., Xu, X., Xia, Y., & Wang, Z. (2018). SERS aptasensor for Salmonella typhimurium detection based on spiny gold nanoparticles. *Food Control*, *84*, 232–237. https://doi.org/10.1016/j.foodcont.2017.07.016.

Malhotra, B. D., & Ali, M. A. (2018a). Functionalized carbon nanomaterials for biosensors. In *Nanomaterials for biosensors: Fundamentals and applications* (pp. 75–103). Elsevier.

Malhotra, B. D., & Ali, M. A. (2018b). *Nanomaterials for biosensors: Fundamentals and applications. In Nanomaterials for biosensors: Fundamentals and applications* (pp. 1–321). Elsevier Inc. Undefined. Retrieved from*http://www.sciencedirect.com/science/book/9780323449236*.

Mansha, M., Khan, I., Ullah, N., & Qurashi, A. (2017). Synthesis, characterization and visible-light-driven photoelectrochemical hydrogen evolution reaction of carbazole-containing conjugated polymers. *International Journal of Hydrogen Energy*, *42*(16), 10952–10961. https://doi.org/10.1016/j.ijhydene.2017.02.053.

Moreno, V., Adnane, A., Salghi, R., Zougagh, M., & Ríos, Á. (2019). Nanostructured hybrid surface enhancement Raman scattering substrate for the rapid determination of sulfapyridine in milk samples. *Talanta*, *194*, 357–362. https://doi.org/10.1016/j.talanta.2018.10.047.

Neto, A. C., Guinea, F., Peres, N. M., Novoselov, K. S., & Geim, A. K. (2009). The electronic properties of graphene. *Reviews of Modern Physics*, *81*(1), 109–162. https://doi.org/10.1103/RevModPhys.81.109.

Ozin, G. A., & Arsenault, A. (2015). *Nanochemistry: A chemical approach to Nanomaterials*. Royal Society of Chemistry.

Pandit, S., Dasgupta, D., Dewan, N., & Prince, A. (2016). Nanotechnology based biosensors and its application. *The Pharma Innovation*, *5*(6, Part A), 18–25.

Patra, J. K., Mahato, D. K., & Kumar, P. (2019). Biosensor technology—Advanced scientific tools, with special reference to nanobiosensors and plant-and food-based biosensors. In *Nanomaterials in plants, algae and microorganisms* (pp. 287–303). Academic Press. https://doi.org/10.1016/B978-0-12-811488-9.00014-7.

Peña-Bahamonde, J., Nguyen, H. N., Fanourakis, S. K., & Rodrigues, D. F. (2018). Recent advances in graphene-based biosensor technology with applications in life sciences. *Journal of Nanobiotechnology*. *16*(1)https://doi.org/10.1186/s12951-018-0400-z.

Ponce, A. G., Ayala-Zavala, J. F., Marcovich, N. E., Vázquez, F. J., & Ansorena, M. R. (2018). Nanotechnology trends in the food industry: Recent developments, risks, and regulation. In *Impact of Nanoscience in the food industry* (pp. 113–141). Argentina: Elsevier Inc.. https://doi.org/10.1016/B978-0-12-811441-4.00005-4.

Priya, T., Dhanalakshmi, N., Thennarasu, S., & Thinakaran, N. (2018). A novel voltammetric sensor for the simultaneous detection of Cd2+ and Pb2+ using graphene oxide/κ-carrageenan/L-cysteine nanocomposite. *Carbohydrate Polymers*, *182*, 199–206. https://doi.org/10.1016/j.carbpol.2017.11.017.

Qiu, H., & Yang, J. (2017). Structure and properties of carbon nanotubes. In *Industrial applications of carbon nanotubes* (pp. 47–69). China: Elsevier Inc.. https://doi.org/10.1016/B978-0-323-41481-4.00002-2.

Rahman, M. M., & Ahmed, J. (2018). Cd-doped Sb2O4 nanostructures modified glassy carbon electrode for efficient detection of melamine by electrochemical approach. *Biosensors and Bioelectronics*, *102*, 631–636. https://doi.org/10.1016/j.bios.2017.12.007.

Rajput, J. K. (2018). Bio-polyphenols promoted green synthesis of silver nanoparticles for facile and ultra-sensitive colorimetric detection of melamine in milk. *Biosensors and Bioelectronics*, *120*, 153–159. https://doi.org/10.1016/j.bios.2018.08.054.

Ramezani, M., Danesh, N. M., Lavaee, P., Abnous, K., & Taghdisi, S. M. (2016). A selective and sensitive fluorescent aptasensor for detection of kanamycin based on catalytic recycling activity of exonuclease III and gold nanoparticles. *Sensors and Actuators, B: Chemical*, *222*, 1–7. https://doi.org/10.1016/j.snb.2015.08.024.

Rawat, M. K., Jain, A., & Singh, S. (2011). Studies on binary lipid matrix based solid lipid nanoparticles of repaglinide: In vitro and in vivo evaluation. *Journal of Pharmaceutical Sciences, 100*(6), 2366–2378. https://doi.org/10.1002/jps.22435.

Sabet, F. S., Hosseini, M., Khabbaz, H., Dadmehr, M., & Ganjali, M. R. (2017). FRET-based aptamer biosensor for selective and sensitive detection of aflatoxin B1 in peanut and rice. *Food Chemistry, 220*, 527–532. https://doi.org/10.1016/j.foodchem.2016.10.004.

Sagadevan, S., & Periasamy, M. (2014). Recent trends in nanobiosensors and their applications—A review. *Reviews on Advanced Materials Science, 36*(1), 62–69. Retrieved fromhttp:/www.ipme.ru/e-journals/RAMS/no_13614/06_13614_suresh.pdf.

Sharma, R., Akshath, U. S., Bhatt, P., Thakur, M. S., & Raghavarao, K. S. M. S. (2017). Gold nanoparticles based enzyme biosensor for the detection of chloramphenicol. *Procedia Technology, 27*, 282–286. https://doi.org/10.1016/j.protcy.2017.04.118.

Shin, W. K., Cho, J., Kannan, A. G., Lee, Y. S., & Kim, D. W. (2016). Cross-linked composite gel polymer electrolyte using mesoporous methacrylate-functionalized SiO2 nanoparticles for lithium-ion polymer batteries. *Scientific Reports. 6*, https://doi.org/10.1038/srep26332.

Shrivas, K., Sahu, S., Sahu, B., Kurrey, R., Patle, T. K., Kant, T., … Ghosh, K. K. (2019). Silver nanoparticles for selective detection of phosphorus pesticide containing π-conjugated pyrimidine nitrogen and sulfur moieties through non-covalent interactions. *Journal of Molecular Liquids, 275*, 297–303. https://doi.org/10.1016/j.molliq.2018.11.071.

Sigmund, W., Yuh, J., Park, H., Maneeratana, V., Pyrgiotakis, G., Daga, A., … Nino, J. C. (2006). Processing and structure relationships in electrospinning of ceramic fiber systems. *Journal of the American Ceramic Society, 89*(2), 395–407. https://doi.org/10.1111/j.1551-2916.2005.00807.x.

Sk, I., Khan, M. A., Ghosh, S., Roy, D., Pal, S., Homechuadhuri, S., & Alam, M. A. (2019). A reversible biocompatible silver nanoconstracts for selective sensing of mercury ions combined with antimicrobial activity studies. *Nano-Structures and Nano-Objects, 17*, 185–193. https://doi.org/10.1016/j.nanoso.2019.01.012.

Su, H., Liu, K. T., Chen, B. H., Lin, Y. P., Jiang, Y. M., Tsai, Y. H., … Lee, C. W. (2019). Rapid identification of herbal toxins using electrospray laser desorption ionization mass spectrometry for emergency care. *Journal of Food and Drug Analysis, 27*(2), 415–427. https://doi.org/10.1016/j.jfda.2018.11.001.

Su, Y. L., & Cheng, S. H. (2018). A novel electroanalytical assay for sulfamethazine determination in food samples based on conducting polymer nanocomposite-modified electrodes. *Talanta, 180*, 81–89. https://doi.org/10.1016/j.talanta.2017.12.026.

Suaifan, G. A. R. Y., Alhogail, S., & Zourob, M. (2017). Paper-based magnetic nanoparticle-peptide probe for rapid and quantitative colorimetric detection of Escherichia coli O157: H7. *Biosensors and Bioelectronics, 92*, 702–708. https://doi.org/10.1016/j.bios.2016.10.023.

Tiwari, J. N., Tiwari, R. N., & Kim, K. S. (2012). Zero-dimensional, one-dimensional, two-dimensional and three-dimensional nanostructured materials for advanced electrochemical energy devices. *Progress in Materials Science, 57*(4), 724–803. https://doi.org/10.1016/j.pmatsci.2011.08.003.

Trevisan, M. T. S., Owen, R. W., Calatayud-Vernich, P., Breuer, A., & Picó, Y. (2017). Pesticide analysis in coffee leaves using a quick, easy, cheap, effective, rugged and safe approach and liquid chromatography tandem mass spectrometry: Optimization of the clean-up step. *Journal of Chromatography A, 1512*, 98–106. https://doi.org/10.1016/j.chroma.2017.07.033.

Xu, J., & Zheng, J. (2019). Quantum dots and nanoclusters. In *Nano-inspired biosensors for protein assay with clinical applications* (p. 67). Elsevier. https://doi.org/10.1016/B978-0-12-815053-5.00003-9.

Wang, W., Liu, L., Song, S., Xu, L., Kuang, H., Zhu, J., & Xu, C. (2017). Identification and quantification of eight Listeria monocytogene serotypes from Listeria spp. using a gold nanoparticle-based lateral flow assay. *Microchimica Acta, 184*(3), 715–724. https://doi.org/10.1007/s00604-016-2028-8.

Wang, P., Wu, L., Lu, Z., Li, Q., Yin, W., Ding, F., & Han, H. (2017). Gecko-inspired nano-tentacle surface-enhanced Raman spectroscopy substrate for sampling and reliable detection of pesticide residues in fruits and vegetables. *Analytical Chemistry, 89*(4), 2424–2431. https://doi.org/10.1021/acs.analchem.6b04324.

Wang, H., Zhao, G., Chen, D., Wang, Z., & Liu, G. (2016). A sensitive acetylcholinesterase biosensor based on screen printed electrode modified with Fe3O4 nanoparticle and graphene for chlorpyrifos determination. *International Journal of Electrochemical Science, 11*(12), 10906–10918. https://doi.org/10.20964/2016.12.90.

Wang, L., Zhu, F., Chen, M., Zhu, Y. Q., Xiao, J., Yang, H., & Chen, X. (2019). Rapid and visual detection of aflatoxin B1 in foodstuffs using aptamer/G-quadruplex DNAzyme probe with low background noise. *Food Chemistry, 271*, 581–587. https://doi.org/10.1016/j.foodchem.2018.08.007.

Wilcock, A., Pun, M., Khanona, J., & Aung, M. (2004). Consumer attitudes, knowledge and behaviour: A review of food safety issues. *Trends in Food Science and Technology, 15*(2), 56–66. https://doi.org/10.1016/j.tifs.2003.08.004.

Wilson, D., Materón, E. M., Ibáñez-Redín, G., Faria, R. C., Correa, D. S., & Oliveira, O. N. (2019). Electrical detection of pathogenic bacteria in food samples using information visualization methods with a sensor based on magnetic nanoparticles functionalized with antimicrobial peptides. *Talanta, 194*, 611–618. https://doi.org/10.1016/j.talanta.2018.10.089.

Winter, C. K. (2017). Pesticide residues in foods. In *Chemical contaminants and residues in food* (pp. 155–169). (2nd ed.). United States: Elsevier Inc.. https://doi.org/10.1016/B978-0-08-100674-0.00007-2.

Wu, L., Li, G., Xu, X., Zhu, L., Huang, R., & Chen, X. (2019). Application of nano-ELISA in food analysis: Recent advances and challenges. *TrAC, Trends in Analytical Chemistry, 113*, 140–156. https://doi.org/10.1016/j.trac.2019.02.002.

Xie, H., Dong, J., Duan, J., Hou, J., Ai, S., & Li, X. (2019). Magnetic nanoparticles-based immunoassay for aflatoxin B1 using porous g-C3N4nanosheets as fluorescence probes. *Sensors and Actuators, B: Chemical, 278*, 147–152. https://doi.org/10.1016/j.snb.2018.09.089.

Yaseen, T., Pu, H., & Sun, D. W. (2019). Fabrication of silver-coated gold nanoparticles to simultaneously detect multi-class insecticide residues in peach with SERS technique. *Talanta, 196*, 537–545. https://doi.org/10.1016/j.talanta.2018.12.030.

Yin, W., Wu, L., Ding, F., Li, Q., Wang, P., Li, J., … Han, H. (2018). Surface-imprinted SiO2@Ag nanoparticles for the selective detection of BPA using surface enhanced Raman scattering. *Sensors and Actuators, B: Chemical, 258*, 566–573. https://doi.org/10.1016/j.snb.2017.11.141.

Zhang, L., Huang, R., Liu, W., Liu, H., Zhou, X., & Xing, D. (2016). Rapid and visual detection of Listeria monocytogenes based on nanoparticle cluster catalyzed signal amplification. *Biosensors and Bioelectronics, 86*, 1–7. https://doi.org/10.1016/j.bios.2016.05.100.

Zhang, H., Xue, L., Huang, F., Wang, S., Wang, L., Liu, N., & Lin, J. (2019). A capillary biosensor for rapid detection of Salmonella using Fe-nanocluster amplification and smart phone imaging. *Biosensors and Bioelectronics*, *127*, 142–149. https://doi.org/10.1016/j.bios.2018.11.042.

Zhao, B., Huang, Q., Dou, L., Bu, T., Chen, K., Yang, Q.,…Zhang, D. (2018). Prussian blue nanoparticles based lateral flow assay for high sensitive determination of clenbuterol. *Sensors and Actuators, B: Chemical*, *275*, 223–229. https://doi.org/10.1016/j.snb.2018.08.029.

Zheng, L., Cai, G., Wang, S., Liao, M., Li, Y., & Lin, J. (2019). A microfluidic colorimetric biosensor for rapid detection of Escherichia coli O157:H7 using gold nanoparticle aggregation and smart phone imaging. *Biosensors and Bioelectronics*, *124–125*, 143–149. https://doi.org/10.1016/j.bios.2018.10.006.

Zhong, M., Yang, L., Yang, H., Cheng, C., Deng, W., Tan, Y.,…Yao, S. (2019). An electrochemical immunobiosensor for ultrasensitive detection of Escherichia coli O157:H7 using CdS quantum dots-encapsulated metal-organic frameworks as signal-amplifying tags. *Biosensors and Bioelectronics*, *126*, 493–500. https://doi.org/10.1016/j.bios.2018.11.001.

Zhou, C., Zou, H., Li, M., Sun, C., Ren, D., & Li, Y. (2018). Fiber optic surface plasmon resonance sensor for detection of E. coli O157:H7 based on antimicrobial peptides and AgNPs-rGO. *Biosensors and Bioelectronics*, *117*, 347–353. https://doi.org/10.1016/j.bios.2018.06.005.

Zou, D., Jin, L., Wu, B., Hu, L., Chen, X., Huang, G., & Zhang, J. (2018). Rapid detection of Salmonella in milk by biofunctionalised magnetic nanoparticle cluster sensor based on nuclear magnetic resonance. *International Dairy Journal*, *91*, 82–88.

Zou, Y., Liang, J., She, Z., & Kraatz, H. B. (2019). Gold nanoparticles-based multifunctional nanoconjugates for highly sensitive and enzyme-free detection of E.coli K12. *Talanta*, *193*, 15–22. https://doi.org/10.1016/j.talanta.2018.09.068.

Subject Index

Note: Page numbers followed by *f* indicate figures, and *t* indicate tables.

Printed in the United States
By Bookmasters